Becoming a
COMMUNITY COUNSELOR

Becoming a
COMMUNITY COUNSELOR

Personal and Professional Explorations

A. Renee Staton
A. Jerry Benson
Michele Kielty Briggs
Eric Cowan
Lennis G. Echterling
William F. Evans
J. Edson McKee
Jack Presbury
Anne L. Stewart

James Madison University

Lahaska Press
Houghton Mifflin Company
Boston • *New York*

Publisher, Lahaska Press: Barry Fetterolf
Senior Editor, Lahaska Press: Mary Falcon
Editorial Assistant: Evangeline Bermas
Senior Project Editor: Margaret Park Bridges
Associate Manufacturing Buyer: Brian Pieragostini
Marketing Manager: Barbara LeBuhn

Cover image: © Dimitri Vervitsiotis / Getty Images

Page 68: The Manifesto: A Guide to Developing a Creative Career by E. Paul Torrance;
foreword by Bonnie Cramond. Copyright © 2002 by E. Paul Torrance. Reproduced with
permission of Greenwood Publishing Group, Inc., Westport, CT.
Pages 197–198: Reprinted with permission from the Diagnostic and Statistical Manual
of Mental Disorders, Fourth Edition, Text Revision, (Copyright 2000). American
Psychiatric Association.

For instructors who want more information about
Lahaska Press books and teaching aids, contact the
Houghton Mifflin Faculty Services Center at
Tel: 800-733-1717, x4034
Fax: 800-733-1810

Or visit us on the Web at www.lahaskapress.com

Printed in the U.S.A.

Library of Congress Control Number: 2003103046

Instructor's examination copy
    ISBN-10: 0-618-73240-3
    ISBN-13: 978-0-618-73240-1

For orders, use student text ISBNs
    ISBN-10: 0-618-37027-7
    ISBN-13: 978-0-618-37027-6

123456789-CRS-10 09 08 07 06

Contents

Chapter 3

Doing Good: Ethical and Legal Issues in Practice   82

Chapter 4

Exploring the Counselor Within: The Facilitative Self   117

Chapter 5

Experiencing Counseling: Concepts, Dynamics, and Change   145

Chapter **6**

Conceptualizing Clients: Individual Assessment   176

Chapter 7

Viewing the Community Kaleidoscope: Embracing Diversity in Counseling   216

Chapter 8

Responding to Change: Lifespan Development   257

Chapter 9

Building on Strengths: Working with Groups   301

Chapter 10

Discovering Options: Career Counseling   335

Chapter 11

Expanding Our Knowledge Base: Research and Evaluation   376

Chapter **12**

Working Behind the Scenes: Consultation and Supervision   397

Name Index   435

Subject Index   437

Preface

It takes a community to write a book about community counseling. As the nine authors of this book, we come from different geographic areas, have diverse backgrounds, and have varied theoretical perspectives, but we share one common value—a deep commitment to the field of community counseling. We have served in a variety of roles in community settings, including counselor, prevention specialist, crisis intervener, outpatient therapist, supervisor, trainer, outreach worker, administrator, and consultant. We have worked in community agencies, hotlines, mental health centers, wellness centers, and in private practices. However, in spite of our training and experience, we have never felt completely prepared; we have often had to "fly by the seat of our pants," and we have made mistakes. As we tell the students in our graduate program, community counseling is an impossible profession for which you will never feel completely prepared and in which nothing is absolutely certain except that you will make mistakes. However, the payoff is that you will be entering a field that is on the cutting edge among the helping professions, you will be participating in innovative programs, and you will be contributing to the well-being of people and their communities.

As you look over this book's contents, you will see that we have covered a great deal of territory. As with all survey textbooks, we did not have the space to really do justice to any particular topic or issue. In fact, writing the book reminded us of some of the vacations our families used to take when we were kids. We would find a spot that was full of wonderful places to explore, but we would soon have to pack up and move along. As we embark on this long trip together across the entire community counseling profession, we encourage you to be patient with the quick overview that we offer. In your future training, you will likely have entire courses that focus on a subject that we sprint through in only a chapter.

THEMES OF THIS BOOK

There are three fundamental themes that thread their way throughout this book. The first theme is that of "profession." Our hope is that this book will help you develop a richer, broader, and deeper awareness of the community counseling profession—its ideas, tools, strengths, challenges, potential, and applications. We will be exploring the wide range of possible roles, issues, programs, and perspectives. This exploration of the profession can be both exhilarating and daunting.

The second theme that runs throughout this book is that of "self." As you prepare to become a member of this profession, you will achieve a richer, broader, and deeper awareness of yourself. As you explore these professional ideas and practice using the tools of the trade, you will gain understanding and insight into your own strengths, dreams, and personal vision. Actively reading this book by reflecting on its key concepts, relating the ideas to your own life, and participating fully in the experiential learning activities is a great way to discover more about yourself. After all, the most important tool you have as a counselor is yourself.

Finally, the third theme is that of "community." Your image of counseling work may be that it is strictly a private process in which you meet with people for their appointments in a quiet office. However, community counseling often involves working in a public arena—the scene of a traumatic event, the home of a troubled family, a neighborhood center, or a town hall. We also remind you to look for connections, interdependence, and opportunities that you may not notice, especially given our society's focus on the individual in isolation, instead of our social fabric.

We wish you the best in your professional development, personal growth, and involvement in your community. We invite you to take risks, to stretch, and to challenge yourself. Erich Fromm said that we are doomed to fail if we spend our lives frantically trying to achieve happiness. Instead, happiness is the by-product of living a full, authentic, and meaningful life. We can bear personal witness that a career as a community counselor can be an important part of such a life.

As you encounter each idea in this book, we urge you to reflect on what you have read, mull it over, sleep on it, and relate it to your own life experiences. That kind of active engagement can often lead to a deeper and richer understanding of concepts and possibilities. Carefully decide what you want to take from the book as you prepare that backpack for your professional journey as a community counselor.

FEATURES OF THIS BOOK

In each chapter, we use a variety of features to help you achieve a deeper understanding of community counseling principles and to gain a real feel for this profession. These features include:

• Chapter Goals

We begin each chapter with a short list of goals to orient you to the key concepts, issues, and strategies covered in the chapter. These goals can serve as beacons to alert you to important material and guide you as you make your way through the book.

- **Defining Moments**

As we were preparing to write this text, we talked with one other, as well as others involved in community counseling, about the defining moments that had a powerful impact on our personal and professional lives. Defining moments are those times when situations and people come together in catalytic ways. These moments heighten our awareness, spur us to reflect on our values, and impel us to revise or renew our commitments. Defining moments are turning points in which our actions then determine the future courses of our careers and lives. We therefore begin each chapter of this text with one counselor's defining moment.

- **Stories**

Many students and colleagues have shared with us their experiences of dealing with the challenges of learning and practicing community counseling. We regularly use these stories to get "up-close and personal" and demonstrate important concepts in action. Hearing the stories of others can expand your horizons by enabling you to benefit from the experiences and discoveries of others.

- **Questions for Reflection**

We pose questions to help you formulate your reactions to the chapter's stories and other activities. Take some time to put your responses into words. Writing is a wonderful way to actively shape your thoughts and ideas.

- **Experiential Learning**

In order for you to truly understand a concept or develop a skill, you must experience it. We regularly give you opportunities to engage in some activity to gain a richer awareness of a principle. The experiential learning may involve performing a task, relating a concept to your own life, or taking part in a structured activity. We encourage you to fully participate in the process. Doing so will help you to truly "get it."

- **Recommended Resources**

At the end of each chapter we recommend books, movies, websites, and other resources to help you learn more about the subject of the chapter. We offer these suggestions because in our own encounters with these works, we have felt a deeper appreciation for some facet of our own humanity and a sense of community with others.

AN INVITATION

This book will not provide you with all the information you will ever need to successfully practice the profession of community counseling. Even if the course could be that comprehensive, much of the information would be out-dated in a few years or irrelevant to your specific counseling role. Instead, we invite you to engage with us in a shared effort to learn more about the ideas, techniques, and strategies of community counseling. You will be learning about the tools of your trade and preparing to practice your craft. The purpose of this book is not to give you the answers, but for us to collaborate, and just maybe, if we're lucky, take off and fly together. Welcome aboard!

SOME WORDS OF THANKS

We wish to thank the many others who have contributed to this book. Students and colleagues in the community counseling field contributed stories, offered suggestions, and gave helpful feedback. They include Tracy Arnold, Ana Castaneda, Harriet Cobb, Kristen Collins, Dee Dunn, Cheree Hammond, Jennifer Hatter, Andrea Hollister, Cindy Hepner, Jill Hufnagle, Salmaan Khawaja, Amanda Kiser, Gary Rafala, Karen Rapp, Neil Rittenhouse, Keith Shank, Mary Smith, Mimi Steele . . . as well as the James Madison University school and community counseling students from 2001 to 2005.

Thank you also to the reviewers who so carefully critiqued the manuscript: Irene Mass Ametrano, Eastern Michigan University; Christopher Faiver, John Carroll University; Eric A. Schmidt, Texas State University–San Marcos; Shawn L. Spurgeon, Western Kentucky University; and David Tobin, Gannon University.

Finally, we wish to thank Barry Fetterolf, Publisher of Lahaska Press, for his interest in helping us to develop the idea for this book. Barry has been an enthusiastic and reliable source of support for us in many ways, and we appreciate his patience and persistence. We also extend our sincere thanks to Mary Falcon, Senior Editor. Her ability to combine humor and pragmatism in a patient and unflappable manner has been vital to this success of this project. Both Barry's and Mary's understanding of the counseling field and of counselors themselves has been a tremendous help to us, and we are grateful to have had them as companions on this journey.

Chapter 1

Putting Ourselves in Context: Professional, Community, and Personal Histories

If you think you're too small to make a difference, you've obviously never been in bed with a mosquito.

Michelle Walker

We know that where community exists it confers upon its members identity, a sense of belonging, and a measure of security. It is in communities that the attributes that distinguish humans as social creatures are nourished.

John W. Gardner

GOALS

Reading and exploring the ideas in this chapter will help you:

- Understand the history, philosophy, and current trends in the counseling profession in general, and community counseling in particular
- Articulate the perspectives and contributions of counseling professionals through a variety of prevention and intervention strategies
- Become more aware of what attracts you to community counseling
- Know the professional organizations and professional identity of community counselors

OVERVIEW

This chapter presents information on the Council for Accreditation of Counseling and Related Educational Program (CACREP) standards relevant for community counseling students, including the role of community counselors, foundations of the field, and trends in the community mental health

movement. Our goal is to introduce you to the history of community counseling, as well as fundamental concepts relevant to your work as a community counselor, including the importance of thinking about yourself and the
context in which you will practice.

Please note that although we use the term *community counseling* in
order to reflect the current thinking in the field, the content of this book
covers topics relevant to those who provide "agency" or "mental health" counseling as well. The unique focus of community counselors on prevention,
holistic conceptualization, and wellness supplements and enhances the core
agency and mental health counseling work of assessment, intervention, and
consultation.

As community counselors, we are especially intrigued with defining moments because they suggest our potential, resilience, interconnectedness, and
worldviews. Community counselors, as well as their clients, often have experiences that become defining moments—those instances in which life decisions are altered or confirmed, forming the foundation for the next stage in
one's personal and professional development. As you read the Defining
Moments features and various stories in this book, we invite you to reflect
on your own experiences and consider where you may be heading as you
embark on your journey toward becoming a community counselor.

___

ANGELA'S DEFINING MOMENT: From Chaos into Clarity

Angela, one of the authors of this book, experienced a dramatic
defining moment as she was trying to make plans for her future. She
was a senior in college, headed home from school on a foggy, gray
Friday afternoon. Ordinarily, she took the interstate, but on this particular occasion, she decided to travel the slower, meandering route
through the mountains bordering the Shenandoah Valley. With very
little traffic and the lush green foliage of the Washington National
Forest all but brushing against her car, Angela's thoughts gravitated
to the choice that confronted her—graduate school or job. This was
a difficult and seemingly monumental decision that many friends
and classmates had managed to make easily, and long before their
senior year.

Angela's reverie was suddenly disrupted. Just as she rounded a
sharp and dangerous curve, she saw a small group of people huddled
together in the middle of the highway. Slamming on the brakes, she
jumped from the car. Someone told her that there had been a terrible
accident up ahead and the road was blocked. Angela asked if the pas-
sengers needed help and a woman warned, "Don't go up there, one
of the drivers is ranting, raving and acting like a crazy man."

For some unfathomable reason, Angela decided to ignore the warning—and the cold knot gathering in her stomach. She walked hurriedly toward the scene of the accident. As she drew closer, she saw a man who was half screaming and half crying. His clothing was torn, blood was streaming down his face, and he looked very much like the villain in a horror movie as he tried to pull a woman on to her feet. It was obvious to Angela that the woman was seriously injured and should not be moved. She could understand why other bystanders were hesitant to approach this man, but she felt a sense of calm and resolve come over her.

Angela moved closer to the man and talked to him in a very slow deliberate way; she suggested that the woman was really too badly hurt to move, and recommended that he should just try to make her comfortable until the rescue squad arrived. The raving man stared at Angela for a long minute, turned his gaze to the injured woman in his arms, and then gently laid her on the ground. A few bystanders, following Angela's lead, tried to make the poor woman comfortable.

Just then the eerie stillness of the forest was shattered by screams of a girl climbing out of a ditch behind the group. It seemed she had been thrown from the car, was relatively unhurt, but thought her mother was dead. The girl alternately cried out to her mother and shrieked accusingly at the bloody man, who was her father.

Without hesitation, Angela moved to the youngster's side, took her hand, and reassured her that an ambulance was on the way. In the meantime, her father began to sob that the accident was his fault, and gave a rambling account of a violent argument that culminated in his wife and daughter fleeing from him. After a harrowing high-speed chase, both cars had skidded off the road.

Angela continued to listen to him, tried to make the semiconscious woman comfortable, and consoled the little girl, whose name was Charity, until the ambulance finally came. The child asked Angela if she would go with her to the hospital, so they followed the ambulance in Angela's car. Angela remained with the girl until her grandparents arrived. Five hours after rounding a curve on that normally peaceful stretch of highway, Angela prepared to resume her journey home.

As she was leaving, Angela was given a hero's reception in the hospital lobby. The word had spread that Angela may have saved the woman's life by keeping her hysterical and guilt-ridden husband from moving her. Angela was also credited with rescuing Charity and sparing her a lonely and traumatic aftermath of the crash.

Although deeply embarrassed by the attention, for days afterwards Angela savored the afterglow of this experience. She had faced a terrible situation and, without hesitation or planning, had made an intervention that altered positively the course of three lives. Angela's decision to become a community counselor coincided with her resolution to swallow her fears and make that long walk up the highway to offer help where it was needed—far from an office, hospital, or agency.

Questions for Reflection

1. What defining moments have you experienced that have created profound changes in your view of yourself or your future?
2. What, specifically, drew you to community counseling?
3. How do you anticipate changing in the next five years?

As a community counselor, you will become skilled at changing your focus of attention. You will learn to take a microscopic view of an individual's inner dynamics, motivations, strengths, and dreams. You will also become proficient at understanding the broader social, cultural, economic, and historical contexts that affect individuals by taking a wide-angle perspective. Both perspectives—the personal and contextual—are essential. The successful community counselor works therapeutically with individuals to achieve personal change, but also intervenes effectively within the community, appreciating how it influences members and recognizing how people can participate in social change.

Besides offering direct counseling, a community counselor also provides a wide range of other services, such as consultation, education, advocacy, crisis intervention, and prevention. In the morning, you may be meeting with a troubled family in their home. At noon, you may be facilitating a support group for survivors of sexual assault. In the afternoon, you may be consulting with members of the clergy on how to respond to a local disaster. Then, in the evening, you may be giving a presentation to a group of parents on how to communicate successfully with their teenage sons and daughters. Such a range of professional duties can be daunting, but also immensely fulfilling. We begin this chapter with a discussion of the importance of community for the counselor.

COMMUNITY

Although definitions of community abound (Rudkin, 2003), it is helpful to know that the word itself comes from the Latin *communitas,* which means fellowship. For our purposes, a community is a particular group whose members are closely linked to one another by a high degree of interdependence and strong sense of identity. These two basic elements—interdependence and identity—are crucial to promoting human growth and development. The community is a special system in which people live together, influence each other, and meet one another's physical, emotional, social, and spiritual needs. Members of especially tight-knit communities feel a profound sense of belongingness, where every single person truly matters to one another and everyone shares in a commitment to stay together (McMillan & Chavis, 1986).

In addition to these ties of interdependence, people strongly identify with their community. Members of a community see themselves not only as an "I," but also as one of "we," intertwined in a broader social fabric. Just as you have your own personal story, communities have their collective narratives, or shared stories, that tell their histories, express their values, celebrate their achievements, honor their traditions, and define who they are (Rappaport, 2000). These stories may be expressed through community meetings, murals, celebrations, cultural festivals, exhibits, community newspapers, community websites, and locally produced television or radio programs. After natural disasters and other community-wide crises, community counselors are now consulting with groups to use these different modalities and media to co-create collective survivor stories that educate the public about resources and celebrate the resilience of the community (Echterling, Presbury, & McKee, 2005).

A successful community is a dynamic system that is constantly changing to address the needs of its members, develop resources, and respond to issues and challenges. Over the years, technology has enabled us to expand our options for gaining a sense of community. Our transportation and communication systems have made it possible for alienated or isolated individuals to find a sense of community with others. In fact, when their place-based communities are inadequate, some people now are turning to virtual communities in cyberspace (Roberts, Smith, & Pollock, 2002).

Pennebaker and his colleagues (Pennebaker, Francis, & Booth, 2001) have made some fascinating discoveries about our rich interpersonal world as members of communities. By studying how people communicate, these researchers have found that our use of language can be a vivid reflection of our social identity. For example, in one study, Pennebaker and Graybeal (2001) found that people's sense of community expands dramatically in times of crisis. When communicating during the week following a highly publicized trauma, people more than doubled their use of the words "we" and "us," while reducing significantly their use of "I" and "me."

Our definition of community presents a notion that goes beyond the individual, pointing out invisible bonds that are real and powerful between people. Given United States society's emphasis on "rugged individualism," you may not fully appreciate how essential a community is to people's health and well-being. Most Western industrialized cultures, particularly the United States, value autonomy, personal achievement, and independence (Sampson, 2000). Counseling and psychotherapy, which have their roots in Western culture, by and large have mirrored these individualistic values (Rudkin, 2003). When traditional counselors describe their intervention goals, they have relied heavily on such terms as *self-esteem, personal growth, self-concept,* and *self-fulfillment.* Even the developmental perspective, which is the cornerstone of the counseling profession, typically has portrayed the ultimate goals of human development as individuation, personal independence, self-reliance, and self-actualization.

In contrast, community counselors believe that focusing only on the individual in counseling work causes us to miss the dynamic richness of the "big picture." For example, the strongest predictor of substance abuse by adolescents is neither their level of self-esteem nor their personal problem-solving abilities, but the degree of abuse by their friends (Hussong & Hicks, 2003). Taking only an intrapsychic view, looking at the inner dynamics of a person, can limit us in appreciating the profound impact of interpersonal systems and interfere with our abilities to design more promising interventions that go beyond the individual.

Communities as Systems

Successful community counselors achieve two fundamental tasks. They serve individuals, groups, and families while also effecting positive influence on the larger community itself. You, as a community counselor, will recognize that any intervention can have an impact on the individual and on the community as a whole.

As a community counselor, your services include promoting personal well-being, enhancing mental health, treating disorders, intervening with troubled families, and preventing future problems. At the same time, you also are working to enhance and enrich the overall vitality of the larger community. Many students begin their graduate training with no idea that their responsibilities will be so far-reaching. Ideally, you will find the prospect to be exciting, as well as sobering.

Three key points are important for you to remember as you think of communities as systems. First, a community is more than a collection of individuals. Communities are interacting units that develop their own norms, cultures, and expectations (Rudkin, 2003). We recommend that you take time now to reflect on the community in which you are living. As a community counselor expected to serve as counselor, advocate, and change agent, you will need to learn to conceptualize your community just as you conceptualize your

EXPERIENTIAL LEARNING

1. Take a look at Figure 1.1. As you can see, there are three individual shapes that are distinctly separate from one another. No one shape seems to have any impact on another. Nothing exciting is going on here between these isolated, individual shapes.

Figure 1.1 Individual Shapes That Have No Connections

2. Now look at Figure 1.2. To gain a feel for how these closely connected shapes have a dynamic influence on one another, try to count the black dots that connect them. As you make this attempt, notice how the entire figure seems to come alive with

black dots quickly appearing out of nowhere and then disappearing just as fast.

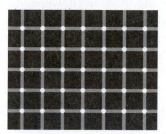

Figure 1.2 Individual Shapes in a Dynamic Context

3. Think of yourself in context. What are some of the invisible, but powerful, connecting bonds between you and your community?

4. How do these bonds influence you?

5. In what ways do you affect these dynamic bonds with others in your community?

clients. We provide specific information regarding community conceptualization in a later section of this chapter.

Second, the subsystems of a community are dynamic and mutually influencing. Subsystems include neighborhoods, churches, agencies, and governing bodies. One subsystem affects the others, which in turn have an impact on the larger system of community. Imagine, for instance, a community in which the city council decided to discontinue funding community mental health services for people struggling with substance abuse. In this case, the governance has made a decision that affects an agency and removes a resource for those with specific needs. What might eventually happen in the community if this chain of events is unaltered? How might this event affect you as a community counselor?

Third, the community is influenced by other systems, including the environment, political climate, and economy. Therefore, predicting the impact of any event in a system becomes a complicated process. Our ideas about cause-and-effect are limiting when we consider the dynamic ways in which systems and their subsystems affect each other (Presbury, Echterling, & McKee, 2002). This idea is captured well in the idea of the Butterfly Effect, a vivid metaphor based on chaos theory (Gleick, 1987) that suggests a butterfly flapping its wings in China might eventually affect the weather in Oklahoma. Small systemic changes, sometimes imperceptible, can create significant, unexpected, and cascading consequences on other systems. Thus, whether or not we notice them, many seemingly minor events can ultimately have a dramatic impact on our clients and communities. However, one encouraging implication of chaos theory for community counseling is that a small, seemingly insignificant, intervention may ultimately result in an extraordinary transformation. Like a gardener who helps seeds achieve their innate potential, your work as a community counselor is to provide the conditions that promote both personal and systemic change. Planting just one seed at the perfect time and under ideal conditions can lead to a bountiful harvest.

Consider the implications that this way of thinking about community has for you as a community counselor. For example, researchers found that economic stressors can undermine an inner-city youth's sense of control, which can lead to clinical depression. However, they also discovered that a family providing a protective haven from stressors can reduce this risk (Deardorff, Gonzales, & Sandler, 2003). With this in mind, community counselors are obligated to work not only individually, but systemically, with families, schools, and agencies within the community.

THE ROLE OF THE COMMUNITY COUNSELOR

At one time, you, as a counselor, could specialize in community agency counseling, a role that defined itself by the site where you provided counseling services. Instead of an asylum or institution that was isolated from the day-to-day activities of people, your primary workplace—e.g., a mental health center, a social services agency—was located within the community itself.

Now, however, the concept of community agency counselor has evolved and broadened to that of community counselor. As a community counselor, you may indeed work in a traditional agency site, but you may also be providing services in disaster assistance centers, emergency rooms, homes of troubled families, schools, or private practice offices. We now define community counselors according to their frame of mind, rather than the site of their workplace. Regardless of their work setting, community counselors co-create strategies to meet the needs of both the person and the community. They conceptualize their clients within the broader context of community. They focus on both preventing and responding to problems in the larger system.

Community counselors maintain four areas of emphasis in their work, all of which relate to the art of conceptualization—how counselors make sense of what is happening.

1. Community counselors focus on *prevention*. The act of preventing problems, or ameliorating the effects of existing problems, is a fundamental aspect of community counseling practice.

2. Community counselors *respond* to client concerns in ways that provide accessible and affordable service to community members in need.

3. Community counselors *consider the interaction between the individual and the community* to be of paramount concern in assessment and intervention.

4. Community counselors *assess the overall functioning of the surrounding community* in their work, and they take action to address problems that interfere with clients' functioning.

Prevent Problems

First, community counselors think in terms of prevention, which is more effective than remediation (Durlack & Wells, 1998). In fact, an emphasis on prevention and the promotion of normal developmental processes is a hallmark that has distinguished counseling as a profession from clinical psychology. Prevention may take a variety of forms, from education and training to individual, group, and family interventions (Repucci, Woolard, & Fried, 1999).

Prevention can be further categorized as primary, secondary, and tertiary (Caplan, 1964). *Primary prevention* includes attempts to promote mental health and decrease mental illness through proactive interventions before people show any signs of disorders. Therefore, successful primary prevention programs reduce the incidence, or new cases, of a problem or disorder. Keeping healthy people healthy is the goal of primary prevention.

Did you ever go to summer camp as a child? For millions of children, experiences such as summer camp are wonderful opportunities for adventures, camaraderie, learning, and memories that can last a lifetime. However, in spite of the fun that kids have at camp, many often feel homesick. Homesickness is certainly a natural, normal reaction for children to have, but it can undermine their ability to cope with separation and novel situations, which are essential parts of personal growth and well-being. An example of a primary prevention intervention designed to reduce this common problem is that of a program developed by Thurber (2005). This inexpensive, multimodal approach included a "sneak preview" orientation brochure for campers, a "Kids Can Cope with Homesickness" booklet for families, practice time away from home, a phone call from a staff member, and specialized staff training. Using a comparison group, the study found that offering novelty reduction, social support, and promotion of personal control significantly reduced the negative emotional intensity of homesickness. Given the uncertain conditions in today's world, these findings have exciting implications for community counselors, who can use these prevention strategies with children who face far more extreme separations, such as immigrants, refugees, and displaced persons (Stroebe, van Vliet, Hewstone, & Willis, 2002).

Secondary prevention involves responding immediately or intervening rapidly once a problem has been identified or a disorder has been diagnosed. The working assumption is that intervention is more effective early in the process when a problem or disorder has not become ingrained or chronic. For example, when Emory Cowen observed that troubled adolescents had started to have school problems early in the primary grades, he organized intensive programs for young children who were beginning to show signs of maladjustment (Cowen & Hightower, 1989). The program involved training parents, using volunteer mentors, providing individual attention, and facilitating support groups. These early and intensive interventions prevented the development of more serious behavior problems in adolescence.

Tertiary prevention, which takes place in any effective treatment, involves interventions that lessen the impact of a problem, reduce the severity of the symptoms, and prevent relapses (Lewis & Lewis, 1989; Rudkin, 2003). The problem has emerged or the disorder has developed, so one cannot prevent its incidence. However, successful counseling not only ameliorates the client's precipitating condition, it also seeks to prevent future problems that pose a high risk for troubled individuals. For instance, if a client's situation continues unimproved, then divorce, job loss, and even death may be the possible consequences. One example of tertiary prevention is the work of Carlo DiClemente (2003) with addicted clients. Before terminating, he prepares clients to prevent relapse by exploring helpful strategies they can use to maintain their recovery.

Community counselors can work preventively in all of these ways, but primary prevention tends to be a salient concern for us. For example, in the immediate aftermath of the September 11 terrorist attacks, many community counselors mobilized resources to provide an array of services to their local communities (Echterling, Presbury, & McKee, 2005; Webber, Bass, & Yep, 2005). These prevention services included community-wide dissemination of information designed to normalize stress reactions, consultation with school systems, and outreach to high-risk populations. Thus, the interventions were aimed not only at helping people deal with their immediate reactions to the attacks, but were designed also to prevent the development of problems and disorders in the future. These powerful community-based interventions combined primary and secondary preventive efforts.

Respond to Problems

When responding to community members' needs at the levels of primary, secondary, and tertiary prevention, community counselors consistently work to ensure that the services they provide are accessible and affordable. Community counselors often work in community agencies, hospitals, and outpatient clinics that provide a range of services, such as individual, group, and family counseling, designed for a wide segment of community members. Many community counselors provide outreach services in which they travel to underserved areas, or they promote their services to specific populations, such as immigrants, the poor, or region-specific minorities, who are not receiving adequate mental health care. Similarly, community counselors in private practice tend to offer evening hours and seek referrals from physicians, outpatient clinics, and social service agencies.

Community counselors have also historically offered low-cost services, often setting their fees on a sliding scale. They usually attempt to fill service gaps in their communities by providing counseling for clients who may be uninsured or underinsured. They are adept at understanding and working with services such as Medicaid, and they are accustomed to helping their clients negotiate the third-party payment system of reimbursement. Most counselors also provide a certain amount of *pro bono* work, meaning they provide services for no fee. In addition to their *pro bono* services, community counselors also typically volunteer their time to serve on the advisory boards of community service agencies, work as victim assistance counselors, or consult with community agencies that have a mental health focus.

Consider the Individual in a Community Context

Whether they are thinking in terms of prevention or response, community counselors conceptualize their clients and themselves in the broader context of the community, and they understand the interactions and mutual influences that exist among these different variables. Individuals are not islands unto themselves. Rather, they are imbedded in a many-layered social fabric (Rudkin, 2003). The only way to effect truly significant change in individuals, and certainly the only way to prevent problems from occurring, is to understand not only the strengths and vulnerabilities of the person, but also the stressors and resources of the surrounding environment. Community counselors then assess the relationship between the individual and the environment to determine how best to intervene. A community counselor needs to be attuned to both intrapsychic and social dynamics as well as to the interactions between the two.

For example, in one small town, community counselors became aware of an increasing need for Spanish-speaking counselors. The town's Latino migrant population was growing, and many Spanish-speaking workers were finding year-round work in local poultry plants. Word was spreading that this town had jobs for Latino immigrants. The mental health community, however, was unprepared. Spanish-speaking clients were struggling to find appropriate services, counselors were asking children who spoke English to translate for their parents, and misunderstandings between agency personnel and clients were leading to ineffective treatment.

In response, a group of mental health workers, including counselors and social workers, developed a conference for local mental health and public health workers that addressed counseling competencies for multicultural populations. These professionals shared the belief that the conference, designed specifically for this community, would prevent a host of problems for both clients and counselors by enhancing provision of services. This intervention was only possible because the mental health workers understood the importance of the community context for their clients.

Assess the Community

When you are counseling an individual, you also are working with your client's community. Counseling a client is one thing, but how do you evaluate how a community functions and how it may affect your client? We suggest you begin by getting to know your community. If you have moved to a different city for your counseling training, look around to ascertain what resources, debits, and challenges you see. What do these community characteristics suggest to you regarding the mental health needs of the community members? If you are not sure, here are a few areas to explore as you begin to understand and form a picture of your community.

- Start by assessing the size, location, employment, demographics, and diversity of your community.

- Become familiar with the community's history—its story. Research both the distant past, such as its founding, and recent events, such as a factory closing or recent influx of urban transplants. Look for evidence of resilience and cohesion in dealing with challenges. A community's story of its development gives you an opportunity to place the current circumstances in its historical context.

- Then look at resources, such as universities, agencies, involved citizen groups, faith-based organizations, or industries that contribute to the economic, cultural, and spiritual vitality of this community.

- Now consider debits, such as unemployment and poverty. Include any problems unique to your area. For example, our local community is struggling with a dramatic increase in the manufacture and use of methamphetamine. The phenomenon is having a distinct effect on our schools, in particular. This relatively rural area is also home to a large number of elderly people who have difficulty traveling to receive mental health services, and a growing population of former migrant workers who have not yet been adequately served by our local mental health agencies.

- Then look for gaps that might include unmet needs, untapped potential, and networks. A university, for instance, has the potential to provide many *pro bono* services, as well as off-site services.

- Finally, assess how much influence a counselor or agency may have. What would it take for a counselor or agency to effectively anticipate and respond to the needs of your community? Obviously, if you are going to have a positive impact on your community, you cannot work alone. It is essential that you collaborate with other professionals, including school personnel, other mental health professionals, medical personnel, faith-based leaders, volunteers, and a diverse group of community members.

The following assignments are designed to help you get a head start on the process of effecting positive change as a community counselor.

- Check with a local hospital or community mental health agency to view any recent community mental health survey data. What do the data suggest to you? If possible, volunteer to assist in gathering and interpreting the data.

- Interview a community counselor. If you find a willing counselor, ask as many questions as you can regarding the counselor's work, including the inherent challenges and rewards.

- Whenever possible, observe counseling sessions, visit board meetings of the community mental health center, and volunteer to assist with outreach programs. Take note of the role of community in these different settings.

- Keep a binder, or develop a webpage, in which you expand on your conceptualization of your community. Explore agency resources, and identify referral options.

THE HISTORY OF COMMUNITY COUNSELING

How are the conceptualizations and interventions of community counselors different from those of other helping professions? For that matter, how did the profession of community counseling evolve? We explore these questions in this section.

Sigmund Freud, Jane Addams, and Frank Parsons

Conjure up a picture of Sigmund Freud. What comes to mind? Inner conflicts? Unconscious fixations? A man with a cigar who sat silently while his client engaged in free association? Now picture an American woman, Jane Addams, a contemporary of Freud, who became a social activist and tireless advocate for the poor and exploited in the late nineteenth and early twentieth centuries. You might picture a woman in Victorian dress working with children and families in the poverty-stricken tenements of urban America. Finally, imagine Frank Parsons, another American who lived during the same era, an idealistic, frail university professor who wrote poetry, loved to play croquet, and originated guidance counseling.

Now imagine a community counselor in twenty-first-century America. What might you see? Perhaps you see a woman who visits a family in their home, working to help parents develop more effective ways of disciplining their children. Maybe you picture a man working at a community agency who provides substance abuse counseling for people with dual diagnoses. Or you may envision a graduate-level intern offering employee assistance counseling over the Internet. Could these people possibly be following in the footsteps of Freud, Addams, and Parsons?

Near the end of the nineteenth century, psychology was emerging as a science that focused on conscious processes. Back then, Freud and his psychodynamic followers created a profound paradigm shift by exploring unconscious dynamics and conflicts. These pioneers also promoted the revolutionary idea that people could be healed as a result of "the talking cure," which inspired the professions of therapy and counseling.

The psychoanalytic approach to understanding and helping troubled people focused on intrapsychic phenomena. The assumption was that meaningful and lasting change begins within the individual's mind. The seeds of change can only take root when they are planted deep in a person's unconscious. At the same time that Freud and his followers, the majority of whom were male, were developing their innovative approaches in Vienna, many Americans took a radically different approach to change (Davis, 1994).

Jane Addams and other activists, many of whom were women, were troubled by the deplorable social conditions that plagued the poor, mentally ill, and homeless in the United States. They decided to change the oppressive environment by beginning the settlement house movement, establishing over 400 programs across the nation. They collaborated with the residents in tenements to build community centers, establish educational programs, and advocate for the enactment of child labor laws. In contrast to the psychoanalysts, these reformers believed that improving social conditions was the necessary catalyst for promoting any significant change in people's lives. From

the perspective of the settlement house activists, dramatic growth is only possible when the environment nurtures and supports the seeds of change. One
of the other consequences of the settlement house movement was the emergence of the profession of social work.

While Freud was refining his psychoanalytic techniques in Vienna and
Addams was founding Hull House in Chicago, Frank Parsons was teaching
university students and developing his ideas about vocational guidance.
Although he grew up in Victorian society, Parsons was an idealist, avowed
socialist, humanitarian, and supporter of women's suffrage. In 1900, he was
fired from what is now Kansas State University after he was accused of being
a political subversive (Pope & Sveinsdottir, 2005). Eight years later, he established the Vocations Bureau at the Boston Civic Service House. Most histori-
ans point to this event as the first instance of professional counseling in a
community setting (Hershenson & Berger, 2001), though nearly two decades
earlier Jesse Davis had become the first school counselor in 1890 (Nystul,
2003).

Fundamental assumptions about the change process form the basis of
most helping professions, including counseling, social work, psychology, and
psychiatry (Nystul, 2003). How did community counseling develop as an integration of psychodynamics, social forces, and human development? Perhaps
the best way to understand these processes is to highlight a few defining moments. Community counseling has its common roots in the ground-breaking
therapeutic work of Freud, in the social reform efforts of Jane Addams, and in
the innovations of Frank Parsons in educating people to achieve their developmental potential. A hybrid of personal therapy, social activism, and education, community counseling has emerged as a profession in its own right—one
that emphasizes human growth, promotes a sense of community, emphasizes
strengths, and builds on resilience.

Of course, any vital profession is both a producer and product of the so-
ciopolitical context in which it occurs. As a result, the community counselors
of today offer services that are dramatically different from those of the
psychoanalyst, settlement home advocate, or professor of over one hundred
years ago. Over the past century, several significant events have substantially
affected the practice of community counseling.

Community Counseling: Where Did We Come From?

Professional counseling has a relatively short, but extraordinarily eventful,
history. Counseling has, within one century, metamorphosed from a few
practitioners who were focused on educational issues and vocational guidance
to a discipline of thousands whose comprehensive approach involves a wide
range of techniques designed to work at both personal and societal levels. Along

the way, the once distinct boundaries between the work of a psychologist, clinical social worker, and counselor have blurred.

You can find counselors in virtually every area of mental health and personal growth work, and it is sometimes difficult to discern any obvious differences between their approach to helping and the techniques that other professionals use. According to the American Counseling Association, as of August 2005, forty-eight states, as well as the District of Columbia and Puerto Rico, had established licensure for professional counselors. As a result, many counselors are able to receive third party payment from insurance companies as they work side-by-side with other mental health providers in agencies or group private practices.

In spite of the large overlap of theories and practices among helping professionals, there are several themes that suggest some distinctions. For example, community counselors typically refrain from using such terms as *patient* and *treatment* because they consider their work to be a collaborative effort between counselor and client—not a procedure that is administered to a passive recipient. In addition, although counselors often intervene with people who have serious psychiatric disorders, their services can be beneficial to anyone who seeks personal growth. Counseling is a developmental process; counselors believe you don't have to be sick to get better. As Hanson, Rossberg, and Cramer (1994) put it, "The purpose of counseling is to provide for the individual's optimum development and well-being" (p. 4).

Another reason why community counselors avoid such terms as *treatment* and *patient* is that they typically operate under the wellness model. Instead of focusing on symptoms of diseases and treating patients for disorders, community counselors emphasize the promotion of wellness by building on the strengths and resources of their clients (Myers, Sweeney, & Witmer, 2000). Interestingly, although the conceptual roots of the counseling profession have always included an appreciation for human development, the trend in the latter part of the twentieth century was to focus on psychopathology. Many counselors had joined psychiatrists, psychologists, and clinical social workers in researching, diagnosing, and treating mental illness. However, a number of theorists and practitioners have gone back to the roots of counseling to explore the upper end of the continuum of human functioning—wellness (Myers & Sweeney, 2005). In fact, Emory Cowen (2000) proposed the pursuit of wellness as a unifying theme, positive goal, and guiding framework for the helping professions.

In the early days of the profession, counselors had two specific functions. First, they provided a system for matching people to occupations for which they seemed best suited. Second, they expanded the role of education by providing guidance to young people for how best to live their lives. The focus of these two approaches was initially on *adjustment*—on getting people to fit well into a democratic society. As the U.S. Office of Education stated in 1950, counseling "better equips all American youth to live democratically with satisfaction to themselves and profit to society as home members, workers, and citizens" (p. 1).

It is ironic that a governmental movement to promote adaptation to national needs and conformity to cultural values served as the catalyst for transforming the focus of counselors from *adjustment* to *growth*. In 1958, the National Defense Education Act (NDEA) was established. The act was in reaction to the Cold War assumption that our country was under threat from the Soviet Union because we did not have enough trained scientists. The Soviets had launched Sputnik, the first space satellite, and legislators worried about a "technology gap." The NDEA was essentially designed to enhance U.S. advances in science, and counselors were trained to identify students with potential and steer them toward careers in science (Hansen, Rossberg, & Cramer, 1994). Many NDEA institutes were set up in the 1960s to train counselors at universities across the country.

Another major historical trend for community counseling began with the last piece of legislation that President John F. Kennedy signed before his assassination—the Community Mental Health Centers Act of 1963. This legislation was the catalyst for the community mental health movement, which promoted deinstitutionalization by treating those with serious psychiatric disorders within their own communities (Rudkin, 2003). During the French Revolution Philippe Pinel liberated the mentally ill, who had been shackled and condemned to endure barbaric conditions in asylums. One hundred and seventy years later, Kennedy began a similarly liberating revolution in the United States by calling for the reintegration of psychiatric patients who had been confined to state mental hospitals back into the community (Levine & Levine, 1970).

For years, the only treatment available to poor individuals had been in public psychiatric hospitals, which were woefully ill-equipped, underfunded, and understaffed. These overcrowded and dehumanizing institutions often became little more than human warehouses, storing the unwanted and the cast-offs of a community unwilling to recognize these individuals as persons who have innate value and inalienable rights. Consequently, after years of hospitalization, the condition of many patients deteriorated so severely that they became "institutionalized" and were no longer able to function independently beyond the hospital walls.

Deinstitutionalization, one of the largest social experiments in the history of the United States (Torrey, 1997), led to a dramatic decline in the number of hospitalized psychiatric patients. In 1963, the inpatient population was over 500,000. Twenty years later, less than 100,000 were hospitalized in public mental hospitals. In spite of these impressive results, deinstitutionalization was by no means an unqualified success. There were also many problems, such as inadequate funding of community mental health services, an increase of homelessness, and poor follow-up of discharged patients.

The new legislation created a nationwide system of community mental health centers to provide five mandated services (Bloom, 1984). The first of these services was inpatient care, which involved traditional mental health services, but took place in smaller programs within the community, instead of in a distant, large, and impersonal state mental hospital. The second service was outpatient care. Before 1963, only a minority of individuals and families could afford the high cost of counseling and therapy services, but for the first time millions of people could have access to individual, group, and family sessions, regardless of their ability to pay for these services. Third, centers were mandated to provide partial hospitalization, which were day programs that offered intensive care for clients who then could return to their homes in the evenings. The fourth was emergency services and crisis intervention. Community mental health centers were expected to become resources when citizens were confronted with psychiatric emergencies and other crises that required immediate intervention. Finally, the centers were charged with the truly revolutionary mandate of providing consultation and education services. We discuss these services in more detail in Chapter 2. Resonating with the values of counselors, the community mental health movement was attempting not only to prevent mental illness but also to promote personal well-being and development.

Along with these innovations in social policy, the decade of the 1960s brought a time of social turmoil and the rise of the human potential movement. Inspired by the existentialist and humanistic literature, and influenced by a culture that embraced an anti-establishment movement, counselors began to transform their professional goals. They saw counseling less as fitting people into slots designed by society, and more about helping individuals become fully actualized. Self-fulfillment, rather than merely adjustment, became the goal.

Both the civil rights movement and the modern women's movement during the 1960s gave voice to years of oppression and advocated for meaningful social change rather than just adjustment to intolerably racist and sexist conditions. Activists questioned prejudiced attitudes, rigid gender roles, and practices of discrimination. The progress in these areas gave encouragement to gay, lesbian, bisexual, and transgendered (GLBT) people, who began to organize politically to advocate for their civil rights. Today, these issues continue to be raised and debated in American communities and are critically relevant to the work of community counselors. A recent study, for example, found that South Asian–American women who experience prejudice are more likely to report higher levels of depressive symptoms (Rahman & Rollock, 2004). Clearly, community counselors need to be aware of these possible consequences and help clients learn skills to combat prejudice.

In spite of the challenges of deinstitutionalization, community-based programs consistently demonstrated their greater effectiveness over traditional inpatient hospitalization (Okin, Borus, Baer, & Jones, 1995). Therefore, as the community mental health movement intensified through the 1970s and early 1980s, the role of counselors broadened in scope and significance. (Hansen, Rossberg, & Cramer, 1994). In particular, community counselors, with their unique combination of relevant knowledge, skills, and values, began to fill an important niche in community mental health centers. During this period, counselor education programs made crucial changes in their training in order to prepare their students to work in community agency settings (Hershenson & Berger, 2001).

COMMUNITY COUNSELING IN THE TWENTY-FIRST CENTURY

Today, community counselors can be found in many settings and operating under a wide range of assumptions regarding their purpose and theoretical orientation. Psychodynamic counselors draw their inspiration from Freudian roots, including the schools of object relations and self-psychology. Others have adopted cognitive behavioral techniques to help clients change their maladaptive ways of thinking and acting. Still others operate with a systems framework to view individual functioning in the context of family and organizational dynamics. More recently, many counselors have adopted the constructivist notions of brief approaches, solution-focused counseling, and narrative therapy. However, the central assumption of most professional counselors remains humanistic, person-centered, and relationship-based. Most counselors still hold in high regard Carl Rogers' assertions about the necessity of a trusting, empathic, and genuine relationship between counselor and client and the presence of core conditions such as unconditional positive regard, congruence, and genuineness for any effective counseling to take place (1961).

No matter what theoretical perspectives may guide their work, community counselors can continue to expect change. For instance, one recent development in practice is providing intensive outreach services. Emergency mental health agencies, family preservation programs, and disaster mental health teams are offering outreach services to people at the site of crises, at a place of refuge, or in the family home. Mobile crisis units, operating twenty-four hours a day, seven days a week, are in place in many jurisdictions across the country. These programs offer free or low-cost emergency counseling throughout the community, providing a combination of telephone hotline and on-the-scene services (Echterling, Presbury, & McKee, 2005). The idea is simple—instead of a counselor sitting back in the office and requiring people to come to the agency for intervention, the counselor goes to them.

This approach has its dangers and special challenges, but actively reaching out as rapidly as possible has and will continue to set the stage for successful community counseling. Additional relevant trends affecting community counseling practice are presented in Chapter 2.

COMMON FACTORS OF SUCCESS IN COUNSELING

What guides how community counselors actually work with their clients? The great psychotherapy and counseling debate over the past decade, according to Wampold (2001), has been between those who subscribe to the "medical model" and those who support the "contextual model."

The medical model approach regards clients as having a specific problem that will respond to a certain treatment-of-choice for that particular disorder. The movement to arrive at empirically-based treatments for each disorder has, in Wampold's view, restricted psychotherapy and counseling to the medical model and obscured the true factors contributing to improvement in clients of counseling and psychotherapy.

The contextual approach focuses on research findings that reveal specific factors that are present in any successful therapeutic endeavor, regardless of the presenting problem of the client. These factors account for nine times more of the variance in outcomes than do the specific ingredients in treatment manuals written for certain disorders. Most important among the common factors of successful interventions is the nature of the therapeutic relationship, or alliance, that is established between the helper and helpee.

Regardless of the approach you take in providing counseling or psychotherapy, it appears that when you intervene with skill and the common factors are present, all theories stand an equally good chance of working. Wampold (2001) stated that someone who gets counseling of any sort is likely to be better off than 79 percent of similar people who try to work things out on their own. Frank and Frank (1991) identified the common factors of successful counseling as:

- An emotionally charged, confiding relationship with a person who seeks to help
- Belief on the client's part that the counselor can be trusted and is able to provide help
- A mutually agreed upon conceptualization of the client's concern and situation

Interestingly, the great counseling and psychotherapy debate over which theory and which therapeutic approach is best has come down to the "Dodo Bird Verdict," which comes from Lewis Carroll's *Alice in Wonderland*. After a confusing race, all the runners demanded that the Dodo Bird declare who had won. The Dodo thought for a long time while the participants waited breathlessly. At last the Dodo declared that *everybody* had won, and *all* must have prizes.

In 1975, Luborsky, Singer, and Luborsky published the results of their meta-analysis of outcomes in counseling, suggesting that there is no significant difference in the effectiveness of the various theoretical approaches to psychotherapy. This is the "Dodo Bird Verdict." All theoretical approaches have won. While this assertion has remained understandably controversial, subsequent studies have confirmed this finding. The Dodo Verdict remains robust (Tallman & Bohart, 1999). While some outcome studies have found an edge for certain therapeutic approaches, there may have been some bias in these results: "When meta-analyses account for the allegiance of the investigator, differences favoring one approach over another largely vanish" (p. 92).

What seems certain is that the field of community counseling will continue to expand and evolve. Community counselors may vary in their styles, theoretical perspectives, and intervention techniques, but they have a shared commitment to help both individuals and communities in dealing with the challenges that confront them. By offering counseling, consultation, education, advocacy, training, supervision, and prevention services, community counselors promote both personal and community resilience.

PROFESSIONAL IDENTITY

Many benefits result from the heritage described earlier. Community counselors can draw upon the research and work of numerous, diverse scholars, including anthropologists, political scientists, cognitive scientists, psychologists, social workers, psychiatrists, and other counselors. They can practice in a variety of settings and use a wide range of interventions, making the most of their personal strengths and providing helping services that are particularly relevant and helpful for specific clients.

A couple of drawbacks, or at least complicating factors, exist as well. Because of the diverse influences on the profession, no two counselors practice in virtually the same way. Consumers of counseling services may therefore be confused about whom to contact for help. Furthermore, counseling specialties have proliferated, resulting in an even more nebulous picture of what it is that counselors actually do. Add to that the fact that some people are called *counselors*—for example, camp counselors and credit counselors—who may have little or nothing to do with the helping professions described above.

Thankfully, the push for certification and standardization helped to clarify expectations for counselors and to establish counseling as a profession. Ritchie (1990) described several criteria for professions. In general, professions

- provide a service that is of social value;
- are based on a common body of knowledge, theory, and skills;
- restrict entry to those with specialized education and training;
- require members to exhibit a minimum level of competency and have supervised internship;
- are legally recognized; and
- have an ethical code.

Although more recent researchers (Gale & Austin, 2003) have complained that counselors lack an obvious and distinct professional identity, in the broadest sense, counseling is certainly a profession. This distinction of profession is important, for it suggests that the potential consumers of our services will be more likely to perceive counselors as competent, ethical, and respected practitioners.

The counseling profession itself assists with the clarification of these expectations through guidelines regarding counseling credentials. Professional credentials for counselors usually include certification and licensure. *Certification* is a process through which counselors indicate that they have had a certain type of training. Certification does not necessarily give the counselor the right to practice counseling for a fee. In order to do so, the counselor must be licensed. *Licensure* is a legal regulation that governs the practice of counseling as well as the use of the title counselor.

As we mentioned earlier, nearly every state currently licenses counselors, which means that counseling professionals throughout most of the United States must have licenses to practice independently. These counselors also can receive insurance and other third-party payer reimbursements for services. These two factors are fundamentally important to ensure the vitality of the counseling profession. If counselors are licensed, then consumers of mental health services can be assured that their counselors have completed a specified program of study and received a certain amount of clinical supervision. Further, these professionals are obligated to uphold the code of ethics established by the American Counseling Association and other relevant organizations. Licensure is therefore one way of protecting the welfare of both individuals and communities. In Chapter 3 we explore the ethical issues that you will face as a community counselor.

The ability to receive third-party payer, or insurance, reimbursement is also extremely important. Imagine Josie, for instance, a woman who is struggling to maintain her self-esteem, as well as her relationship with her husband, when she is laid off from her job of twenty years. She decides to see a helping professional. She is covered under her husband's insurance, so she calls the insurance company to see what referrals they can offer. If counselors are not licensed in her state, her husband's insurance will only pay for services offered by psychologists, psychiatrists, or licensed social workers. The only way for the profession of counseling to continue to grow is to ensure that counselors are recognized as legitimate, well-trained professionals who offer a unique and necessary service.

If you have not already done so, take time now to find out what your state requires of you. For example, according to the American Counseling Association (2004), in order to become a Licensed Professional Counselor in Virginia, one must complete sixty semester hours or ninety quarter hours of graduate study and earn a graduate degree in counseling or a related field from an institution that meets certain curricular requirements. In addition, Virginia licensure applicants must complete 4000 hours of post-graduate supervised experience, with 200 hours of supervision, and pass a licensure examination. On the other hand, to become a Licensed Professional Counselor in Texas, one must complete a graduate degree in professional counseling or a related field that includes forty-eight graduate hours and a 300-hour practicum. Texas applicants also must complete 3000 hours of post-master's supervised experience and meet other requirements in order to become licensed.

Keep in mind, also, that licensure requirements can change. You will need to keep careful records of your counseling practice and to check that your supervisors meet state requirements. We talk about this issue more in Chapter 12; for now it is good practice to carefully document your experience. Creating and maintaining a professional portfolio is an excellent way for you to begin the process of documenting your work experience while charting your professional development goals.

So, imagine that Josie is fortunate enough to live in a state that has counselor licensure. She receives a list of referral options from her husband's insurance company that includes counselors, licensed social workers, and psychologists. Whom should she see? How will she decide? In an ideal world, community members would be well informed about the type of services that different helping professionals provide. Then, they could choose a helper based on their own preferences and needs. In reality, though, many people making the decision to seek mental health care rely on the advice of friends. Others think about what they have seen in television and movies and, understandably, may be reluctant to seek help.

Portrayals of Counselors in the Media

Notice how counselors and therapists are often portrayed in mass media. Strikingly, in the world of movies, it is nearly impossible to find a counselor or therapist who is consistently ethical, professionally committed, and routinely competent. Instead, movies have depicted counselors and therapists as wounded healers, incompetent fools, or malevolent controllers.

A popular example is the movie *The Prince of Tides*, in which a successful but unhappy therapist, played by Barbra Streisand, has sex with a man who met with her to help his hospitalized sister. An alarmingly high number of movies present counselors and their clients developing romantic, sexual relationships in the course of their work together; rarely is there any mention that such behavior is a serious breech of ethics (Gabbard & Gabbard, 1999).

Another troubling example is the therapist portrayed by Robin Williams in the popular movie *Good Will Hunting*, which is often cited as a positive portrayal of a helping professional (Koch & Dollarhide, 2000). The Williams character is authentic, empathic, and caring—but he also slams his client against a wall and threatens him. It is disturbing that few critics and viewers have expressed objections and concerns regarding such outrageously unprofessional behavior.

If potential clients rely on this type of information for help in making decisions about seeking mental health care, it is a wonder we have any clients at all! And it is no wonder that we sometimes have to spend some time with new clients to educate or re-educate them about what counseling is and how it works. Clearly, professionalism in counseling is fundamental, not only for the well-being of our clients, but for the sake of the profession itself.

So, back to the question of Josie seeking mental health services. Whom should she see? Before making a referral for Josie, we should consider several issues. According to Gelso and Fretz (1992), counselors tend to focus on "assets and strengths regardless of the degree of disturbance . . . , and the interaction between the person and his or her environment" (pp. 7–9). Counselors tend to see their goals as promoting greater well-being rather than reducing pathology, and they often focus on enhancing strengths and resources, rather than reconstructing personality. Of course, some community counselors work with seriously mentally ill clients who have been deinstitutionalized and receive services in community mental health agencies.

The foci listed above also describe counseling psychologists, at least in practice. One difference between a Licensed Professional Counselor (LPC) and a licensed counseling psychologist, however, is their level of training. In most states, the educational requirement for an LPC is a master's degree. Licensed counseling psychologists must have a doctoral degree and will likely have more training in research than the LPC. In addition, counseling essentially emerged from educational settings and many counselor education programs are housed in Schools of Education. Counseling psychology is a specialty within the field of psychology and is considered, by some, to embrace a scientist/practitioner model with a heavier emphasis on the scientist role than some counselors would claim.

The similarities between these professions can create confusion not only for consumers, but also for the professionals themselves. Gale and Austin (2003), for instance, stated that professional counselors lack a specific identity. Earlier, Goodyear (1984) addressed this issue, saying, "It is important, then, that we do not forsake aspects of our profession that are uniquely ours as we struggle to become recognized as legitimate providers of mental health services" (p. 5).

Ideally, Josie should have the chance to learn more about the specific expertise and training of a number of mental health professionals. Then she could choose the helper who is right for her. We do not live in an ideal world, of course, and referrals are often haphazard. The reality for Josie is that we cannot, with any degree of certainty, assert that Josie's issues are more appropriate for a counselor, rather than a clinical social worker or clinical psychologist. In fact, the interventions of a particular counselor, social worker and clinical psychologist may look more alike than those of three LPCs, depending on their orientations and practice.

The key point is that, disregarding individual differences among practitioners, counseling is not watered-down psychology. Counselors fill a specific niche in our communities with their emphasis on prevention, positive well-being, and education. Within this profession, specialties and variety abound. Although we share a common foundation, the ways in which we work are as diverse as we are. The table below outlines distinctive features of counselors, psychologists, and social workers.

Table 1.1 Comparison of the Educational Requirements, Professional Focus, License, and Typical Work Settings of Counselors, Social Workers, and Psychologists

Profession	Education	Focus	License	Typical Work Settings
Counselors	Master's degree in counseling or related field	Individual, family, and group counseling	Usually Licensed Professional Counselor or Licensed Marriage and Family Counselor	Community mental health agencies, hospitals, private practice, college centers, career counseling centers
Clinical Social Workers	Master's degree in social work	Individual and family counseling with an emphasis on collaboration with social service agencies	Usually Licensed Clinical Social Worker	Hospitals, social service agencies, private practice
Counseling and Clinical Psychologists	Ph.D., Ed.D., or Psy.D.	Counseling and psychotherapy; assessment and evaluation	Often Licensed Clinical Psychologist	Hospitals, community agencies, university counseling centers, private practice

EXPERIENTIAL LEARNING

1. Take some time now to consider what attracted you to counseling as opposed to clinical psychology or social work.

2. Now envision your future as a community counselor.

- What will you be doing?
- Where will you be working?
- What clients will you be serving?
- What values, goals, and dreams will be guiding you?

Professional Organizations

As you refine your interest in the counseling profession, find out more about the American Counseling Association (ACA), which is the parent organization for professional counselors in the United States. What we now know as ACA was initially established as the American Personnel and Guidance Association (APGA). This organization was developed in 1952 in order to better organize counseling, guidance, and personnel interests that were initially represented by four distinct organizations: The National Vocational Guidance Association, the National Association of Guidance and Counselor Trainers, the Student Personnel Association for Teacher Education, and the American College Personnel Association (History of ACA, n.d.).

As we mentioned earlier, several events then made a significant impact on the development of counseling as a distinct profession. The first major event was passage of the National Defense Education Act (NDEA). School counseling and guidance programs benefited as the government pumped more money into education. As a result, the importance of counseling and guidance became more evident. Then, in 1963, when the Community Mental Health Centers Act was passed counselors found more job opportunities and a broader scope of practice as they moved away from strictly school and career settings (Bloom, 1984).

By then, APGA had developed a code of ethics and Gilbert Wrenn had written about counselors as experts in developmental issues. In the next ten years, counselors continued to expand their scope of practice and began to emphasize specialties, such as mental health counseling and community counseling. Licensure requirements were enacted in some states, and APGA began to push beyond its emphasis on guidance and personnel.

Then, in 1981, the Council for Accreditation of Counseling and Related Educational Programs (CACREP) was formed, which identified training standards for counselor education programs. The National Board for Certified Counselors (NBCC) was formed in 1983. The NBCC administered a counselor examination and then certified, on a national level, the counselors who passed. At this time, APGA governance realized that the scope of counselors had changed, and APGA became the American Association for Counseling and Development (AACD). The next ten years saw considerable growth as counselor specialties continued to proliferate. In 1992, AACD became the American Counseling Association, which is now the world's largest association that exclusively represents professional counselors.

Currently, ACA provides leadership training, advocacy, and other membership services, such as defining professional and ethical standards for the profession. ACA also supports accreditation, licensure, and national certification efforts across the country and represents the interests of counselors to Congress and federal agencies. ACA has nineteen divisions and divisional affiliates, which include:

Association for Assessment in Counseling

Association for Adult Development and Aging

Association for Creativity in Counseling

American College Counseling Association

Association for Counselors and Educators in Government

Association for Counselor Education and Supervision

Association for Gay, Lesbian, and Bisexual Issues in Counseling

Association for Multicultural Counseling and Development

American Mental Health Counselors Association

American Rehabilitation Counseling Association

American School Counselor Association

Association for Spiritual, Ethical, and Religious Values in Counseling

Association for Specialists in Group Work

Counseling Association for Humanistic Education and Development

Counselors for Social Justice

International Association of Addiction and Offender Counselors

International Association of Marriage and Family Counselors

National Career Development Association

National Employment Counseling Association

As you look through this list, which divisions appeal most to you? What work settings attract you? Take some time to visit the ACA webpage at **www.counseling.org** and explore the organization. This organization is intended to represent you and can provide numerous benefits to you as a professional counselor.

WHAT IT TAKES TO BE A COUNSELOR

As a community counselor, your most important tool is yourself. Chapter 4 will invite you to examine and explore who you are as a person. At this point, we set the stage by suggesting some adjectives that describe the ideal community counselor: skilled, flexible, collaborative, committed, ethical, person-centered, community-focused, and—most important—self-aware.

Working as a counselor is a calling that entails hardships as well as rewards. Your training is an ideal time to investigate how you will deal with the challenges and how you will reap the benefits. When we screen applicants for our training programs, we often hear repeatedly that students feel compelled to become counselors. They love helping people, are good listeners, and feel that counseling is their calling. Their enthusiasm and excitement are palpable, and their potential seems boundless.

However, after they begin the training program, something happens. They receive feedback about how they present themselves and how that affects their ability to help others. They watch videotapes and listen to audiotapes of themselves. They engage in practice counseling sessions in which they draw a blank and have no idea what to say. Then they watch the videotapes of those sessions in the company of their peers and instructors. They have a peer counseling session and think they were wonderful, and then hear from their professor or peers that they missed the boat. That is when, for many, the stress of self-discovery and counseling practice takes its toll.

ETHICAL AND LEGAL ISSUES IN PRACTICE

The importance of ethical and legal practice in community counseling is paramount for ensuring the ongoing vitality and growth of the profession. We discuss ethical and legal issues in detail in Chapter 3, but for now we encourage you to go to the ACA website and read the ACA Code of Ethics and Standards of Practice. The ACA ethical code covers a wide range of behaviors that encompass fundamental aspects of community counseling, such as the need for counselors to maintain productive, honest relationships with other professionals; the demand that counselors practice within the scope of their own competence; and the expectation that counselors exhibit multicultural competence in their work with clients.

Furthermore, community counselors are required to understand their licensure requirements, state legal obligations, and agency policies. The only way to ensure that you are practicing ethically and legally is to be aware of and meet the professional expectations of community counselors. If you have not already done so, read the regulations regarding the practice of licensed

Keshia's Story

Keshia was in the second year of her training program. She had struggled emotionally in her Process of Counseling class but felt she had faced and dealt with some of the personality traits that negatively affected her counseling. Her perfectionism, for instance, and the discomfort she felt receiving feedback were less intense now than they had been when she entered the training program.

Now she was in the fifth week of her practicum class. She was seeing actual clients for the first time and was gaining some sense of counseling self-efficacy. Keshia knew she could "show up and have something to say," which was more than she could have said last year at this time.

Then she hit a wall. She found herself experiencing a negative reaction to a client and was confused about why she felt so ineffective with him. In her supervision session, as she explored the effect that countertransference could have on her practice, Keshia began to feel overwhelmed and discouraged. That night, she thought about other times in her life when she had had similar negative reactions to people. These musings led her to examine how she related to men in general. By the time her boyfriend called her late that evening, she felt anxious and exhausted. She wondered if she was able to relate to men at all.

The next day, she went back to her supervisor and said, "I think I've had it with all this introspection. I'm tired. I'm sick of the scrutiny. Also, I can't get this client out of my head! How am I going to deal with people who have problems on a regular basis? I can't take all my clients' worries home with me every night. And not only that, now that I know all this stuff about myself, I can't go back to the way I used to be. I don't think I was prepared for this. My relationships with other people are being affected by this training. Maybe I should just go and work in retail. I want my old way of being back."

Keshia processed her feelings with her supervisor, who helped her explore how she was changing. Together, they identified the positive aspects of Keshia's developing skills, such as her ability to listen empathically and conceptualize. They agreed that becoming immersed in counseling training is a life-changing experience. Keshia likened it to how she felt when she learned to drive a car. As she sat behind the wheel for the first time, she became aware of the awesome responsibility she had, how many things she had to pay attention to, how she had never before realized what driving was really like, how she'd never feel the same as a passenger again, and how her dependence on others was now permanently changed. Like learning to drive, learning to be an effective counselor offered a level of independence and agency that she had never experienced before.

The personal demands of counselor training can be intense. Keshia agreed to seek counseling at the university's counseling center and determined to continue to explore her personal and

(continued)

(Keshia's Story, continued)

emotional reactions to her training. She felt that, in order to be proactive and prevent burning out later, she had to use her training experience to fully delve into her own personal dynamics.

Questions for Reflection

1. How do you think you will deal with the scrutiny and feedback that are requisite components of counselor training?

2. What ways of being, or personal characteristics, do you want to hold on to as you learn to be an effective counselor?

3. What is the most challenging feedback that you have received?

4. How do you plan to respond effectively to this feedback?

---

professional counselors in your state. These regulations should be available via links provided on your state's governmental webpage. (As of August 2005, only California and Nevada have not yet licensed professional counselors.)

CONCLUDING THOUGHTS

We've given you much to consider as you begin your training experience. Where do you fit in your community? What is unique about you? What do you have to offer? How will you influence, and be influenced by, the continuing evolution of the counseling profession? Chapter 2 is designed to give you a glimpse into the lives of community counselors as you learn more about community counseling as a vibrant and challenging profession.

RECOMMENDED RESOURCES

In order to get a better sense of the systemic, wellness, and humanistic influences on community counseling, we suggest you read, or reread, the following:

Anderson, R. E., Carter, I., & Lowe, G. R. (1999). *Human behavior in the social environment: A social systems approach* (5th ed.). Hawthorne, NJ: Aldine de Gruyter.

Myers, J. E., & Sweeney, T. J. (Eds.). (2005). *Counseling for wellness: Theory, research, and practice.* Alexandria, VA: American Counseling Association.

Rogers, C. R. (1961). *On becoming a person: A therapist's view of psychotherapy.* Boston: Houghton Mifflin.

For an idea of how community change in general occurs, you may want to read:

Homan, M. S. (2004). *Promoting community change: Making it happen in the real world.* Belmont, CA: Brooks/Cole.

Other Resources

This list may not be quite what you're expecting. To complement the articles and books that you read in the professional literature, we're providing here a few resources that are a little less traditional. Consider the following:

To Kill a Mockingbird. This novel by Harper Lee is a wonderful evocation of both a child's view of the world, as well as a vivid portrait of a community dealing with a profound challenge to its oppressive traditions. The book enables the reader to truly appreciate how one person can make a powerful difference in a community.

I Know This Much Is True. This book is powerful in portraying the impact of mental illness on a family. Author Wally Lamb captures the richness of both the personal and systemic dynamics.

The Heart Is a Lonely Hunter. Carson McCullers did a magnificent job of creating a paradox of someone who is experienced as a wonderful listener, but who is actually deaf. The story also gives poignant testimony to the interrelatedness of a small community.

Along with everyone else, you've probably seen the classic movie *It's a Wonderful Life,* which showed the impact of one individual on the well-being of his community. You may also want to view other movies that give expression to the complexity and interconnectedness of a dynamic community. For example, *Sunshine State,* directed by John Sayles, offers a multifaceted depiction of the interactions and interplay of ethnic and social class subsystems within a Florida community. Another movie, *The Sweet Hereafter,* is a compelling representation of the wide-ranging effects of a school bus accident on a small town.

Organizations. The community counseling profession has organizations at the state, regional, and national levels. Below is a list of related national associations. All have developed websites that provide excellent information regarding resources, training and employment opportunities, and current issues in the profession.

American Association for Marriage and Family Therapy (AAMFT)
> 1133 Fifteenth Street, N.W., Suite 300
> Washington, DC 20005-2710
> 202.452.0109
> **www.aamft.org**

American Counseling Association (ACA)
> 5999 Stevenson Avenue
> Alexandria, VA 22304-3300
> 703.823.9800 or 800.347.6647
> **www.counseling.org**

American Mental Health Counselors Association (AMHCA)
> 801 N. Fairfax Street, Suite 304
> Alexandria, VA 22304
> 703.548.6002 or 800.326.2642
> **www.amhca.org**

Council for Accreditation of Counseling and Related Educational Programs (CACREP)
5999 Stevenson Avenue
Alexandria, VA 22304
703.823.9800 ext. 301
www.cacrep.org

National Board for Certified Counselors (NBCC) and Affiliates
3 Terrace Way, Suite D
Greensboro, NC 27414-7699
336.547.0607
www.nbcc.org

In addition, if you have not already done so, consider joining your state branch and local chapter of the American Counseling Association. These groups can help you develop a network of professional colleagues, provide professional development opportunities, and help you stay informed regarding proposed legislation that may affect your scope of practice and insurance reimbursement. Joining these state and local groups is also good practice in professional advocacy.

REFERENCES

American Counseling Association. (2005). *ACA Code of Ethics.* Retrieved August 22, 2005 from http://www.counseling.org/Content/NavigationMenu/ RESOURCES/ETHICS/ACA_Code_of_Ethics.htm

American Counseling Association (2004). *State licensure chart.* Retrieved August 5, 2005 from http://www.counseling.org/Content/NavigationMenu/ RESOURCES/LICENSUREANDCERTIFICATION/Licensure_and_Certi.htm

Bloom, B. L. (1984). *Community mental health: A general introduction* (2nd ed.). Monterey, CA: Brooks/Cole.

Caplan, G. (1964). *Principles of preventive psychiatry.* New York: Basic Books.

Cowen, E. L. (2000). Community psychology and routes to psychological wellness: Some opportunities and some limiting factors. In J. Rappaport & E. Seidman (Eds.), *Handbook of community psychology* (pp. 79–99). New York: Kluwer Academic/Plenum Press.

Cowen, E. L., & Hightower, A. D. (1989). The Primary Mental Health Project: Thirty years later. *Prevention in Human Services, 6,* 225–257.

Davis, A. F. (1994). *Spearheads for reform: The social settlements and the progressive movement, 1890–1914.* New Brunswick, NJ: Rutgers University Press.

Deardorff, J., Gonzales, N. A., & Sandler, I. N. (2003). Control beliefs as a mediator of the relation between stress and depressive symptoms among inner-city adolescents. *Journal of Abnormal Child Psychology, 31,* 205–217.

DiClemente, C. C. (2003). *Addiction and change: How addictions develop and addicted people recover.* New York: Guilford.

Durlack, J. A., & Wells, A. M. (1998). Evaluation of indicated preventive interventions (secondary prevention) mental health programs for children and adolescents. *American Journal of Community Psychology, 26,* 775–802.

Echterling, L. G., Presbury, J., McKee, J. E. (2005). *Crisis intervention: Promoting resilience and resolution in troubled times.* Upper Saddle River, NJ: Prentice Hall.

Frank, J. D., & Frank, J. B. (1991). *Persuasion and healing: A comparative study of psychotherapy* (3rd ed.). Baltimore: Johns Hopkins University Press.

Gabbard, G. O., & Gabbard, K. (1999). *Psychiatry and the cinema* (2nd ed.). Washington, DC: American Psychiatric Press.

Gale, A. U., & Austin, B. D. (2003). Professionalism's Challenges to Professional Counselors' Collective Identity. *Journal of Counseling and Development, 81,* 3–10.

Gelso, C. J., & Fritz, B. R. (1992). *Counseling psychology.* Orlando, FL: Holt, Rinehart & Winston.

Gleick, J. (1987). *Chaos: Making a new science.* New York: Viking Penguin.

Goodyear, R. K. (1984). On our journal's evolution: Historical developments, transitions, and future directions. *Journal of Counseling and Development, 63,* 3–8.

Hanson, J. C., Rossberg, R. H., & Cramer, S. H. (1994). *Counseling: Theory and process.* Boston: Allyn & Bacon.

Hershenson, D. B., & Berger, G. P. (2001). The state of community counseling: A survey of directors of CACREP-accredited programs. *Journal of Counseling & Development, 79,* 188–193.

History of ACA. (n.d.). Retrieved August 3, 2005, from http://www.counseling.org/Content/NavigationMenu/INSIDEACA/INSIDEACA1/HISTORY.htm

Hussong, A. M., & Hicks, R. E. (2003). Affect and peer context interactively impact adolescent substance use. *Journal of Abnormal Child Psychology, 31,* 413–426.

Koch, G., & Dollarhide, C. T. (2000). Using a popular film in counselor education: *Good Will Hunting* as a teaching tool. *Counselor Education and Supervision, 39,* 203–209.

Levine, M., & Levine, A. (1970). *The social history of helping services: Clinic, court, school, and community.* New York: Appleton-Century-Crofts.

Lewis, J., & Lewis, M. (1989). *Community counseling.* Pacific Grove, CA: Brooks/Cole.

Luborsky, L., Singer, B., & Luborsky, L. (1975). Comparative studies of psychother-apies: Is it true that "everyone has won and all must have prizes"? *Archives of General Psychiatry, 32,* 995–1008.

McMillan, D. W., & Chavis, D. M. (1986). Sense of community: A definition and theory. *Journal of Community Psychology, 14,* 6–23.

Myers, J. E., & Sweeney, T. J. (Eds.). (2005). *Counseling for wellness: Theory, research, and practice.* Alexandria, VA: American Counseling Association.

Myers, J. E., Sweeney, T. J., & Witmer, J. M. (2000). The wheel of wellness coun-seling for wellness: A holistic model for treatment planning. *Journal of Counseling and Development, 78,* 251–266.

Nystul, M. S. (2003). *Introduction to counseling: An art and science perspective* (2nd ed.). Boston: Allyn & Bacon.

Okin, R. L., Borus, J., Baer, L., & Jones, A. L. (1995). Long-term outcome of state hospital patients discharged into structural community residential settings. *Psychiatric Services, 46,* 73–78.

Pennebaker, J. W., Francis, M. E., & Booth, R. J. (2001). *Linguistic Inquiry and Word Count (LIWC 2001): A computerized text analysis program.* Mahwah, NJ: Erlbaum.

Pennebaker, J. W., & Graybeal, A. (2001). Patterns of natural language use: Disclo-sure, personality, and social integration. *Current Directions in Psychologi-cal Science, 10,* 90–93.

Pope, M., & Sveinsdottir, M. (2005). Frank, we hardly knew ye: The very personal side of Frank Parsons. *Journal of Counseling and Development, 83,* 105–115.

Presbury, J. H., Echterling, L. G., & McKee, J. E. (2002). *Ideas and tools for brief counseling.* Upper Saddle River, NJ: Prentice Hall.

Rahman, O., & Rollock, D. (2004). Acculturation, competence, and mental health among South Asian students in the United States. *Journal of Multicultural Counseling and Development, 32,* 130–141.

Rappaport, J. (2000). Community narratives: Tales of terror and joy. *American Journal of Community Psychology, 28,* 1–24.

Repucci, N. D., Wooland, J. L., & Fried, C. S. (1999). Social, community, and pre-ventive interventions. *Annual Review of Psychology, 50,* 387–418.

Ritchie, M. H. (1990). Counseling is not a profession—yet. *Counselor Education and Supervision, 29,* 220–227.

Roberts, L. D., Smith, L. M., & Pollock, C. (2002). Mooing till the cows come home: The search for sense of community in virtual environments. In A. T. Fisher, C. C. Sonn, & B. J. Bishop (Eds.), *Psychological sense of community: Research, applications, and implications* (pp. 223–245). New York: Kluwer Academic/Plenum.

Rogers, C. R. (1961). *On becoming a person: A therapist's view of psychotherapy*. Boston: Houghton Mifflin.

Rudkin, J. K. (2003). *Community psychology: Guiding principles and orienting concepts*. Upper Saddle River, NJ: Prentice Hall.

Sampson, E. E. (2000). Reinterpreting individualism and collectivism: Their religious roots and monologic versus dialogic person-other relationships. *American Psychologist, 55,* 1425–1432.

Stroebe, M., van Vliet, T., Hewstone, M., & Willis, H. (2002). Homesickness among students in two cultures: Antecedents and consequences. *British Journal of Psychology, 93,* 147–168.

Tallman, K., & Bohart, A. C. (1999). The client as a common factor: Clients as self-healers. In M. A. Hubble, B. L. Duncan, & S. D. Miller (Eds.), *The heart & soul of change: What works in therapy* (pp. 91–131). Washington, DC: American Psychological Association.

Thurber, C. A. (2005). Multimodal homesickness prevention in boys spending 2 weeks at a residential summer camp. *Journal of Consulting and Clinical Psychology, 73,* 555–560.

Torrey, E. F. (1997). *Out of the shadows: Confronting America's mental illness crisis.* New York: John Wiley & Sons.

U.S. Office of Education. (1950). *Report on the national conference on life adjustment.* Washington, DC: Author.

Wampold, B. E. (2001). *The great psychotherapy debate: Models, methods, and findings.* Mahwah, NJ: Erlbaum.

Webber, J., Bass, D. D., & Yep, R. (Eds.) (2005). *Terrorism, trauma, and tragedies: A counselor's guide to preparing and responding* (2nd ed.). Alexandria, VA: American Counseling Association.

Chapter 2

Living the Life: Practical Realities of Community Counseling

We all live in suspense from day to day; in other words, you are the hero of your own story.

Mary McCarthy

Can't nothing make your life work if you ain't the architect.

Terry McMillan

GOALS

Reading and exploring the ideas in this chapter will help you:

- Gain a sense of the daily life of community counselors in various settings
- Gain an understanding of the challenges and opportunities facing community counselors, such as managed care and technology
- Glean suggestions for thriving as a community counselor
- Anticipate trends that will affect the practice of community counselors

---

OVERVIEW

This chapter presents information on the role of community counselors in various practice settings, organizational dimensions of institutions in which community counselors practice, general characteristics of human services programs and networks, psychopharmacology and counseling, and the role of advocacy, managed care, and creativity in community counseling.

As you read through this text you will find that each chapter presents a view of a segment of community counseling. In this chapter we introduce the experience of community counseling to you. What does the work of community counselors actually look like? How do they spend their days? More importantly, you may be wondering, *Am I going to enjoy this work? Can I find a place for myself as a community counselor?* These questions will be answered, at least in part, by the particular setting in which you practice. The answers to these questions also lie in your own skills, needs, and interests.

The milieu of the community counselor is incredibly diverse, so here we provide an overview of work settings. We also present excerpts from three counselors' journals to offer you the opportunity to understand their experiences, just as you will attempt to listen to, empathize with, and conceptualize your clients' experiences. After the journal excerpts, we provide more detailed information about specific issues those counselors face.

LENNIE'S DEFINING MOMENT: The Epiphany

Lennie, one of the authors of this book and an experienced community counselor, has developed a wealth of experience in responding to individual and community crises. In his efforts to research crisis response and intervention, he has traveled extensively to work with clients and agencies in the United States and abroad. Recently he decided to squeeze in a brief vacation in Ireland prior to continuing his international research. The following is his recollection of an early morning revelation:

"On the first day of our vacation in Ireland, my wife and I checked into a charming little Bed and Breakfast along the Ring of Kerry. The scenery was ruggedly beautiful and, after being cramped on a trans-Atlantic flight for so long, I decided to go for a run. Barry, the owner of the B & B, suggested a route that included spectacular sights, steep hills, and a little beach nestled among the rocky terrain. The run proved to be wonderful, but dangerous. The narrow road could barely accommodate two cars, let alone a runner, and the traffic included mammoth-sized tour buses. The stone walls that bordered the road were quaint and picturesque, but they left no escape for a hapless runner who may have to share the road with large vehicles. Maybe the most troubling was the fact that the traffic traveled on the left side, so I had to constantly remind myself to run on the right so that I would face the traffic.

"I was in this slightly disoriented, vigilant state of mind when I finally made it to the steep descending path that would take me to an isolated cove. Ahead and below, I could see large rocks, a bit of sand, the water . . . and a very large dog looking up straight at me. My only choice, it seemed to me, was to stop running, assume a non-threatening posture, and offer a friendly greeting in my most soothing tone of voice. The dog, still eyeing me, moved even closer.

Then, when he got within striking distance to me, the big dog dropped a stick at my feet and looked up into my eyes imploringly. As we made eye-contact, I suddenly understood. I picked up the stick, threw it out into the ocean, and savored the sight of the dog galloping off in hot pursuit. He retrieved the stick, ran back joyfully, dropped it at my feet once again, and looked up at me expectantly.

"That nameless dog and I had a wonderful time playing together. When I reluctantly began my run back, my new Irish friend was playing with a girl and her father. This encounter seems an apt metaphor for the experiences of community counselors. As I ran back to the inn the words of Teddy Roosevelt came to me—'Speak softly, but carry a big stick.'

"Of course, Roosevelt was referring to the need for acting with diplomacy, but being well-armed. Ideally, as a community counselor, you'll also be well armed. Your 'stick' will include the tools that create a solid foundation for your counseling practice: your comprehension of theory, skills, and process, and your understanding of yourself and your clients. And, just as I had no idea what to expect from the dog, you'll have no idea what challenges and joys you might encounter with every new contact you make and every new client you encounter."

Questions for Reflection

1. As you envision your future work as a community counselor, what do you most fear you'll encounter?

2. In the past, how have your fears either limited you or perhaps encouraged you toward personal revelations?

WORK SETTINGS OF COMMUNITY COUNSELORS

As we mentioned in Chapter 1, the work of community counselors has changed dramatically over the past forty years, and the process of change is continuing. In the early 1960s, then-President John F. Kennedy named poverty as a factor in mental illness and called for the establishment of enhanced community prevention efforts (Hartley, Bird, Lambert, & Coffin, 2002). In 1963, the Mental Retardation Facilities and Community Mental Health Centers Construction Act (PL 88-164), commonly known as the CMHC Act, was passed. This act eased the responsibility of the state hospital system and enhanced services for deinstitutionalized patients by supporting the development of community mental health centers. These centers received federal grant funding and were expected to provide the five essential services we outlined in Chapter 1: outpatient, inpatient, consultation/education, partial hospitalization (such as day treatment programs), and emergency/crisis intervention (Wagenfeld, Murray, Mohatt, & DeBruyn, 1994). Thus, the typical setting for much community counseling work was formed.

Community Mental Health Centers have changed since 1963, and many have faced significant obstacles. The original Act provided funding for construction of centers, for example, but not funding for staffing those centers. Further, initial grants were intended to be temporary. Community mental health centers have therefore struggled for financial solvency since they were first developed (Dorwart & Epstein, 1993).

In addition, although one expectation of the CMHC Act was that agencies would provide services for low-income clients, the guidelines regarding those services were minimal. Amendments to the CMHC Act increased expectations of community mental health centers and resulted in pressure for agencies to serve deinstitutionalized patients and other "priority patients," specifically those who are seriously and persistently mentally ill and/or severely emotionally disturbed children (Schnapp, Bayles, Raffoul, & Schnee, 1999). As a result, community mental health centers are often strapped to provide sufficient services to significant populations within the community, and prevention and education services are at times sacrificed. The evolution of community mental health centers highlights the importance of professional as well as client advocacy skills among counselors. Advocacy is discussed in more detail later in this chapter, as well as in Chapter 7.

As community mental health centers have changed, counselors have adapted. They flourish in our communities, providing community mental health services in a variety of settings.

Outpatient Counseling

Outpatient counseling services usually include providing individual, family, and group interventions in order to help people improve their general levels of adjustment and functioning. Clients seeking services in outpatient settings range from the "worried well," people who are essentially high functioning but who have one or more significant areas of concern, to individuals who struggle with persistent mental illness.

Inpatient Counseling

Inpatient counseling services are usually offered in local or state hospitals operating in partnership with community agencies. Counselors who offer inpatient services usually expect to work intensively with patients with the intention that the patient will leave the hospital as soon as possible. After leaving the hospital clients are usually the recipients of a series of services coordinated through counselors and social workers.

Day Programs

Day programs, the work site for many community counselors, provide a variety of services, such as individual, group, and recreational therapy, in addition to medication management and life-skills training, for individuals who do not need complete hospitalization but require intensive assistance to cope with their mental health needs and adjust to life in society. Day programs include *partial hospitalization programs,* which usually offer a fairly structured program for clients needing a greater level of care, and *intensive* or *structured outpatient programs,* for clients whose struggles are less acute and who can therefore manage with less assistance.

Consultation/Education Services

Consultation/education services are often seen as the specialty of community counselors, so it's unfortunate that these important services sometimes take a back seat to secondary and tertiary prevention, or direct intervention. However, many community counselors devote significant time to providing consultative and educational services to clients, clients' family members, and other agency personnel. Some agencies also support primary prevention to the degree that they encourage their counselors to provide educational workshops and programs for the community. Most agencies, however, require their counselors to provide a specific number of billable hours, meaning hours that will be reimbursed by clients, insurance, or other funding sources. Unless an organization contracts for these services from the agency, or an agency receives grant funding to provide such services, consultation and education are not usually paid for by entities outside the agency. Therefore, many agency administrators view consultation and education services as volunteer or pro bono work. Some counselors have therefore become skilled at writing grants that support their consultative and educational service.

Emergency/Crisis Intervention

Emergency/crisis intervention services allow community members twenty-four-hour access to help. Community members experiencing acute emotional or mental distress can contact these community agencies to receive immediate crisis intervention assistance. Many counselors find their first full- or part-time jobs working with emergency services. Although the experience is valuable, the work is challenging and can quickly lead to counselor burnout. Similarly, many beginning counselors are hired to provide *substance abuse services* in order to help clients deal with addiction, dependence, abuse, and recovery. Substance abuse services may be offered in outpatient or inpatient settings and may require a significant amount of family work and interprofessional collaboration.

Case Management Services

Most community counselors are quickly introduced to case management services. Counselors engage in case management in order to gain access as efficiently as possible to the most relevant resources for clients. In doing so, their goals are to prevent the development of additional problems for the client and enhance the client's chance to live successfully and independently. When working as case managers, counselors often assist their clients in dealing with other health professionals, such as physicians, home health workers, and psychiatrists. They may also ensure that clients receive timely and well-informed access to community services such as subsidy programs for low-income individuals. The line dividing case management from social work services is narrow, and, in many ways, from the perspective of the client that dividing line becomes irrelevant. Effective community counselors learn quickly how to secure a variety of services in the best interests of their clients.

Residential Programs

Community counselors also work in residential programs, which offer supportive services to clients who, for a variety of reasons, are not able to live independently in the community. Residential programs include homes for clients who have recently been released from the hospital but who need significant structure and support, group homes for adolescents who have been involved with the court system and who have not yet been approved for return to home or foster care in the community, homes for individuals with mental retardation or developmental delays, and homes that offer substance abuse counseling and recovery services in a residential setting.

Other Settings

Community counselors work in many other settings as well. They provide school-based mental health services, stepping in to provide more intensive therapeutic services for students than the school counselor or school psychologist will provide. They staff employee assistance programs, working for corporations or hospitals to provide counseling and referral services for employees. Community counselors also work in private practice, often joining with other counselors, social workers, and psychologists to provide services within their specific range of competence and training.

DAYS IN THE LIVES

The journal excerpts that follow reflect experiences of three community counselors: Kelly, who works in an in-patient setting; Barry, who works in private practice; and Catherine, who works with the Head Start Program. As you read you may be surprised, or even intimidated, by some of their experiences. We provide their stories so that you can get a glimpse of how these counselors spend their days. Later in the chapter, we expand on specific themes from their journals that are likely to be relevant for you in your work. Keep in mind that these journal excerpts do not reflect the totality of experiences for community counselors—they are essentially snapshots. Remember, too, that your experience as a community counselor will be your own creation.

___

KELLY'S JOURNAL

> Kelly works at a state psychiatric hospital for children. Her job as the substance abuse counselor includes running five substance abuse groups per week, seeing individual clients who have extensive substance abuse histories, attending treatment reviews and treatment planning meetings, and promoting smoking awareness for events such as The Great American Smokeout.

October 16

Today was a hectic day because I was working on my presentation to the Tobacco Settlement Foundation, which gave the grant for our substance abuse program. Next week I will be going to another county to explain our program, show how we have used our funding, and meet other grantees. I compiled some of the data we had been collecting about patient attendance and motivation toward quitting drug use. Then I put together a PowerPoint presentation. This was challenging because I also had to juggle several new admissions to the hospital that needed to be evaluated before group.

During group supervision the substance abuse team discussed some of the more difficult cases and how to best offer services. We are always working on coordinating our efforts. At times it can get confusing because our patients all need special services. Some can handle groups; others with behavior problems or psychoses benefit more from individual sessions.

After that, I did several substance abuse evaluations, administering the SASSI (Substance Abuse Subtle Screening Inventory) and the PRQ (Problem Recognition Questionnaire) to assess motivation, and I completed a clinical interview. Following the patient's interview, I referred her to the Substance Abuse program and placed her in my group.

Then, I attended "shift exchange" on one of the units. I try to attend these every day, because this is when first shift reports to second shift and the clinical staff regarding how the patients have done during that day. I check to make sure none of my group members have been aggressive or have had any other problems. Then I know whether or not they are safe to be in my group. This is also a good check-in point with the doctors about coordinating treatments and observations.

I ran my first group of the day with adolescents on unit 4. After that group, I had a break for dinner. It was the first time I relaxed in six hours, and I was exhausted. It's amazing how quickly I process all that happens in the hospital and how crisis becomes so normal. I am constantly in a state of alert. Patients become aggressive and suicidal on a daily basis. The stressors of the patients are astronomical, ranging from mental illness, being in a new and tense environment, living with other patients with illness, family issues, pending legal charges, and so much more. My job as counselor does not happen in a closed session. I'm "on" during every interaction with every patient.

Following the break, I led another group very similar to the first. After doing case notes I was finished for the day.

October 18

In my job I have faced so many challenges. It is difficult for me to even describe how fast-paced the acute crisis hospital setting can be. My case load includes suicidal patients whom I spend time with all day. At times the patients become aggressive, and that adds another element of worry about my own safety. At first, it was difficult for me to process the stories and the needs of the patients. There is little time to think between each case, and eventually I started getting a little hardened. Now, abuse, substance abuse, and terrible family situations seem normal to me. I am not sure how I feel about this, but I know it has allowed me to leave work at work and feel competent knowing that my emotions are not driving my counseling.

Another struggle in my job has been being a part of a treatment team. I work closely with psychiatrists, psychologists, nurses, social workers, and recreation therapists. We must coordinate all our efforts and have the same patient goals in mind in order for the patients' treatment to be successful. This can be difficult when people's backgrounds cause them to have different points of view. In my role as counselor, I find that I have very little power in the hierarchy despite the fact that I seem to know the patients very well. I am constantly fighting to be heard, and I'm learning to find my voice in these meetings.

Despite the challenges and stress, I love my job. I find it exciting and immensely rewarding. While others worry about medicine and diagnosis, I work hard to provide a safe place for the patient to explore feelings and needs. Because my clients are inpatients, and in distress, the simple gesture of spending a few minutes to check in with them each day is rewarded with gratitude. It is obvious that my presence makes a difference. The job is also constantly changing. With the average patient's stay being three to four weeks, I have had the opportunity to work with many patients, see many different types of treatment, and never get bored.

I wish when I was in my graduate training program that I had paid more attention to the information presented about the clinical side of counseling. I always felt a little "above" the medical model, so I was a bit uncomfortable at first when people here talked exclusively about treatment planning, diagnosis, and medication management. I have worked hard to learn to communicate with doctors and understand things from a medical model point of view. However, sometimes I'm not sure how I really feel, even now, about the medical model. Do I buy into the model? I'm not sure. Interprofessional collaboration was also a big adjustment for me. Learning how different professionals approach the same client has been interesting. I would also have liked to have learned more about psychopharmacology. I have learned a lot from listening in on psychiatrists' recommendations. I have found that the medication affects the way clients are able to participate in therapy and can confound their treatment. However, I still feel underprepared and a little self-conscious when I try to talk with other professionals about medications.

Thankfully, I do feel that my graduate program prepared me to succeed at my job. I have never doubted my counseling ability or my work with clients. I have also been able to deal with difficult issues because the program encouraged me to seek counseling for my own concerns.

Questions for Reflection

1. Clearly, Kelly faces many demands in her work. As you read her journal, what were your reactions to her work day?

2. What parts of her job do you think you would enjoy? What aspects would be less appealing to you?

3. Kelly mentions several topics she wishes she would have explored while in graduate school. What experiences can you create for yourself *now* in order to be best prepared for the work you plan to do?

BARRY'S JOURNAL

Barry is a licensed professional counselor who has been in private
practice for five years. He also works as a "counselor in residence" for
a graduate counseling training program at a nearby university.

Tuesday

Our office manager left two weeks ago on maternity leave. It has
been difficult without someone to call the insurance companies, run
the bills, remind us about the treatment plans, and keep the bills
paid. Now, with HIPAA (Health Insurance Portability and Accountability Act) regulations, we need to be extremely cautious about
how we control and protect information about our clients. Maintaining confidentiality is a challenge in a small town.

My first client today was a new intake. I love ironies. He makes
his living as a clown. A clown in therapy is the kind of thing that
keeps my work interesting. At the end of our session he told me he
was encouraged about therapy and felt hopeful about working with
me. These kinds of experiences still make me feel good and give me
hope.

Now I'm off to the local Head Start program to do mental health
screenings. I noticed when talking with teachers that they are often
appalled by stories they hear about kids and how they are treated
by their families. I wonder if I'm somewhat desensitized to this by
now. In many ways what's important is the child or client in front of
me. I can't get too caught up in how horrible their parents are, or
how bad their past has been. I've got to stay with the person I'm
with now, and focus on their reality and their potential. I may be
desensitized, but I have not lost my empathy.

Lunch next with my wife, who is also my therapy partner. We
don't get to do this often. We are usually too busy scheduling thirty
clients per week. Sometimes we staff cases; other times we talk
about how to juggle our kids' schedules. I don't think I ever realized
how fast-paced a private practice can be. Before my wife and I
started this practice I was working in a community agency. I liked
my work but wanted more autonomy. We wrote a huge list of pros
and cons for private practice before I quit my job—I wish I could
find that list now to see how accurate we were! One of the best
things about this practice is the fact that everything I do is intentional. I do my work with purpose. I'm not filling out paperwork for
other people or justifying what I do. I feel like it's me and my

clients, working in a streamlined and often intense partnership. What a relief after working with social service agencies for so long.

I had a no-show today. At one point this would make me panic. I'd worry how I was going to pay the bills, what if other clients didn't show, etc. Now, I have to admit that sometimes it feels like a relief. I have time to do paperwork and return phone calls. I spent a great deal of time today trying to remember how to post insurance payments. Without an office manager I'm reminded how much time is spent doing non-clinical work.

Wednesday

First client at 8 A.M. Nice young boy who has good social skills and only one problem: He has a mother with Borderline Personality Disorder. His father has custody, but mom terrorizes the family and is beginning to harass me now. I have set good boundaries with her, but she persists with calls and e-mails. I fear she is building a case to go back to court. This type of struggle definitely takes a toll on me.

After a few more clients there is more of the business stuff. I needed to post the insurance checks, print out the Head Start screenings, and return a mountain of calls. The calls are primarily from new referrals, and follow-up calls for school observations and other exchanges of information. I also sent out e-mails to counselors across the state about the pending legislation regarding Medicare reimbursement for counselors. I was formerly the president of our state clinical counselors association, so I still keep abreast of current legislative news that affects counselors. It drives me crazy that social workers and psychologists can be reimbursed by Medicare for providing services to clients, but counselors can't be. I know that when legislation was first introduced regarding this issue counselors were only licensed in about twenty-five states. Now, though, almost every state has licensure, and the training for LPCs and social workers is certainly equivalent. There's no reason to leave LPCs out of this loop. I get a little hot and bothered by this type of thing. I think it's my responsibility to make sure counselors work together to make sure we're taken care of. Maybe one day I'll take a part-time job as a lobbyist!

I notice as I look back over what I've written that I've focused on difficult issues. I have seen several clients today and felt that our sessions went very well. A thirty-year-old man who is struggling with his fiancé over a guilt-filled revelation about a past incident in his life. . . . A man who is struggling with changing his own behavior and alcoholism. . . . The kind of work that reminds me why I do what I do.

Thursday

I got a bit of a jolt today—I heard that a large group from the Washington, D.C. area is coming in to open a mental health practice to serve this and surrounding areas. A little competition is good, I guess, but I admit I felt mildly nervous when I heard this. I've been reading so much lately about e-counseling. Would that be a reasonable endeavor for us? Frankly, I can't imagine not having the face-to-face contact with my client. Reading back over this journal has also made me aware that my ability to express myself in writing is not nearly as keen as my oral communication skills. I wonder if other counselors have the same concern? The ethical issues also seem immense. At the same time, though, I feel there is a need, and definitely interest, in e-counseling. My wife and I are going to have to talk about this. The learning in this job is never-ending.

Monday

I'm working at the university today. My job is to teach, see clients so that students can observe me, and provide supervision for counseling graduate students. I am struck by the difference in atmospheres between the university and my office. The pace at school is slower, and not having to respond to people's needs one after another is wonderful for me. I had planned to broaden our income sources so I wouldn't be so dependent on insurance reimbursement, and this teaching and supervision work fits the bill. Not only is it a good business move, but it refreshes me to be out of the office and have the chance to interact with other professionals. I had forgotten how important that was to me when I was working in the public sector. I also think that I may end up supervising some of these students once they've graduated and are working on their residency requirements for licensure. I never before thought about providing supervision, but that's another way to expand the practice and diversify a little. Diversify! Who would ever have thought that I'd use words like that to describe my work? Being in private practice does require a bit of an entrepreneurial spirit. It's probably not for everyone, but I can't imagine anything else I'd rather be doing.

Questions for Reflection

1. Before leaving his job in a community agency, Barry developed a list of "pros and cons" regarding opening a private practice. Create your own pro and con list for the type of counseling job you'd like to have. Discuss your list with your peers.

2. Barry writes that being in private practice requires an entrepreneurial spirit. In light of this observation, how suited do you believe you
are for private practice work?

CATHERINE'S JOURNAL

Catherine works as a counselor for Head Start. In addition to completing behavioral screenings for children in Head Start classrooms,
she provides play therapy to children who have been identified as
needing extra attention. This is Catherine's second year after
graduation.

3/31

Today is Monday, and as usual it has been a whirlwind. I have
FINALLY finished mental health screenings on all classes. Let's see—
seventeen students per class—and I am in charge of eight classes, so
that makes 136 students. Whew. I am glad it is over. It's difficult,
since I don't think that the screenings are that effective. It was hard
to justify spending my time on these screenings when there were
some behavioral crises going on.

Just spoke to my fellow case manager. My supervision was just
cancelled. It is okay, though, because I have two weeks of paperwork to complete and parents to contact. One thing about paperwork—it always seems I am behind. It's not so much that I am disor-
ganized (I will admit that plays a part in it); it's more that there
never seems to be enough time. In my job I travel all day, so it's
difficult to stay on top of anything that doesn't feel critical.

4/3

This is the first day I have been in my office longer than five minutes
since my last entry. Instead of doing paperwork, I contacted parents.
I actually was able to connect with all of them, which is a rare and
true blessing. Today has been a very emotional day though. On my
way to a play therapy session my supervisor called with a crisis at a
school. A child that I have been working with has increased his
aggressive behaviors (at times he needs to be held up to thirty minutes). He was hitting, kicking, and trying to bite other students and
the teacher. We have a behavior plan in place. Part of the plan includes calling this child's mother and having her work with the
school in helping her son deal with his feelings. Good idea—but I
believe this mother is very inappropriate with him. She also uses
corporal punishment, which I believe is ineffective with this child.

In the past, instead of staying with him, she takes him home. Who knows what happens when they get home? All I do know is that his tantrums have increased in frequency and length, and I know that he is hurting even more than when I first met him. Last week his mom told me that when she found out he kicked his teacher she went home and kicked him "so he could see how it feels." It is SO DIFFICULT to work with parents who just don't know how their actions are impacting the child.

So today my supervisor calls and I go to the school and take my client out for a play therapy session. In walks the principal to let me know that his mother was coming to pick him up. My client was doing well until that point, but then he began to cry, saying "she's going to punch me." I felt so awful and powerless. The principal had decided the child should go home (for the safety of other children) yet I feared strongly for the safety of my client. The entire energy of the classroom has been tense lately. So I sat with my client and said little, just reflecting his feelings. I then helped him get his things ready. I sat with him in the office and in walked mom. It was awful. She screamed, ripped up a book, and threw it away. She threatened him. I hated it. I could feel the tears begin to well in my own eyes. I did sit out with her for a bit and try to calm her down and process what would be an appropriate consequence for him. We talked about how to manage her anger and disappointment. Unfortunately, she was not in a place that she could be receptive to the conversation. Well, I am feeling tired and disappointed now. I feel like I let my client down. I have to continually work on keeping myself centered, focused, and aware of the limits of my power with my clients.

4/11

Well, a lot has happened with this little boy since my last entry. I didn't feel I could write everything down at the time, because the whole thing was ugly and hard to witness. When I tried to intervene with the mom and the little boy, the mom yelled, "What do you know?! You don't have children!" The gist of the story is that Child Protective Services (CPS) was called. CPS is now beginning an investigation of emotional abuse with this family. Since CPS has intervened, the mom has cursed at me and threatened my life. I'm having nightmares. Sometimes I lie in bed and think about my cases and reflect on sessions and what I would want to do differently or next session. I pray for my families. It carries on into my dreams. That is always a huge red flag for me. I am still working on boundaries between my home life and work life.

4/13

I have spoken with the little boy's mother and finally reached a place where she felt heard and could understand my reasons for intervention as well. It was very difficult because she wanted to know who called CPS regarding her and her child. I usually want to be very transparent and genuine with my clients and their families. However, this woman was threatening, and she has a violent history. I did not want to be involved in affirming or denying her, as I don't want to participate in her process of blaming others. However, it felt like I was being dishonest as well. I didn't really have anyone to process this with afterward either. I tried to call my supervisor and ended up processing with a colleague (thank goodness). I'm still incredibly concerned for the little boy. It must be so hard for him to live the way he's living right now. I'm getting ready to go to supervision now.

Back from supervision. The principal wants to expel the little boy from school since his mother won't follow any of our recommendations. I see both sides. Other children are being put at risk if he is lashing out. However, I am not sure that this mother is ever going to get help for herself or learn how to manage her relationship with my client. So if he leaves the program, that means he won't have any structured, safe environment. I suppose time will tell.

4/17

I have just a few minutes to write before my next session. I have been thinking of some areas in which I wish I had more training. Well, some areas that I definitely need to continue to work on are:

1. Boundary issues. My first job was an in-home counselor (5 hours/week with each family in the family's home). Boundaries were very difficult. In my current job boundaries continue to be difficult. My role as a consultant to the teaching team, parents, and with the children is sometimes hard to balance. What exactly *is* my role?

2. Insurance companies. Medicaid. The problem is that I am focused on being present, in the moment, and process oriented, and then I remember that I have to keep notes in a certain style and complete formal paperwork. This seems so far removed from what I'm actually doing every day. Fulfilling some of the requirements seems ridiculous.

3. Play therapy. Not all supervisors are like my university supervisors! I could use more concrete feedback regarding my play therapy skills.

4/25

Things I love about my job:
- Working with children!
- Playing
- Ongoing learning
- Flexibility—I control my own schedule
- My schedule (8:00–3:30)

Things I don't particularly like:
- School politics
- Insurance companies (who sometimes seem to know very little about mental health)
- The fact that paperwork is never-ending
- I don't have anyone to really process with at work

5/5

I've been thinking about trust—sometimes it takes MONTHS to gain rapport and eventually trust with a family. I was quite naïve in school. I thought that I could exhibit qualities of openness, compassion, being present, active listening . . . and that would be enough. Of course those things are important to have and strive for, but there is *work* involved in gaining the trust as well. It takes time, as these individuals have been hurt so much before. And, even though I don't work for social services anymore, I still remind clients of all of the past pain that occurred as a result of their prior relationships with social services or Child Protective Services. As a counselor I am associated with, and even represent, all social service agencies. I have to leave my ego at the door, go in, and stand in for all their past hurts. Then comes the trust (hopefully). This is such hard work, but I really do love it. The gains I receive far outweigh the challenges and stress.

5/6

So far today has been low key. I spent the morning observing a couple of children at school. There is only one more month of school left. Yahoo! Then I went to the library to do some research. Next came taking those mental health screenings to the teachers. I am getting ready to meet with a teacher and a family service worker (like a social worker for the family) to consult about a child and build a plan for success. Then I am done for the day.

Questions for Reflection

1. Although Catherine records very stressful events in her journal, she indicates that the rewards of her job outweigh the challenges she experiences. What rewards do you believe you will need in your work in order to compensate for the stresses you'll encounter?

2. Catherine writes that she is working to maintain boundaries and keep herself centered in her work. How do you take care of your emotional and mental health needs now? How will you plan to do so in your work as a community counselor?

Kelly, Barry, and Catherine have similar graduate training but very different careers. Such are the lives, and choices, of community counselors. Although their work is different, these counselors' journals present several salient issues that you will undoubtedly encounter in your work. More information follows on the topics of working with others, advocacy, third-party reimbursement, understanding medications, counseling and technology, and, perhaps most important, working creatively in order to avoid counselor burnout. We end with a discussion of counseling trends and ethical and legal concerns in practice.

WORKING WITH OTHERS

Kelly and Catherine mentioned struggling with aspects of interprofessional collaboration. They're not alone. As we've been writing this book, we've been discussing the content with community counselors, counselor educators, students, and interns. We've heard loud and clear, over and over again, the need to address the topic of dealing with "politics."

What do we mean by politics? We're not referring to one's affiliation as a Democrat or Republican, but instead to the numerous ways in which agencies operate behind the scenes, including their invisible networks of power and clout. Lauren, for instance, shared this story about her internship:

> My supervisor told me that the social worker in my agency was cold
> and difficult to work with, and the psychologist was brilliant and in-
> credibly helpful. My supervisor encouraged me to stay away from
> the social worker and shadow the psychologist. My experience has
> been exactly the opposite! The psychologist has been unapproach-
> able in many ways, and the social worker has been a lifesaver. She
> has intensive training with attachment issues, so I asked my supervi-
> sor if I could join the social worker's child treatment team one day a
> week. My supervisor said no, right off the bat, for no apparent

reason that I could discover. I think he just doesn't want me to be around the social worker.

Annie, a recent graduate, said:

Now that I've been working for several months, I'm learning a lot about how this agency really works. I figured out, for instance, that around here you can't just go to the director with an idea. First you have to check it out with your supervisor, and then if the supervisor thinks it's a good idea the supervisor then takes it to the director. You may or may not get credit for the idea. To do it any other way is considered jumping ranks, which gets you in trouble.

Greg initially refused to play this game. He said:

When I was first hired I was cocky. I knew that there were power games going on behind the scenes, but I didn't care. I was hired because of my ability to work with clients, not because of my ability to schmooze my peers. I refused to worry about whose toes I was stepping on. After awhile I realized, though, that I was feeling isolated. People really didn't like me. As a result it was hard for me to reach out when I needed help.

After a year at a community agency, Andy said:

When I first started working here everyone wanted to tell me who to like, how certain people were going to treat me, and who I was likely to have trouble with. I tried to take all that information and just push it aside. I think you get what you look for, so I decided to look for good things to happen. In many ways, that's exactly what happened. Most of my relationships are positive and professional. However, I have to admit, I was unprepared to bump up against what feel like undiagnosed, or at least untreated, personality disorders among the staff. The histrionic, the narcissistic, the borderline— we've got them all! What I'm learning is that my relationships with my peers are sometimes the most stressful part of my job.

I've developed a plan that helps me negotiate these relationships while keeping my sanity and my integrity. When I imagined being a community counselor I didn't think this would be how I'd spend my energy. I feel a little disappointed by how things really are, but in general, I really do enjoy my work, and I do enjoy most of my colleagues.

These experiences are not intended to suggest that you're destined to have trouble with your colleagues. Renee, for instance, found in one of her first jobs that the climate of the community agency where she worked was warm, inviting, and collaborative. In fact, the agency was a welcome respite from the competitive feel of her graduate program. She trusted her colleagues and formed lasting, supportive relationships with them. Ideally, you'll also experience the joy of working with colleagues whom you respect and trust. You should, though, be prepared to work at your relationships with your peers. You'll also need to understand the unspoken rules of communication and power brokerage that might go on in your agency.

We offer the following suggestions as you prepare to build and maintain healthy professional relationships with your colleagues:

Maintain appropriate professional boundaries. When you first begin your internship or job, you're likely to experience times when you feel overwhelmed, confused, or irritated. You'll want to vent, or process, how you feel. In our experience, people rarely regret the angry or frustrated words that they *don't* say, so practice reasonable constraint when complaining. Choose your confidants carefully, and then choose your words even more carefully.

Observe the system prior to intervening. If you've determined you have the solution to what's plaguing the agency, or an idea for how to better manage client care, do your research and present your ideas thoughtfully. In other words, before rocking the boat, try to figure out who's steering it and where they're going. Then, as you understand the leadership and direction of the system, you'll be better able to work effectively within that system (Lundberg, 1993; White & Loos, 1996).

Acknowledge the importance of collegial relationships. Your peers are an important part of your work. They may be invaluable resources to you. Building and maintaining relationships with your colleagues is therefore critical. You may want to set aside time, or at least reserve energy, for anticipating and responding to the needs of these relationships (Schein, 1993).

Know your limits. Unfortunately, some people will work in agencies that feel sick. The counselors are dissatisfied, the leadership is ineffective, and the work environment is toxic. For example, agencies that allow discrimination, sexual harassment, or other inappropriate uses of power are breeding grounds for dysfunction. People who are overworked and undercompensated tend to accelerate toward burnout more quickly than the average counselor. You'll need to determine what work environments you'll accept. If you're in a situation that seems to be sick, or that is making you sick, you'll likely have two choices: Leave or change the system. The wisest, healthiest, happiest counselors are those who know their limits and respond appropriately to those limits.

Knowing your limits also means knowing when you have reached the boundaries of your competence. According to the ACA Code of

Ethics (2005), ethical counselors practice only within their area of exper-tise (C.2). They keep up with relevant trends in the field, and seek pro-fessional development opportunities regularly. Knowing your limits is one significant way to help you avoid counselor burnout.

Get help. Seek consultation or counseling as needed. Even if you move as quickly as possible from agency work to private practice, you'll need to learn to work with other professionals. Create space in your professional development plan for discovering your preferred work style and learning what type of colleague you are. The people with whom you work will thank you.

ADVOCACY

In his journal Barry discussed his efforts in advocating for professional coun-selors in the state. Advocacy in counseling usually takes the form of speaking up on behalf of clients (Kiselica & Robinson, 2001) or speaking up to further the good of the profession. The first type of advocacy, client advocacy, tends to feel natural for counselors. As a community counselor you will become aware very quickly that your clients' personal struggles are always mediated by their environments. You will have the power, systemically and personally, to speak out for your clients to ensure that their needs are taken into consid-eration by policymakers, caregivers, and legislators (Toporek, 2000).

For many counselors, this form of social justice comes fairly easily. Peo-ple who are focused on others—people like counselors—may find it difficult to speak up for themselves but can often find a way to stand up for others. Furthermore, finding your voice as an advocate may seem quite natural to you, for it requires the wise use of your counseling skills. As an advocate you will use your ability to listen, empathize, and influence. You will also rely on your ability to conceptualize, both individually and systemically, to ensure that you respect your clients' autonomy and wishes. As an advocate you will be speaking on behalf of your client, not for your client. You will be adding your voice, rather than taking away the voice of your client (Toporek & Liu, 2001).

According to Lewis and Bradley (2000), effective client advocacy will empower clients while changing environmental structures so that they are more responsive to clients' needs. Thus, client advocacy requires that the counselor: (1) accurately conceptualize the client and the client's environ-mental context; (2) build effective working relationships with agencies and individuals who affect the client's life; (3) include the client whenever possible in clearly articulating the client's needs; (4) suggest appropriate environmental changes that include actions such as developing programs, initiating or changing policy, and educating the community; and (5) evaluate the effectiveness of their advocacy efforts (Lee & Walz, 1998). This type of advocacy may take a variety of forms to address any number of issues or causes.

In one city, for instance, counselors realized that the local Community Services Board (CSB) was unable to adequately serve a large number of potential clients. These community members were poor and did not fit the criteria of "priority population," in that they were not necessarily seriously mentally ill. Counselors discovered that many of these people were receiving psychotropic medications from physicians and from the local free clinic but were receiving no supportive mental health services. In response, counselors talked with staff at the free clinic and administrators at the CSB to determine how these agencies perceived the needs of this client group. The counselors also visited the free clinic and talked directly with the clients themselves.

Over time, the counselors who first investigated this problem took action to improve the situation. They identified counselors in the community who were willing to provide low-cost and pro bono counseling services. Then, they disseminated "fact sheets" to clients at the free clinic, which detailed the benefits of counseling, listed available counselors and counseling centers, and highlighted warning signs for depression and alcoholism. Counseling students from a nearby university visited the free clinic each week to sit with clients in the waiting room and ensure that clients understood their rights and opportunities to receive mental healthcare. Community counselors also talked with the staff of the free clinic regarding the needs of this specific population, emphasizing the stress that accompanies poverty, unemployment, and inadequate education. The counselors then contacted their state legislators to inform them that constituents were being inadequately served by the current mental health system. They lobbied for counselors' right to be reimbursed by Medicare and worked with the state branch of the American Counseling Association to educate policy makers in the state regarding mental health needs in their communities. Finally, they kept in contact with the clients and agencies involved to assess the ongoing effectiveness of their efforts.

In this case, client advocacy overlapped with a second type of advocacy—advocating for the profession. For many counselors, advocacy for the profession feels like a distinct, and perhaps even alien, endeavor. Unfortunately, many counselors are hesitant to let others know what counseling is and what counselors do. As a result, counselors tend to be paid less and reimbursed at lower rates than social workers, a group of professionals with very similar levels of training and experience. (Check out the Bureau of Labor Statistics website at **www.bls.gov** for more information regarding professional compensation.) If we want to ensure the vitality and relevance of our profession, we as community counselors must find our voices. Perhaps we also need to find our professional pride, so that we can speak with authority regarding the benefit of counseling and the skills of counselors.

The ACA has produced resources to help community counselors attempting to advocate for the profession. Information available on the ACA website, **www.counseling.org,** includes brochures regarding public awareness strategies for counselors, facts about professional counseling services, and advocacy competencies for counselors. Further, the public policy link on the ACA website provides up-to-date information on pending legislation and policy that affect not only clients but counselors. By clicking on relevant links, counselors can immediately send prepared e-mail messages to the appropriate legislators. Some state branches of ACA have similar links on their webpages. These sites make it incredibly easy for counselors to join their voices, speak up, and be recognized.

We believe that although it's never too late to learn, developing advocacy skills while in your graduate training program is ideal. You'll have peers with whom to practice and faculty and supervisors to serve as mentors for you. The following lists of advocacy activities are not exhaustive but will serve as suggestions for you as you prepare for the role of community counselor as advocate.

Advocacy Activities

Client Advocacy

- Attempt to fully conceptualize your clients' experiences and situations. As you put yourself in your clients' shoes, try to determine what external, environmental obstacles may exist that could be ameliorated or addressed by you or your community agency.

- Discuss your advocacy ideas with your supervisors and peers. Ensure that you are empowering clients through your advocacy, not taking your clients' power away.

- Look at the policies of the agencies where you work or hope to work. Are they reasonable? Inclusive? Relevant to clients' needs?

- What group or groups of clients are marginalized in your community? Who can help them? How can you help them?

Professional Advocacy

- Become well versed in singing the praises of community counseling. Be able to explain to interested others what counseling is, how it works, and how counselors are trained.

- Be aware of pending legislation and governmental policies at the state and federal levels that will affect counselors. You can do this easily by visiting the ACA webpage and following appropriate links for public policy. Then, contact your legislators and policy makers to let them know how you feel. ACA resources will provide sample letters to legislators, letters to editors, press releases, and public service announcements.

- Join ACA and the local chapter and state branch of ACA. Join ACA divisions that interest you. Talk with other counselors about how you can mobilize and make sure counselors' needs are represented.

- Conduct a service project with your peers, such as giving a talk on depression at a local factory or library. Be sure that your audience members understand that you represent professional community counselors.

Advocacy Skills

Regardless of the type of advocacy in which they engage, counselors will find that they are required to be resourceful, effective communicators who can facilitate difficult dialogues. They must also be well-informed experts who understand how to gather and interpret data to provide persuasive arguments. Effective advocacy demands that counselors understand systemic influence, power differentials, and client strengths (Toporek & Liu, 2001).

Advocacy is therefore a demanding and time-consuming endeavor. Many community counselors work in agencies in which they are not adequately compensated for their advocacy work. As one counselor put it, "Advocacy comes out of my hide. My supervisors don't see how client and professional advocacy positively influences this agency and my clients." This counselor therefore began to demand that her advocacy efforts, which included giving drug prevention talks at schools, lobbying at the state capitol, and networking with community agencies, be included in her job performance evaluation each year. Her supervisor conceded, and the counselor now feels that her advocacy work is taken seriously by her agency and recognized by her peers.

Advocating for your clients and for your profession is one way to ensure that you and the counseling profession stay vital and relevant in a rapidly changing society. We must be aware of the issues and trends that surround us, for they are bound to influence our clients, ourselves, and our practice.

UNDERSTANDING MEDICATIONS

Kelly mentioned several concerns about her work, including her understanding of medications. When we first began to work in community agencies we quickly learned that we needed to know more about the psychoactive medications that are recommended for various mental disorders. Most community counselors find that many of their clients will be taking these medications. Counselors usually work with physicians who prescribe such drugs, and clients will regularly report their experiences with these meds. It is, therefore, necessary that you become familiar with the families of drugs that are used for certain categories of mental disorders. In fact, the use of medications with counseling is now considered to be a general standard of care for many mental disorders (King & Anderson, 2004).

In this section, we offer a brief listing by category of some of the meds in use at the time of this writing. But, as York and Cooper (2001) stated, "New psychoactive drugs are being discovered and are daily added to current medications. Any listing becomes obsolete as soon as it is printed" (p. 325). With this in mind, we believe that you can at least begin to think about how medications are prescribed for different diagnoses of mental disorders.

Mood Disorder Medications

A confusing aspect of drug lists is that all medications are known by two designations: one is the brand name and the other is the generic name. For example, the generic name of the drug most people know as Prozac is Fluoxetine HCL. Physicians will often use the generic designation, while your clients will usually refer to their medications by brand name. Beyond this, drugs are organized by class. For example, medications that are commonly prescribed for depression fall into the class of Selective Serotonin Reuptake Inhibitors (SSRIs), so some physicians may refer broadly to "an SSRI" rather than specifying "Celexa" or "Paxil." See Table 2.1.

These antidepressants are based on the notion that people who are depressed do not have sufficient levels of the neurotransmitter serotonin available at certain locations at the synapses in their brain. You may remember that the synapse is a gap between the neurons where neurotransmitters carry

Table 2.1 SSRI Class of Mood Disorder Medications

Brand Name	Generic Name
Celexa	Citaloprom hydrobromide
Lexapro	Escitalopram oxalate
Luvox	Fluvoxamine
Paxil	Paroxetine HCL
Prozac	Fluoxetine HCL
Zoloft	Sertaline HCL

messages from one neuron to the next. After the neurotransmitter has done its job, it is taken up again by the neuron that produced it and "reloaded" for the next firing of the neuron. SSRIs are intended to slow the reuptake process so signal transmission between neurons lasts longer. This description is an over-simplification of the process, but it gives a rough idea of how the medication may be helpful. Several SSRIs have also been found to be useful in the treat-ment of Obsessive Compulsive Disorder. In particular, Luvox (Fluvoxamine HCL) is specifically intended for such use, but Paxil, Prozac, and Zoloft also seem to be helpful in such cases.

In addition to SSRIs for depression, there are monoamine oxidase in-hibitors (MAOIs) and Tricyclic antidepressants. MAOIs (brand names: Nardil, Parnate, and Elderpryl) are not used much any more because they can be dangerous. For instance, someone can have a very bad reaction if he eats aged cheese or drinks red wine or beer while taking MAOIs. Also, this type of medication should not be used along with any other form of antidepressant. If you have a client who is taking an MAOI, you should consider contacting the prescribing physician for information to give your client regarding this drug.

Examples of the other class of medications for depression, known as Tricyclic antidepressants, are represented in Table 2.2. Like the SSRIs, Tricyclic medications are thought to increase the level of available neurotransmitters in the brain. These meds are often seen as undesirable by clients because of cer-tain side effects. For example, many people experience dry mouth, weight gain, and decreased sexual desire and ability to perform sexually. People on Tricyclic medications might become even more depressed by these negative side effects.

Additional antidepressants currently in use that are neither SSRIs nor tri-cyclics are listed in Table 2.3. See the section entitled "Mood Stabilizers" in this chapter for drugs that help mood disorders that specifically include mania.

Table 2.2 Tricyclic Class of Antidepressants

Brand Name	Generic Name
Ascendin	Amoxapine
Elavil	Amitriptyline HCL
Norparmin	Desipramine HCL
Tofranil	Inipramine HCL
Zyban	Bupropion

Table 2.3 Additional Antidepressants

Brand Name	Generic Name
Desyrel	Trazodone HCL
Effexor	Veniafaxine HCL
Serzone	Nefazodone HCL
Wellbutrin	Bupropion HCL

Table 2.4 Benzodiazepine Class of Antianxiety Drugs

Brand Name	Generic Name
Ativan	Lorazepam
Dalmane	Flurazepam
Librium	Chlordiazepoxide
Restoral (Restoril)	Temazepam
Serax	Oxazepam
Tranxene	Chlorazepate Diapotassium
Valium	Diazepam
Xanax	Alprazolam

Anxiety Disorder Medications

People experiencing anxiety are usually prescribed medications that are specific to anxiety symptoms. However, some of the above-mentioned antidepressants will work for anxiety as well, because people often exhibit mixed symptoms of anxiety and depression. There are many antianxiety drugs in current use which are classified as benzodiazepines—central nervous system depressants. Benzodiazepines that are currently popular are shown in Table 2.4.

These drugs are essentially intended to sedate or calm anxiety. The problem with many antianxiety drugs is that they are addictive. Sudden withdrawal of their use can be quite dangerous. People who use alcohol along with benzodiazepines are doubly at risk. Imagine pushing a spring and compressing it with each dose of these antianxiety drugs, and you can see that sudden withdrawal would produce a dramatic release of energy that could overwhelm or even kill some people. Withdrawal from antianxiety drugs must be gradual. Often, because of the dangers of such drugs, physicians will prescribe a medication like BuSpar (Buspirone Hydrochloride). BuSpar is not as effective in calming anxiety as some of the other drugs, but it has fewer side effects and is less dangerous. Sometimes, physicians will prescribe beta blockers for anxiety. These were originally designed as medications for people with heart conditions to lower their blood pressure but have also been found to be useful with some cases of anxiety.

Psychotic Disorder Medications

Antipsychotic drugs are prescribed for people who suffer from hallucinations, delusions, and general thought confusion. Some of the earliest drugs that appeared on the market back in the 1950s and 1960s were a class of medications known as phenothiazines or "neuroleptics." They included Thorazine (Chlorprimazine HCL), Stelazine (Trifluopemazine), Prolixin (Fluphenazine) and Melloril (Thioridazine). While still in use today, these antipsychotics can cause tardive dyskinesia—a Parkinsonian-like set of symptoms that may include stiffness of the neck and body, tongue thrusting, strange facial expressions, and a shuffling gate—when taken for long periods of time. More recently, atypical antipsychotic medications have been introduced that have may have fewer side effects than the phenothiazines. Examples of typical antipsychotic medications are listed in Table 2.5.

In some cases these drugs have proven to be more effective than Phenothiazines with schizophrenic patients, but they may produce serious side effects—some similar to the phenothiazines. There is some thought that an excess of the neurotransmitter dopamine is implicated in schizophrenic disorders. However, lack of dopamine in certain areas of the brain causes Parkinson's Disease. Thus, some researchers believe that giving psychotic patients antipsychotic drugs presents a double-bind situation.

Newer drugs may be on the way that will alleviate this problem. According to York and Cooper (2001), newer atypical antipsychotic drugs are being developed that may be as effective while causing fewer side effects. This is

Table 2.5 Atypical Antipsychotic Medications

Brand Name	Generic Name
Abilify	Aripiprazole
Clozapine	Clozaril
Geodon	Ziprasidone
Risperdal	Risperidone
Seroquel	Quietiapine
Zyprexa	Olanzapine

important, because many people with psychotic disorders, when released from the hospital, will cease taking their medications because the side effects are so uncomfortable.

Psychostimulants

Community counselors who work with children are particularly advised to learn more about psychostimulants. Psychostimulants are controlled, amphetamine-like drugs that affect how the brain responds to impulses by controlling neurotransmitters. They are currently used for the treatment of attention-deficit/hyperactivity disorder (ADHD). These medications do have abuse potential and can induce side effects such as loss of appetite, insomnia, slowed growth, and mood changes (Barkely, 1990). Some parents and child advocates fear that children who begin taking drugs such as psychostimulants will be more likely to abuse drugs in the future, and some worry about the use of any drug that is developed for adults and then marketed for children. Although there are no long-term benefits of the drugs for the manifestation of ADHD, children do usually show marked improvement in their ability to concentrate and moderate their behavior when they begin taking these drugs. Community counselors are advised to explore parental and children's reactions to taking these drugs, and be prepared to serve as children's advocates to physicians and schools. See Table 2.6 for examples of psychostimulants prescribed for treating ADHD.

Mood Stabilizers

Mood stabilizers are what clinicians call the various drugs usually prescribed to treat bipolar disorder. The key to these drugs is the need to successfully treat manic episodes without inducing depression. The drugs, which include anticonvulsants, are believed to work by affecting neurotransmitters, but bipolar disorder is a complex phenomenon that is still not fully understood (Goodwin, et al., 2003). These drugs take time in order to be effective, and they require frequent monitoring. People who are taking Lithium must have

Table 2.6 Commonly Prescribed Psychostimulants

Brand Name	Generic Name
Adderall	Adderall
Cylert	Pemoline
Dexedrine	Dextroamphetamine
Ritalin	Methylphenidate

Table 2.7 Commonly Prescribed Mood Stabilizers

Brand Name	Generic Name
Depakote	Divalproex Sodium
Eskalith	Lithium
Lamictol	Lamotrigine
Lithobid	Lithium
Tegratol	Carbamazepine

their blood levels checked regularly because of possible toxicity if the Lithium level is too high. Patients taking Depakote must have liver studies performed every six months to ensure that they are not at risk. In addition, side effects of these drugs can include weight gain, which can be distressing for many clients, and thirst. Examples of mood stabilizers are listed in Table 2.7.

We have offered these lists of medications to familiarize you with some of the types of drugs you will encounter in your work with clients in your community agency. These lists are in no way comprehensive and, as stated above, are likely to be out-of-date as you read this. However, the major categories of disorders remain fairly stable, and the good news is that development of drugs with increased effectiveness and fewer side effects is in the works.

In many cases, taking drugs will allow clients to become more amenable to counseling. Someone who is in a manic state, or who is catastrophically depressed, is not in a good place to profit from counseling. Once stabilized, people can often overcome their difficulties through a combination of counseling and drug therapy.

You will also need to try to keep up with the newer drugs on the market. Some easy ways to do this are to go on the Internet and contact sites that offer information on efficacy, contraindications, and the side effects of various drugs. The search engine **www.google.com** is a good place to start. Also, **www.mentalhealth.com** and **www.webmd.com** are useful sites. Your community agency will probably have a *Physicians' Desk Reference* (PDR) that gives descriptions of all drugs in current use. The PDR is also a good source if your client is in possession of a prescription drug the identity of which is unknown. Often, teenagers will bring drugs to school from their parents' medicine cabinet and sell them or pass them around, not knowing what they are. The PDR has photographs of all drugs, so that you can look them up according to their color and markings to determine their identity. Parents and school administrators may regularly contact you for such information.

Kelly described feeling self-conscious about her relative ignorance when discussing medications, as well as her overall hesitation regarding the "medical model." Keep in mind that the physicians with whom you are in contact will have their favorite medications and will regularly prescribe the same ones. This practice will limit the types of drugs with which you come in contact. You do not have to memorize the PDR or know every medication that is in use. Most of what you will learn will be from conversations with colleagues. Don't hesitate to ask questions, and be prepared to do your own research regarding medications. Know that you will become more familiar with medications as you gain more experience.

At the same time, however, as a community counselor you are a member of a team. Your decisions regarding client care will be informed by and in turn influence the decisions of professionals such as physicians, social workers, and occupational therapists. Therefore, you are expected to understand the potential implications of your clients' use, or misuse, of their medications. Clients may confess to you, for instance, that they have stopped taking their medication, or, because their anxiety is suddenly worse, they have begun to "double up" on doses. During those times you are obligated to understand and discuss with your clients the need for careful adherence to their physician's recommendations. In your sessions with clients you may discover that side effects are becoming unreasonable for the client, or the client is simply unlikely and/or unwilling to take her medication. If so, you as the client's counselor are expected to be an advocate and discuss with her treating physician these obstacles to treatment adherence (King & Anderson, 2004). This type of treatment team involvement is typical and vital in the work of community counselors.

COUNSELOR SELF-CARE

After presenting Kelly's, Barry's, and Catherine's journals, it is fitting that we discuss one of the most relevant themes of community counseling—taking care of ourselves as professionals. All three counselors described stressors that affected their daily lives. Catherine in particular described the effect that stress had on her personal life.

The work of community counselors demands complex and critical thinking, emotional availability, physical energy and stamina, assertiveness, and, depending on the work setting, hypervigilance in responding to client needs and demands. These job requirements, coupled with the level of responsibility that counselors feel for their clients, can quickly combine to create an exhausting situation. Additionally, if we consider that many community counselors receive relatively low pay when they first enter the field and face daunting amounts of paperwork, it is no wonder that counselors are at risk for experiencing intense levels of work-related stress.

Skovholt, Grier, and Hanson (2001), identified several work-related "hazards" that can negatively affect counselors (p. 169), including the fact that counselors must consistently be empathic and sensitive while dealing with clients who have what appear to be unsolvable problems. Counselors sincerely want to help their clients reach their counseling goals but are faced with the reality that the clients themselves, as well as numerous other factors such as family and environmental support, may be the ultimate determinants of success. Further, the definition of "success" in counseling is often ambiguous and elusive.

Preventing Burnout

Fortunately, many community counselors have learned how to deal with the stress of their jobs. They face their work with realistic expectations of themselves and others, and they are able to be assertive regarding their own and clients' rights. Unfortunately, however, many counselors arrived at this healthy approach to their work after initially struggling with counselor burnout.

Burnout can be described as a type of professional exhaustion, in which the demands of work create levels of emotional and mental fatigue great enough to interfere with one's ability to effectively engage in that work (Iacovides, Fountoulakis, Kaprinis, & Kaprinis, 2003). For counselors, burnout often takes the form of being unable to connect with clients, and feeling unsuccessful and overwhelmed with the task of helping (Skovholt, Grier, & Hanson, 2001). The counselor's inherent inability to control the outcome of his or her interventions compounds the exhaustion. If untreated, burnout may evolve into depression and other manifestations of illness.

Ideally, most counselors will learn in their graduate training to be watchful for the signs of burnout. The dawning realization that a counselor feels unusually emotionally unsettled or distraught, anxious, depressed, physically spent, and unable to think creatively of how to respond to everyday situations suggests that burnout may be occurring. The ways to respond to burnout are practical and intuitively appealing, but in order to be successful counselors must be willing to recognize the problem and be sufficiently motivated to take action.

The most obvious way to begin addressing counselor burnout is to develop an action-oriented plan for making personal and professional changes. By systematically assessing their current functioning, much as they might assess a client, counselors can identify their own strengths and weaknesses and then formulate their own plan. Specific areas to assess include the following:

Physical wellness: Is the counselor eating properly and finding time for some type of exercise?

Emotional wellness: Is the counselor attending to his or her own intrapersonal and interpersonal needs by receiving sufficient family and communal support? Is the counselor taking time to explore her or his long-term personal goals, including the desire to connect emotionally with significant others? How often does the counselor feel genuinely happy? How often does the counselor feel overwhelmed or angry?

Boundaries: Is the counselor able to be assertive enough to say no to unrealistic work-related demands? Is he able to fully experience and enjoy life away from work without allowing anxiety about work to detract from the present moment?

Self-awareness: How well does the counselor know herself and her personal needs? Is she able to reflect upon and explore what motivates her, what challenges her to strive for success, and how she chose to become involved in the helping profession?

The answers to these and related questions should suggest appropriate interventions. Some counselors, especially those who rely on validation from external sources, are able to find some relief from burnout by enhancing their own sense of professional competence and efficacy. Engaging in professional development opportunities and keeping abreast of recent research are relatively easy, and at times engaging, ways to bolster one's sense of professional competence (Skovholt, Grier, & Hanson, 2001).

In addition, scheduling time into the day to ensure that the counselor's own physical and emotional needs are met is crucial. The tricky aspect of this suggestion is that counselors often let their job demands come first. They attempt to justify unhealthy behavior by telling themselves, "I need to get to work a little earlier this morning, so I won't exercise today. Actually, I won't pack my lunch either. I'll just get crackers and soda from the vending machine." Once this cycle is created, it becomes harder and harder for some counselors to stop, set limits regarding work, and establish a self-care plan for themselves. The cycle is exacerbated by the fact that few jobs in community counseling will require the counselor to set realistic boundaries for herself. On the contrary, if the counselor is willing to do the work, the work will continue to grow, and, in many cases, the more successful the counselor is, the more work she will receive.

In response, Skovholt, Grier, and Hanson (2001), suggest that counselors create a "professional greenhouse" at work (p. 174). The professional greenhouse provides the counselor with the conditions necessary for optimal growth. For many counselors, these conditions include striking a personal/professional balance, eliciting the help of supportive peers and mentors, working for and/or with effective leaders, and trying to have fun throughout the day. Some counselors have expanded on this idea by building in time for their own individual counseling, massage, and exercise before, after, or even during their work week. Further, counselors can ensure that they are realistic in their own appraisal of their work situations. As we mentioned before, some work settings are so problematic that the counselor's best option may be to leave and find another job. This option may sound drastic, but counselors must be prepared to weigh the drawbacks of any job against the benefits.

Maintaining Creativity

We believe that one of the best ways to take care ourselves, both personally and professionally, is to stay connected to our own inherent creativity. In order to be able to perturb and improve your client's world through the creative process of counseling, you must, yourself, maintain your own creative stance regarding life. Ordinary living, rigid counseling, and repetition compulsion in your own style of living will result in your facing the same types of situations that your client brings to you.

Every client who comes to you is unique. This means that if you tend to see all clients as diagnostic categories and all concerns as categorical, you will not be exercising your own creative processes with these clients, and you will miss their uniqueness. If your approach to counseling becomes formulaic, you will lose the sense of awe for people that brought you to the profession in the first place. A major part of staying vital in your profession is to stay creative.

E. Paul Torrance conducted a twenty-two-year longitudinal study of people in various professions who had been able to maintain their creativity over many years (Millar, 2002). From this research, Torrance (2002) identified certain important factors and offered a seven point "manifesto" which you might find helpful as you attempt to preserve your creativity. We offer the following suggestions with Torrance's permission.*

"1. Don't be afraid to fall in love with something and pursue it with intensity.

2. Know, understand, take pride in, practice, develop, exploit, and enjoy your greatest strengths.

3. Learn to free yourself from the expectations of others and to walk away from the games they impose on you. Free yourself to play your own game.

4. Find a great teacher or mentor who will help you.

5. Don't waste energy trying to be well rounded.

6. Do what you love and can do well.

7. Learn the skills of interdependence." (pp. 10–11).

---

*Posters of Torrance's Manifesto are available from The Torrance Studies of Creative Thinking, Aderhold Hall, College of Education and Psychology, University of Georgia, Athens, Georgia 30606.

EXPERIENTIAL LEARNING

- Look back through your journal and/or other written exercises you've completed since you've started your training experience. What strengths and challenges do you see that will affect your work as a community counselor? How will you address the challenges and build upon the strengths? How will you ensure that you continue to tap into your creativity?

- Take time now to develop a short- and long-term professional development plan. Be as creative and specific as possible, and include dates for the completion of each activity. Share your plan with a peer, and then check back with each other periodically to offer encouragement and assistance.

Remember that taking care of yourself is not a journey that must be taken alone. Learn the skills of collaboration. Share your talents, and borrow talents from others. Being a team player has many rewards. Give up the notion that you must be competitive in order to stand out. You will be more respected if you generously give of your creativity and seek the contributions of others in the work that you do.

TRENDS IN THE FIELD OF COMMUNITY COUNSELING

One constant in the work of community counselors is change. Sources for funding community agencies shift, policies are revised, standards of practice evolve, job expectations are renegotiated, supervisors leave, and, of course, clients come and go. In addition to this evolution at the agency or institutional level, community counselors can also count on broader, societal changes that affect expectations of practice. We can't predict all the changes that will affect community counselors in the future, but we can provide several suggestions that may influence your ongoing explorations in your training program.

For instance, the effects of the September 11 terrorist attacks in the United States continue to reverberate through our society. These attacks highlighted the need for crisis and trauma responses, and for ongoing preventive strategies that promote mental health across the lifespan (Echterling, Presbury, & McKee, 2004). Crisis intervention and resolution work is a natural fit for many community counselors who are trained to look for strengths and emphasize wellness rather than focus on pathology and illness.

The emphasis on wellness, long the domain of counselors, has also recently received more emphasis in the popular press as well as in professional journals, thanks in part to the work of the proponents of brief, solution-focused therapy and the writings of Martin Seligman regarding positive psychology (Peterson & Seligman, 2004; Seligman, 2002). Further, the continued popularity of Eastern approaches to healthcare have reminded counselors to take a more holistic view of clients and include spiritual and physical aspects of wellness in their definitions of mental health. Although the medical model, with an emphasis on diagnosis and pathology, still informs community counseling practice, many counselors are recognizing, often with relief, that their emphases on clients' strengths and options are being reinforced by current research.

The need to connect counseling interventions with such research has been and will likely continue to be of concern to community counselors. Effective and ethical client treatment relies on the counselor's awareness and understanding of new, empirically supported treatment strategies (Granello & Witmer, 1998). Gone are the days (if, indeed, they ever existed in the first place) in which counselors received their degrees and then practiced for years, pausing now and then to glance through a professional journal. Increasingly, states are requiring that their licensed counselors meet demands for ongoing professional development. Ideally, counselors will respond to this call by choosing to engage in more practitioner-oriented research themselves. Not only will accountability and outcomes-based data be helpful to counselors seeking reimbursement from third-party sources, counselors' findings from their daily practice can contribute significantly to the community counseling field.

Further, taking a macro view of the United States as a community on a grand level reveals that the individuals in this country still struggle with issues of social justice. Often, our responses to diversity in the United States reveal layers of distrust, ignorance, and fear. A glance through almost any newspaper suggests that the effects of racism, heterosexism, xenophobia, and classism will continue to plague our clients, and perhaps ourselves, for some time. Although individual reactions to these concerns vary depending on the counselor's own beliefs and values, the job of the community counselor includes the need to promote positive community change (Toporek & Liu, 2001). Therefore, community counselors can expect to be called upon to work directly and indirectly to promote policy and legislative changes that will further social justice and enhance our communities for everyone.

Finally, two significant trends have affected the community counseling field and will likely continue to encourage—or force—counselors to examine and perhaps change the ways in which they practice. The first, third party reimbursement, has sparked controversy and occasional revolt among counselors. The second, the use of technology in counseling, is proving to be just as controversial. Both of these trends seem to hold potential for eventually improving the provision of service to clients. Currently, though, many community counselors face these developments with skepticism and grudging acceptance.

Practical Issues—Third-Party Reimbursement

Both Barry and Catherine bemoaned paperwork and partnerships with insurance companies and Medicaid. However, such systems are apparently here to stay. Although some community counselors in private practice choose to see only "self-pay" clients, meaning clients who pay directly for their counseling without asking for reimbursement from insurance companies, most counselors learn quickly that third party reimbursement is standard practice in agencies. Third party reimbursement for counseling services means that an insurance company or health maintenance organization pays a portion of the fee for counseling services rendered to a client. Most managed care systems are health maintenance organizations (HMOs) or preferred provider organizations (PPOs) (Glosoff, 1998). Government-funded programs, such as Medicaid or Medicare, are also organized systems of managing and supporting healthcare. HMOs charge a monthly fee for coordinating and providing comprehensive healthcare. PPOs are groups of practitioners who contract with employers or insurance companies to provide health services. Clients who use PPOs for service pay a higher fee if they see a practitioner who is not a part of the PPO network. Medicaid and Medicare are government-funded programs intended to assist with costs for healthcare, including mental healthcare. Medicaid pays for medical services for qualifying people with low incomes. Medicare pays for healthcare for qualifying people age sixty-five or older and some people under age sixty-five with disabilities.

Currently, Medicare does not always reimburse for the services of state-licensed professional counselors. However, the American Counseling Association legislative consultants are lobbying to ensure that licensed professional counselors will be reimbursed by Medicare for providing approved mental health services. Fortunately, thanks to the efforts of ACA lobbyists and counselors across the country, licensed community counselors are usually eligible for reimbursement by the vast majority of managed care and insurance companies in their states.

Counselors usually apply to the managed care and insurance companies by providing evidence of their licensure and qualifications. Then, if approved, counselors are assigned a provider number and receive information about how to seek reimbursement for services. Some companies are "counselor-friendly," meaning their policies are reasonable and their employees are accessible and helpful. Other companies are more difficult to work with, demanding extensive paperwork and offering what can feel like a micromanagement approach to the client's care.

Managed care systems were created to contain medical costs and monitor client care (Winegar, 1993). Thus, managed care systems pay for only specific types of services that meet particular criteria. Treatment for some diagnoses, e.g., personality disorders, may not be reimbursed by managed care systems. Further, treatment is expected to be time limited, and counselors are often encouraged to refer clients to relevant support groups such as Alcoholics Anonymous or Al-Anon for supplementary client care. Managed care systems attempt to monitor client care by reviewing counselors' treatment plans and requiring updated records and frequent communication between counselors and the reimbursing agency (Anderson, 2000).

Clearly, managed care has dramatically affected community counselors. For instance, counselors are finding that managed care systems often advocate brief interventions and, in particular, cognitive-behavioral approaches to client care (Cooper & Gottlieb, 2000). In theory, managed care can help clients gain access to an array of medical services and can ensure that providers are competent and thorough. In reality, however, many counselors report feeling constrained and frustrated by managed care systems. Counselors have struggled to be recognized as authorized providers, and some have felt that the gatekeepers who approve treatment are insufficiently trained (Glosoff, Garcia, Herlihy, & Remley, 1999). Counselors who rely on managed care reimbursement have to keep very detailed paperwork, some of which seems redundant and excessive. Many of these counselors have had to adjust their therapeutic approaches, and some feel they are required to release information in manners inconsistent with typical expectations of client confidentiality (Glosoff, 1998).

Managed care systems also present counselors with potential ethical dilemmas. Counselors are expected to fully conceptualize their clients and then provide relevant treatment. When managed care organizations limit the number of treatment sessions and mandate specific treatment modalities, however, client care is in some ways removed from the client expert—the counselor—and given to a company. In order to be reimbursed, counselors feel forced to comply with guidelines that may seem questionable to them, and client welfare may thus be compromised (Danzinger & Welfel, 2001). In addition, once client information is shared with a managed care organization, that information is out of the counselor's hands. Some counselors therefore provide extensive informed consent documents to their clients to ensure that the implications of their release of information forms are fully understood by clients (Copper & Gottlieb, 2000). Further, as Davis and Meier (2001) point out, in some cases providers have been held legally liable for the actions of the HMO for which they worked. This seems a nightmarish situation for the counselor, but such incidents are likely to occur again in the future.

Third party reimbursement is a critically important issue for community counselors. Although managed care has brought perhaps more than its share of dilemmas to the profession, counselors rely on third party reimbursement for their livelihood. Community counselors are therefore encouraged to investigate and fully understand their rights and obligations when working with managed care systems. Ideally, counselors will also practice their advocacy skills in speaking out against bureaucratic policies that unnecessarily restrict client care.

Counseling and Technology

One of Barry's concerns was the need to retain a stable client base. He therefore wondered about the possibility of e-counseling. E-counseling, also known as cybercounseling or webcounseling, is a reality. The June 2005 edition of *Counseling Today,* the American Counseling Association's monthly newsletter, devotes several articles to technology and its impact on counselors. This form of counseling is likely to affect you in the future.

In the early 1960s, Joseph Weisenbaum, an MIT professor, developed a computer program that he called ELIZA (Rothfeder, 1985). Half-jokingly, Weisenbaum designed ELIZA according to his understanding of how Carl Rogers (1961) might respond to input from his clients. It was immediately clear to all but the most naive observers that ELIZA could not handle conversations in natural language. For example, if the user typed something like, "I believe that necessity is the *mother* of invention," the program would respond with, "Tell me more about your family." However, to Weisenbaum's surprise, people who heard about his cybernetic counselor began to request sessions with the machine. Weisenbaum's own secretary would occasionally stay after work to consult with the computer program about her personal issues.

Some have predicted that, through the application of artificial intelligence, computers may eventually be able to take over many of the functions of counselors. That day, if it ever arrives, is far into the future. However, Moore's Law states that computer efficiency doubles every eighteen to twenty-four months. Computational power is increasing exponentially, so that the capabilities of computing will continue to expand beyond our imagination (Kurzweil, 1999). This means that nearly everything we can envision doing with a computer will probably be a reality in your lifetime.

To date, there are dozens—perhaps hundreds—of websites that offer counseling over the internet. Some examples of these websites include Here2listen.com, Etherapy.com, 4therapy.com, Cybershrink.com, Helphorizons. com, and Counseling.com. An organization called the International Society for Mental Health Online (**www.ismho.com**) has been established as a clearinghouse for online counseling information, and counselors can become certified by having their credentials checked through the Mental Health Net (**www.cmhc.com/check**), which will provide a certification check symbol on the counselor's website once the counselor's degree, license or certification, and other professional information have been reviewed. For a yearly renewal fee, about $20 in 2004, the counselor can continue to display the credential check symbol, attesting to his or her professional legitimacy. Helphorizons.com provides various services to cybercounselors, such as setting up appointments, billing, and other virtual office management assistance. New terms have entered our nomenclature. The alternative to face-to-face (FTF) counseling is now known as computer mediated (CM) counseling. The number of computer mediated counseling sessions performed by virtual counselors is expanding daily.

Will you go virtual? Michael Feeny (2001) asserted that the future of counseling will include immense numbers of online therapy sessions. Feeny stated that estimates of online contacts between counselors and clients ranged between 5,000 and 25,000 per day. Most contacts were through e-mail, private chats, web-based teleconferencing, and instant messaging. As of 2001, more than 60,000 counseling sessions had taken place by way of television and computer links, and the term "mental health" had produced more than 900,000 hits on the AltaVista search engine. As people become more sophisticated in the use of the Internet and computing technology continues to improve while decreasing in price, more and more clients may seek help via this route.

According to Feeny, clients appreciate a number of advantages when engaging in counseling by e-mail. The absence of visual cues helps a client to feel less inhibited, and the sense of anonymity encourages more candid and honest responses. Further, virtual communication alleviates pressure to perform in session and provides sufficient time to create thoughtful responses.

Until such time as we all acquire more powerful computers with streaming audio and high-resolution video technology, making it possible to do virtual face-to-face counseling, most cybercounseling communication will be text-based. However, counselors who can create conditions of warmth and acceptance in person may have some problem doing so online. Bloom (2001) stated that new cybercounseling techniques must be developed in order to use the existing technology effectively. For example, Bill Lubart (in Feeny, 2001), who has a website called Here2listen.com, uses certain strategies to communicate nonjudgmental and caring messages to his clients. He employs the now common emoticons: :-) to communicate a smile, the :-(for a frown, and ;-) for a wink. He also uses abbreviations such as: "good 4 u."

Murphy and Mitchell (1998), who offer counseling services over the web at a site called Therapyonline.ca, stated that an online counselor needs to use two self-disclosure techniques that they labeled *emotional bracketing* and *descriptive immediacy*. Bloom (2001) offered an example of emotional bracketing, suggesting that it would look something like this:" 'It has been several weeks since I heard from you, John [concern, worry] and I would very much appreciate it if you could at least acknowledge this e-mail [feeling pushy, demanding]' " (p. 200). Descriptive immediacy requires the counselor to share his or her reactions while writing, such as "As I read your description of the assault, I felt tense and vigilant myself."

Using the traditional postal service, White and Epston (1990), pioneers in face-to-face-forms of narrative counseling, would regularly write to clients between counseling sessions with great results. Obviously, one advantage of a letter or e-mail message is that the client can read and reflect on it several times. After a face-to-face counseling session, a client has to rely on his or her memory to recall the counselor's words. However, as much as we may appreciate receiving correspondence from a friend, relative, or lover, it's never as good as face-to-face contact. Virtual relationships may be convenient, but they have limitations and even serious drawbacks.

For example, what if you were counseling by personal chat or e-mail a person who represented herself as a twenty-one-year-old bank teller but turned out to be a fourteen-year-old high school student? What is your responsibility and liability if your online client commits suicide? Can you form an adequate clinical judgment regarding your client's strengths, medical condition, or readiness for counseling through text communication? Will your professional liability insurance cover online counseling activities? If you are licensed in one state, and your client is in another state, or even country, have you put your licensure in jeopardy? One example of this concern, cited by Bloom (2001), is that Licensed Professional Counselors in Texas are prohibited from providing treatment intervention through electronic media, when that medium is the primary means for maintaining the counseling relationship (p. 189).

The ACA Code of Ethics (2005) addresses the ethical use of technology in counseling, and the American Counseling Association (ACA, 1999) and the National Board of Certified Counselors (NBCC, 1998) have published Internet counseling guidelines. The various guidelines complement existing codes of ethics and include the following standards:

• Preservation of the integrity of the counselor/client relationship

• An emphasis on privacy and client rights to confidentiality

• Informed consent

• Client safety

• Quality of the hardware and software in use (using secure websites, for instance, rather than nonsecure sites)

- Providing sufficient attention to cultural issues
- Appropriate local backup measures in case of emergencies

In an examination of 136 web-based counseling sites in 2003, not one of the sites complied completely with the NBCC Standards (Heinlen, Welfel, Richmond, & Rak, 2003).

Clearly, we have not yet fully realized the legal, ethical, and pragmatic issues involved in e-counseling. More research must be conducted to determine the relative efficacy of online versus face-to-face counseling (Heinlen, Welfel, Richmond, & Rak, 2003). Further, the proliferation of Internet counseling guidelines does not fully address the particular concerns of using technology in counseling (Baltimore, 2000).

The computer has brought many advantages to the practicing counselor in the form of record keeping, report writing, and correspondence with other professionals. Now, the technology has brought us into an era of change that presents many challenges. For those of us who have been trained in the traditional face-to-face methods, we may find ourselves resisting this change. But online services provided by cybercounselors are already being offered to millions of clients in one form or another. Perhaps it is time to rethink our conception of the counseling relationship (Bloom, 2001).

Just as Joseph Weisenbaum's secretary fell under the spell of the computer counseling program ELIZA, untold numbers of people now seem ready to seek counseling services by way of the Internet. Perhaps this should not be surprising to us, since at the time of this writing eight million people have also paid to seek a mate on the Internet dating service Match.com, which is only one of dozens of matchmaking sites on the Internet. Connections that once required intimate contact between people have now become mediated, virtual relationships—removed from real touching. Can this be a good thing? Can we learn, as Barry said, to be as effective in our written expression as we are in person? Only time will tell.

ETHICAL AND LEGAL ISSUES IN PRACTICE

The varied duties of community counselors suggest that there are numerous ethical and legal concerns for counselors. In fact, anticipating all the potential ethical or legal questions a counselor may encounter is impossible. For example, the Health Insurance Portability and Accountability Act (HIPAA) of 1996 is an example of a relatively new law that changes expectations regarding standards of care in health service. HIPAA has several implications for healthcare providers, including the establishment of national standards for electronic transactions regarding client healthcare information, requirements for safeguarding the privacy of health information, and clear statements regarding

---

EXPERIENTIAL LEARNING

1. Join with a peer and conduct a counseling role play using instant messaging or e-mail. Experiment with techniques such as emotional bracketing and descriptive immediacy.

2. Discuss the benefits and obstacles you encountered in your e-counseling session.

3. How might client demographics (age, gender, ethnicity, socioeconomic class) affect if and when clients choose to use e-counseling?

---

client rights to access and control their own records. HIPAA will affect you, so take time now to investigate this act. More information is available at the U.S. Department of Health and Human Services Office of Civil rights website (**www.hhs.gov/ocr**) or the Centers for Medicare and Medicaid Services websites (**www.cms.hhs.gov** and **http://www.hipaa.org**).

To facilitate your efforts to meet counseling's ethical standards, we encourage you to know and understand the ACA and related ethical codes and standards of practice, seek consultation and/or supervision regularly, ensure you never practice in isolation, and keep abreast of changing regulations, laws, and policies. More specific information regarding ethical and legal aspects of community counseling practice are provided in Chapter 3.

CONCLUDING THOUGHTS

What will your life as a community counselor offer you? How will you impact your clients and your community? What changes are in store for you, both personally and professionally? Your training experience will give you the tools and skills to create a place for yourself as a community counselor. Never forget, though, that you—your self, your "you-ness"—are the key ingredient in the counseling relationship. As Barry said in his journal, "The learning never ends."

RECOMMENDED RESOURCES

The *Journal of Mental Health Counseling,* published by the American Mental Health Counselors Association (AMHCA), a division of the American Counseling Association, provides an array of articles relevant for community counselors. The AMHCA webpage is also very helpful: **www.amhca.org.**

For more information on managed care in counseling, you may want to read:

Stout, C. & Grand, L. (2004). *Getting started in private practice: The complete guide to building your mental health practice.* New York: Wiley.

If you're interested in learning more about managed care, consider:

Mechanic, D. (1998). *Mental health and social policy: The emergence of managed care* (4th ed). Boston: Allyn & Bacon.

Certainly, you'll want to look through the ACA and the American Mental Health Counselors Association websites, paying particular attention to public policy information and resources for members. The ACA newspaper *Counseling Today,* published monthly, contains articles that address a range of issues that are likely to affect you in your work as a community counselor. Counselors for Social Justice also has helpful resources on its website, **www.counselorsforsocialjustice.org.**

We also believe that some of your best resources are the members of your current learning community. We encourage you to join with your instructors and peers to discuss the profession of counseling, to share your dreams, and to urge each other on toward your goals.

Other Resources

As you prepare for your life as a community counselor you are essentially beginning a new way of life. You may want to read *The Water Is Wide,* by Pat Conroy, and watch *To Sir with Love,* with Sidney Poitier. Both detail the lives of teachers discovering how their work has the potential to change their own and others' lives.

REFERENCES

American Counseling Association. (2005). *ACA Code of Ethics.* Retrieved August 22, 2005 from http://www.counseling.org/Content/NavigationMenu/RESOURCES/ETHICS/ACA_Code_of_Ethics.htm

American Counseling Association (1999). *Ethical standards for internet on-line counseling.* Alexandria, VA: Author.

Anderson, C. E. (2000). Dealing constructively with managed care: Suggestions from an insider. *Journal of Mental Health Counseling, 22,* 343–353.

Baltimore, M. L. (2000). Ethical considerations in the use of technology for marriage and family counselors. *The Family Journal, 8*(4), 390–393.

Barkley, R. A. (1990). *Attention deficit hyperactivity disorder: A handbook for diagnosis and treatment.* New York: Guilford.

Bloom, J. W. (2001). Technology and web counseling. In H. Hackney (Ed.), *Practice issues for the beginning counselor* (pp. 183–202). Boston: Allyn & Bacon.

Cooper, C. C., & Gottlieb, M. C. (2000). Ethical issues with managed care: Challenges facing counseling psychology. *The Counseling Psychologist, 28,* 179–236.

Danzinger, P. R., & Welfel, E. R. (2001). The impact of managed care on mental health counselors: A survey of perceptions, practices and compliance with ethical standards. *Journal of Mental Health Counseling, 23,* 137-150.

Davis, S. R., & Meier, S. T. (2001). *The elements of managed care.* Belmont, CA: Wadsworth.

Dorwart, R. A., & Epstein, S. S. (1993). *Privatization and mental health care: A fragile balance.* Westport, CT: Auburn House.

Echterling, L., Presbury, J., & McKee, J. E. (2004). *Crisis intervention: Promoting resilience and resolution in troubled times.* Upper Saddle River, NJ: Merrill/Prentice Hall.

Feeny, M. (2001). Better than being there. *Psychotherapy Networker,* March/April, *25,* 31-70.

Glosoff, H. L. (1998). Managed care: A critical ethical issue for counselors. *Counseling and Human Development, 31,* 1-16.

Glosoff, H. L., Garcia, J., Herlihy, B., & Remley, T. P. (1999). Managed care: Ethical considerations for counselors. *Counseling and Values, 44,* 8-16.

Goodwin, F. K., Fireman, B., Simon, G. E., Hunkeler, E. M., Lee, J., & Revicki, D. (2003). Suicide risk in bipolar disorder during treatment with Lithium and Divalproex. *The Journal of the American Medical Association, 290*(11), 1467-1473.

Granello, P. F., & Witmer, J. M. (1998). Standards of care: Potential implications for the counseling profession. *Journal of Counseling and Development, 76,* 371-380.

Hartley, D., Bird, D. C., Lambert, D., & Coffin, J. (2002, November). *The role of community mental health centers as rural safety net providers.* (Available from the Maine Rural Health Research Center, Edmund S. Muskie School of Public Service, University of Southern Maine Desk, PO Box 9300, Portland, ME 04104-9300).

Heinlen, K. T., Welfel, E. R., Richmond, E. N., & Rak, C. F. (2003). The scope of web-counseling: A survey of services and compliance with NBCC standards for the ethical practice of webcounseling. *Journal of Counseling and Development, 81,* 61-69.

Iacovides, A., Fountoulakis, K. N., Kaprinis, St., & Kaprinis, G. (2003). The relationship between job stress, burnout and clinical depression. *Journal of Affective Disorders, 75,* 209-221.

King, J. H., & Anderson, S. M. (2004). Therapeutic implications of pharmacotherapy: Current trends and ethical issues. *Journal of Counseling and Development, 82,* 329-336.

Kiselica, M. S., & Robinson, M. (2001). Bringing advocacy counseling to life: The history, issues, and human dramas of social justice work in counseling. *Journal of Counseling and Development, 79,* 387-397.

Kurzweil, R. (1999). *The age of spiritual machines: When computers exceed human intelligence*. New York: Penguin Books.

Lee, C. C., & Walz, G. R. (Eds.). (1998). *Social action: A mandate for counselors*. Alexandria, VA: American Counseling Association.

Lewis, J., & Bradley, L. (Eds.). (2000). *Advocacy in counseling: Counselors, clients, and community*. Greensboro, NC: ERIC Counseling and Student Services Clearinghouse.

Lundberg, C. C. (1993). Knowing and surfacing organizational culture. In R.T. Golembiewski (Ed.), *Handbook of organizational consultation* (pp. 535–547). New York: Marcel Dekker.

Millar, G. (2002). *The Torrance kids at mid-life: Selected case studies of creative behavior*. Westport, CT: Ablex Publishing.

Murphy, L., & Mitchell, D. (1998). When writing helps to heal: E-mail as therapy. *British Journal of Guidance & Counselling, 26,* 21–32.

National Board of Certified Counselors. (1998). *A set of standards for on-line counseling* [Online]. Available: http://www.nbcc.org/ethics/wcstandards.htm

Peterson, C., & Seligman, M. (2004). *Character strengths and virtues: A handbook and classification*. Washington, DC: Oxford University Press and American Psychological Association.

Rogers, C. R. (1961). *On becoming a person: A therapist's view of psychotherapy*. Boston: Houghton Mifflin.

Rothfeder, J. (1985). *Minds over matter*. New York: Simon & Schuster.

Schein, E. H. (1993). Legitimating clinical research in the study of organizational culture. *Journal of Counseling and Development, 71,* 703–708.

Schnapp, W. B., Bayles, S., Raffoul, P. R., & Schnee, S. B. (1999). Privatization and the rise and fall of the public mental health safety net. *Administration and Policy in Mental Health, 26*(3), 221–225.

Seligman, M. (2002). *Authentic happiness: Using the new positive psychology to realize your potential for lasting fulfillment*. New York: Free Press.

Skovholt, T. M., Grier, T. L, & Hanson, M. R. (2001). Career counseling for longevity: Self-care and burnout prevention strategies for counselor resilience. *Journal of Career Development, 27,* 167–176.

Toporek, R. L. (2000). Developing a common language and framework for understanding advocacy in counseling. In J. Lewis & L. Bradley (Eds.), *Advocacy in counseling: Counselors, clients, and community* (pp. 5–14). Greensboro, NC: ERIC Counseling and Student Services Clearinghouse.

Toporek, R. L, & Liu, W. M. (2001). Advocacy in counseling: Addressing race, class, and gender oppression. In D. Pope-Davis & H. Coleman (Eds.), *The intersection of race, class, and gender in multicultural counseling* (pp. 385–416). Thousand Oaks, CA: Sage.

Torrance, E. P. (2002). *The manifesto: A guide to developing a creative career*. Westport, CT: Ablex.

Wagenfeld, M., Murray, D., Mohatt, D., & DeBruyn, J. (1994). *Mental health and rural America, 1980–1993: An overview and annotated bibliography* (No. NIH Publication no. 94-3500). Rockville, MD: Office of Rural Health Policy, Health Resources and Services Administration.

White, L. J., & Loos, V. E. (1996). The hidden client in school consultation. *Journal of Educational and Psychological Consultation, 7,* 161–177.

White, M., & Epston, D. (1990). *Narrative means to therapeutic ends.* New York: W. W. Norton.

Winegar, N. (1993). Managed mental health care: Implications for administrators and managers of community-based agencies. *Families in Society: The Journal of Contemporary Human Services, 74,* 171–178.

York, M. W., & Cooper, G. D. (2001). *A unifying approach to the theories and practice of psychotherapy and counseling.* Boston: Allyn and Bacon.

Chapter 3

Doing Good: Ethical and Legal Issues in Practice

Do the right thing for the right reason.

Steven Covey

GOALS

Reading and exploring the ideas in this chapter will help you:

- Adopt basic ethical principles
- Understand ethical decision-making models
- Identify relevant ethical and legal guidelines for community counselors
- Grasp the overall relevance of ethical issues in community counseling

OVERVIEW

This chapter covers ethical standards and applications of ethical and legal considerations in community counseling. Simply put, counselors are expected to behave ethically. Our clients expect this of us, as do our supervisors, members of our communities, our legislators, and members of our licensure and certification boards. The behavior seems simple, and the expectation seems reasonable. Why, then, would counselors commit ethical violations, thereby risking their licenses and reputations, and negatively affecting client welfare? Why do we hear stories about counselors who date their clients, breach confidence, abuse substances, and get entangled in quagmires of unhealthy and inappropriate behaviors?

We don't have the answers for these questions. We do know, however, that many licensed counselors who have committed ethical violations have had fine training. They have graduated from CACREP-accredited programs. Yet they have made mistakes, sometimes grave mistakes, which typically reflect, at the very least, poor judgment. Knowledge of ethical principles and guidelines is obviously insufficient to ensure appropriate practice.

We believe that counselors must know themselves, understand their weaknesses, and have the capability to ask for help when needed. This chapter is therefore intended to offer a broad view of ethical principles and issues, as well as legal considerations for community counselors, while encouraging you to begin or continue your process of self-exploration. We discuss this process of self-exploration in more detail in Chapter 4. Having accurate self-knowledge and understanding of the expectations of ethical practice is the best way to ensure that you will be an ethical community counselor.

FRED'S DEFINING MOMENT: Common Sense Versus Ethics and the Law

The following is an actual case. The names of the counselor and clients have been changed.

Fred, a Licensed Professional Counselor, had worked for five years in a community agency that specialized in child, adolescent, and family counseling. He specialized in family work and had a busy case load. He felt competent in his skills and confident in his ability to respond appropriately to his clients' needs.

Fred's defining moment began one Friday morning when he met the Parks family for the first time. He ushered the family into his office and arranged the chairs so that they could all sit in a circle. Ray, the father, was the first to speak: "We're here because I made a stupid mistake." Fred requested a more specific explanation. Ray revealed that he had gone into his stepdaughter Lauren's bedroom one night and touched her genitals while she was sleeping. However, nine-year-old Lauren had only been pretending to sleep, and the next morning she told her mother about the incident.

Ray and Joan had been married for three years. They described their marriage as "working well," although they confessed that their sex life was not completely satisfactory. Joan reported that Ray seemed to need sex more frequently than she desired. "It's probably my fault," said Joan, "if I had been more responsive, he wouldn't have done it."

Ray and Joan were both college-educated and seemingly intelligent people. Ray worked as a police detective and Joan was a legal secretary. They lived and worked in a small town about twenty miles from the mental health center. They explained that there was a mental health facility in their town, but they knew some of the personnel who worked there and they wanted to avoid a hometown scandal. Lauren reported that nothing like what had happened had ever occurred before, and Joan stated that she believed this was true. Ray protested that he had been drinking that night and that he "didn't know what had come over him." He vowed that it would never happen again.

In every state, mental health providers are legally bound to report instances of child abuse to the proper authorities. Fred knew this; he had only recently attended a daylong workshop on child abuse. The workshop presenter had detailed the procedure for reporting suspected incidents and the method that Social Services used to "found" a case of child abuse. The presenter lamented that the case load for child protective services workers was unreasonably large and that the percentage of "founded" cases was quite small. A founded case exists when investigation determines without a doubt that child abuse has taken place. Fred had asked the worker what happens after a case is founded. "Well, most of the time, unless there is imminent danger to the child, we would refer the perpetrator back to you for counseling." Fred rolled his eyes and thought, "Yeah, bureaucracy."

Fred told Ray and Joan that he was mandated to report child abuse cases to Social Services. Ray began to sob, and Joan pleaded with Fred not to report Ray. Joan said that the report would be the end of his law enforcement job and that if word got out they would probably have to move.

Fred felt torn. On the one hand, he knew that the law was clear about reporting such cases. On the other hand, he was sure that reporting would sever his relationship with the family and end his chance of being helpful to them. Since, as the child protective services worker had said, it was likely that the family would eventually be referred for counseling, Fred decided to work efficiently, bypass Social Services, and contract for multiple family therapy sessions with Ray, Joan, and Lauren.

After working with the family for about six months, they all agreed that things were going well. No repeat of Ray's sexual abuse of Lauren had taken place, and the parents reported that their relationship had improved "in every way." At that point, it seemed reasonable to all concerned that the family counseling could be terminated. Then, about a year later, a representative from the State's Attorney's office came to speak with Fred. He said that Ray had once again touched Lauren "inappropriately" and that Joan had called Social Services and reported the incident. Furthermore, Joan had told the Social Services worker that Fred had known about a similar situation happening months before. The attorney wanted to know why Fred had not reported this knowledge of the previous event to the proper authorities.

Certainly, Fred's decision to go ahead and work with the family was within the bounds of common sense. Furthermore, at a certain level, Fred was complying with the ethics of his profession to keep confidential the issues of his clients. Moursund and Kenny (2002) wrote that this ethical consideration is as old as the Hippocratic Oath, which states that the helping person should pledge to keep confidential the client's stated concern: "[I]f it be what should not be noised abroad, I will never divulge, holding such things to be holy secrets" (pp. 226–227).

The problem facing Fred was that common sense, ethics, and the law do not always line up well. While he felt he had acted ethically in the best interest of his clients and that he had exercised reasonable judgment under the circumstances, his choosing to skirt the legal mandate resulted in the kind of trouble that no counselor would ever want to experience.

Questions for Reflection

1. What would you have done in Fred's situation when the family first presented the abuse?

2. How do you think Fred's behavior affected his relationship with the little girl? With her mother? With the father?

3. Fred's decision to not report the father made sense to him at the time, but he failed to fully anticipate the consequences of his actions. What ideas would you suggest to Fred to ensure that he didn't make the same mistake again? Should Fred be sanctioned?

ETHICS AND THE LAW

Fred's situation illustrates the overlap between ethical and legal principles for community counselors. The ACA Code of Ethics (ACA, 2005) states that confidentiality does not apply if disclosure of information is required to prevent harm. Furthermore, as a licensed counselor in his state, Fred is a mandated reporter, meaning that he is legally obligated to report child abuse. In this case the ethical and legal expectations gibe.

Legal and ethical expectations are distinct, however, regarding their general purpose. Laws are generally developed by courts, tradition, and legislation (Remley, 1985). They dictate what is legal or just in a society, usually enforced by some penalty or punishment, but they do not necessarily define what is ethical or moral. On the other hand, professional ethics address our expectations for how people make decisions and how they behave toward each other (Anderson, 1996; Kottler, 2000). Ethics are often prescriptive in nature and describe minimal expectations for responsible, professional behavior. Ethical codes often include specific standards of practice that further operationalize expected ethical behaviors. Ethics approaches more closely the concept of morality, which usually involves a judgment about what one considers broadly to be right or wrong. Typically, morality includes one's overall sense of acceptable behavior.

These distinctions become most interesting when the concepts of ethics, law, and morality intersect. For instance, consider the practice of moonshining. Some people distill their own alcohol at home and sell it. This act is illegal. Some people, such as those who abstain from alcohol for religious reasons, would also label the practice immoral. If a counselor distills alcohol at home, or buys alcohol from a moonshiner, is she acting unethically? (You may want to read the ethical codes prior to making your decision.) If you can't conceive of moonshining, think instead about using seat belts. According to the Insurance Institute for Highway Safety, as of 2005, forty-nine states required drivers to use seat belts. So, if a counselor drives without her seat belt, she's breaking the law. Is she acting immorally? Unethically?

To complicate matters, conflicts sometimes exist between ethical and legal expectations for practice. What if, for instance, a counselor is court-ordered to reveal her case notes? Although her ethical codes obligate her to maintain client confidentiality, if she does so in this situation she could be found in contempt of court. What should she do? The easy answer is to first determine whether she lives in a state that recognizes clients' right to privileged communication with counselors. Even if she does, however, she should realize that the ways in which courts interpret laws can change over time or according to circumstance and may therefore overrule or amend the state's legal protection of confidentiality (Vacc & Loesch, 2000).

One of our students who was also a practicing attorney used to say, "People can try to sue for almost anything," and in many ways he's right. This is not to suggest that community counselors are constantly at the mercy of a litigious society. Courts must find legitimacy in a case in order to hear that case, and simply being sued does not mean the counselor has failed to behave legally or ethically. However, we do believe that forewarned is forearmed, to use a militaristic metaphor, so we encourage you to be well informed regarding not only your ethical codes but also the legal parameters affecting your various roles as a community counselor.

Moonshining and seat belts may seem far removed from counseling practice, but these types of discussions reveal the philosophical nature and ambiguity of the study of ethics. Thinking about such issues now, and talking about them with your professors and peers, will help you not only to better understand ethical and legal issues, but will assist you in developing a stronger sense for how to assess your own behavior.

ETHICAL PRINCIPLES OF THE COUNSELING PROFESSION

Often when describing ethics people tend to think about aspirations—what our ideal behaviors would be in any given situation. For counselors, our ideal behaviors usually center on protecting the welfare of our clients. Thus, we rely on several basic principles to guide our practice. These principles are foundational for most helping professions and are the basis of our ethical codes (Kitchener, 1984).

Nonmaleficence—doing no harm. The first order of business in helping others is to make sure you are not adding to their problems. Most people come to counseling broken and bruised by life. As counselors we want to make sure we do not add to their pain. Therefore, we must always ask ourselves if there is any potential for harm in the helping relationship or the treatment plan we are offering.

Beneficence—contributing to the welfare of others. This principle guides us in our desire to help others. Most community counselors go into the field because they want to help others to become more healthy and whole. So we must continually ask ourselves if the course of action we are taking with our clients is the most beneficial path to take.

Fidelity—conducting one's self with integrity, trustworthiness, and faithfulness. We seek to be faithful and true to the best practices we know as community counselors. Acting with fidelity means that we keep our promises.

Autonomy—allowing individuals to be free to act and make choices for themselves. Community counselors attempt, whenever possible, to allow clients to make decisions regarding their treatment and their lives. This principle also informs our beliefs about client rights to confidentiality and informed consent. There is an additional consideration regarding autonomy that can confound our basic understanding of ethical principles: The concept of respecting autonomy illustrates the profession's theoretical grounding in Euro-American cultural traditions. In Western culture, autonomy is a value of paramount importance. Many Western cultures promote individual autonomy, and as counselors, we tend to respect and value the idea that clients must be free to choose for themselves. Keep in

EXPERIENTIAL LEARNING

Read the following and answer the questions. Compare your answers with those of your peers.

You are in your seventh week of your supervised practicum experience, and this particular client has seen you for four sessions. You believe you have established great rapport with the client, who is struggling with a difficult relationship. You sense that the client trusts you and appears willing to share very sensitive details. Today's session went well, and you feel the client is almost strong enough to make the decision to leave what appears to be a very unhealthy relationship. The client is just a few years older than you, and you like this person, enjoying spending time with the client in each session.

After writing up your case notes, you stop by your clinic mailbox to see if you have any messages. The administrative assistant snickers as you pull an attractively wrapped gift from your box. "Who is this from?" you ask. "Open it and see," you are told. To your amazement it is a beautiful, heavy gold necklace. You know it is a costly gift. Attached is a card from your client, thanking you for all your help. The note ends with "Maybe we can do lunch soon!" You freeze. "Is my supervisor in?" you inquire. "No, he's gone for the day," the assistant replies.

What concerns, if any, would you have about receiving the gift and note?

Who would you talk to?

What would you do?

mind that for many people influenced by eastern cultural values, their approach to decision making may be more collectivist in nature. They will often need to consider how their decisions will affect extended family members and their social circle of friends.

Justice—fairness, balance, and equity. The actions we take with clients must be guided by fairness and equality. Our treatment must be consistent and fair, regardless of ethnicity, race, sexual orientation, philosophical values, age, or physical disability. Justice for all does not necessarily mean one size fits all. To be fair requires that we recognize that different life situations create different demands on our clients. We therefore respond in recognition of our clients' unique contexts, realizing that their realities and worldview may be distinct from our own.

Even if you do not have a copy of the ACA Code of Ethics handy, you can always recall these basic principles to guide your initial assessment of potentially tricky ethical questions (Granello & Witmer, 1998). Consider these principles as you read through the Experiential Learning exercise.

ETHICAL CODES

Ethical codes are developed from ethical principles by professional organizations in order to legitimize the profession and promote expectations regarding appropriate behavior (Swanson, 1983). These codes are designed to guide practitioners toward ethical conduct, establish appropriate standards of practice, and facilitate accountability in practice (Herlihy & Corey, 1996). When you become a member of any professional helping organization, you agree to abide by that organization's ethical code.

As a community counselor, you are most likely to adhere to the American Counseling Association's (ACA, 2005) Code of Ethics, and perhaps the American Mental Health Counselors Association Code of Ethics (AMHCA, 2000). AMHCA, a division of ACA, does not specifically represent community counselors, but its overall focus on the practice of counseling is appealing to many community and agency counselors. The National Board for Certified Counselors (NBCC, 2005) has also produced its own codes of ethics. The ACA, AMHCA, and NBCC codes are all readily accessible on the Web at these addresses, respectively: **www.counseling.org; www.amhca.org;** and **www.nbcc.org.** If you belong to all of these organizations, which codes do you follow? All of them. Although this situation is not ideal because of the potential for confusion, currently there is no one universal code for all counselors (Remley & Herlihy, 2001).

Ethical codes such as ACA's, AMHCA's, and NBCC's are usually revised regularly in order to address changes in societal expectations as well as ensure ongoing cultural sensitivity. The ACA Code of Ethics (2005), for example, is the most recently revised of the abovementioned documents, having been approved and published in August 2005. Further, most organizations, including those mentioned above, have additional resources, such as casebooks, texts, and continuing education opportunities, to help members understand their ethical obligations. The ACA has also developed Standards of Practice (1995) to supplement the ethical codes. The standards offer specific descriptions of what is considered minimal, mandatory behavior (Granello & Witmer, 1998). As of the fall of 2005, the 1995 Standards of Practice have not yet been updated to reflect changes in the 2005 Code of Ethics. They nevertheless have utility as pragmatic guides to expectations of acceptable, ethical behavior.

Because the American Counseling Association is the parent organization of AMHCA, we focus here specifically on the ACA Code of Ethics (2005). The ACA Code addresses eight broad areas:

Section A: The Counseling Relationship. This section covers the counselor's need to protect client welfare, respect diversity, protect client rights, and avoid dual relationships. This section also includes a specific prohibition regarding sexual intimacies with clients. The importance of advocacy, including client consent and confidentiality, is also covered in this section. End-of-life care for terminally ill clients is addressed, including expectations for quality of care and counselor competence. The last three topics in this section include guidelines for setting fees, terminating and making referrals, and using technological applications in counseling.

Section B: Confidentiality, Privileged Communication, and Privacy. This section covers one of the most fundamental issues in counseling— the client's right to privacy. The section addresses multicultural/diversity considerations regarding client rights as well as exceptions to confidentiality, and provides information regarding confidentiality in specific work situations, such as working with groups or minor clients. This section also specifies how counselors are expected to maintain records. (Obviously, there is no escaping the demand for paperwork.) The section concludes by covering the need for anonymity in research and testing and the respect for privacy in consultation.

Section C: Professional Responsibility. This section covers the broad area of professional competence, stating clearly that counselors are expected to practice within the limits of their own competence, receive supervision regarding new areas of practice, only accept jobs for which they are qualified, and be responsible for attending to their own effectiveness. This section also describes the need for continuing education and includes a prohibition against providing counseling services when impaired. Additional topics covered in this section include the expectation of accurate advertising and professional qualifications. For instance, counselors should only advertise their highest educational degree earned in counseling or a related field. Thus, a person who has a master's degree in counseling and a doctoral degree in art should not refer to herself as Jane Smith, PhD when advertising her counseling services. This section also provides a very comprehensive specification that counselors avoid discrimination based on factors such as age, culture, disability, ethnicity, race, religion/spirituality, gender, gender identity, sexual orientation, marital status/partnership, language preference, and socioeconomic status. The section concludes by covering counselors' responsibilities to the public and to other professionals.

Section D: Relationships with Other Professionals. This section covers counselors' relationships with employers and employees, including confidentiality and the need to establish professional and legal expectations. This section also specifically addresses consultation, including the importance of consultant competency and informed consent in consultation.

Section E: Evaluation, Assessment, and Interpretation. This section describes the primary purpose of assessment and emphasizes the need to protect client welfare during assessment procedures. Topics include competence to use and interpret tests, informed consent regarding assessment; release of information; proper diagnosis; choosing appropriate tests; conditions of test administration; recognizing the significance of diversity in assessment; test scoring and interpretation; assessment security; obsolete assessments; and assessment construction. This section concludes with counselor obligations and client rights regarding forensic evaluation.

Section F: Teaching, Training, and Supervision. This section is particularly relevant for counselor educators and students. Topics include counselor supervision and client welfare; counselor supervision competence; supervisory relationships—including boundary issues, supervisor responsibilities, and evaluation; remediation; and endorsement in supervision. In addition, Section F covers responsibilities of counselor educators, student welfare, student responsibilities, evaluation and remediation of students, and roles and relationships between counselor educators and students. The final category in this section emphasizes the need for multicultural/diversity competence in counselor education and training programs. Many students find this section to be especially interesting as they evaluate the structure of their own training program.

Section G: Research and Publication. This section covers the broad area of research responsibilities, including the appropriate use of human subjects in research, informed consent, avoidance of deception, confidentiality, relationships with research participants, reporting results, and publication of research.

Section H: Resolving Ethical Issues. The final section outlines expectations that counselors understand and follow their ethical codes, and provides recommendations for responding to conflicts between ethical and legal responsibilities. This section also specifies that if counselors find that other counselors are behaving unethically, they take appropriate action by consulting and attempting to resolve the issue directly with the other counselor. If the informal resolution is impossible or unsuccessful, or if the violation has or could substantially harm others, counselors are expected to contact state or national ethics committees. Throughout this process the counselor is expected to protect the confidentiality rights of those concerned.

The ACA Code of Ethics concludes with a glossary, which defines terms such as advocacy, diversity, and forensic evaluation.

This very basic description does not do justice to the comprehensive nature of the ACA Code of Ethics. We strongly recommend that you take time now to read through the ACA's and other related organizations' Codes of Ethics and the ACA Standards of Practice. If you have any questions about professional expectations, address them in class with your instructor and peers. Don't wait until you're faced with a confusing or surprising ethical situation.

It seems clear that at the heart of these ethical guidelines is the belief that counselors should do what they can to ensure client welfare. These guidelines may seem straightforward, but enacting them is sometimes challenging. The codes aren't sufficiently specific, for instance, to suggest ethical behavior in every situation. Further, the codes do not, and in fact can not, address every possible ethical dilemma or question that may arise (Remley & Herlihy, 2001). Ethical codes often don't thoroughly cover the nuances of effective multicultural practice (Pedersen, 1997), and may become dated as soon as they are approved. Society changes too quickly for documents such as ethical codes to keep pace, especially considering that the process of revising ethical codes usually involves months of information gathering prior to the actual rewriting process, usually followed by review by an attorney and approval by the organizational entity. Ethical codes also do not address the emotional burden of ethical dilemmas. At times, living up to one's ethical and legal expectations can be a daunting task.

"Elliot's Workout," described on the next page, reveals one of the difficulties inherent in responding to ethical and legal situations. Expectations for ethical and legal practice are clear in this case: Elliot needed to call CPS. However, actually making that call, while managing the family's reaction, was frightening for Elliot. Thus, simply knowing the ethical codes does not guarantee that acting ethically is easy.

In some cases, we may fear what will happen as a result of our decision to intervene. If we call CPS, for instance, will parents retaliate against their children after CPS workers conduct an investigation? Will we be confronted personally? In other cases, we may feel uncertain or confused about how to proceed. What chain of action will we set in motion if we work to involuntarily commit a client we fear is suicidal? If a client threatens to kill someone because she's so frustrated, is she serious? Should we intervene? During a play therapy session a child makes comments that could be construed as sexually suggestive. Has the child been abused? We hear from an acquaintance that his therapist has asked him out for a date. Should we confront the therapist?

ETHICAL DECISION MAKING

Thankfully, we do not have to face questions such as these alone. Help is always available to us from our supervisors, colleagues, licensure and certification boards, and from organizations such as the American Counseling Association. Remley and Herlihy's model of professional practice (2001) is a good way to

Elliot's Workout

Elliot was in the second semester of a field placement experience in a family counseling center. He felt reasonably competent and was beginning to truly enjoy his work. Elliot's newest family clients consisted of a rambunctious group that included Mom, Dad, a twelve-year old boy, ten-year old girl, and eight-year old twin boys. The family had come to counseling for conflict and anger management, and Elliot had found their communication style to be sarcastic and confrontational. Midway through their second session Dad left the counseling room to go the bathroom. While he was gone the ten-year old girl revealed that Dad had recently hit the twins with a belt. Elliot felt his hands start to sweat. "Is that right?" he said clumsily to no one in particular.

"Big deal," the twelve-year-old said. "He kicked the crap out of me the other day. I fell all the way down the basement stairs. You don't see me whining about it."

Elliot looked with alarm at Mom, who sat silently and looked back at him. She seemed to be waiting to see what Elliot would do. Dad re-entered the room.

Get me out of here, thought Elliot as he looked helplessly at the video camera in the corner of the room. He knew his supervisor and peers were watching the session on the television monitor in the office, and he prayed silently that they would enter the room and save him somehow.

They didn't.

"What's going on?" Dad demanded. "Why did you all shut up when I came in the room?"

Before you continue reading, think about what you would do if you were Elliot. What, specifically, would you say?

Elliot took several deep breaths and looked cautiously at Dad. "Well," Elliot said slowly, "We were talking about something that seemed difficult—at least it was difficult for me. The kids were telling me about your hitting them with a belt and kicking them." At that point the little girl jumped up and ran to her mother. "Don't say anything!" she shouted at Elliot. "Just be quiet about it!" Elliot was startled, and he began to feel even more panicky. Dad, who had settled into his chair when he first entered the room, now stood up slowly, his face turning red. He proceeded to call Elliot a liar, and told the family to get up and leave.

Elliot stayed seated. He sincerely feared that Dad might hit him and wanted to be prepared to defend himself, but he intuitively felt that if he stood up he would escalate Dad's anger. Instead he said softly, "Is this what happens at home when you get mad?"

Dad started yelling at Elliot, waving his arms and shaking his fist. "I'm feeling really intimidated by you right now," Elliot said, "I need to let you know you're getting to me. I know you remember, though, that last week, when we first met, I told you that I would protect your confidentiality except for certain situations. This is one of those situations. I'm concerned about these kids' welfare. I'm concerned about all of you."

Dad continued to yell, the daughter and twins began to cry, Mom sat silently

(continued)

(Elliot's Workout, continued)

shaking her head, and the twelve-year old put his face in his hands. "I'm going to call Child Protective Services, and I want you to know that now," Elliot said. "If you want, you can make the call with me. You all came here for a reason. Look around! You're not happy with the way things are. Let's make it right." At that point Dad called Elliot a "little punk," knocked over the coffee table, and left the counseling room. Thankfully, Elliot's supervisor was able to talk with Dad before Dad left the building. Elliot then helped the other family members process the situation prior to calling Child Protective Services. Mom joined Elliot and talked with the CPS worker on the phone.

Questions for Reflection

1. How well do you think Elliot handled this situation? What, if anything, would you have done differently?

2. What reactions do you have to the idea of confronting parents regarding child abuse, calling Child Protective Services, or intervening to protect your client's welfare?

---

begin conceptualizing your role as an ethical practitioner. In their view, counselors begin with a thorough understanding of themselves and their beliefs. They understand the ethical and legal expectations of the profession, and they understand the process of ethical decision making. They are then informed by consultation, supervision, ongoing professional development, relevant laws, their codes of ethics, and the policies of the agencies in which they work. Therefore, the counselor sees himself or herself as an intentional decision maker working within the broader context of a supportive system.

Ethical Decision-Making Models

The particular ways in which counselors go about answering ethical questions and resolving ethical decisions vary, but several decision-making models have been proposed that can be helpful for community counselors. Cottone and Claus (2000) provide a review of several models. We have chosen to provide a basic overview of two models to give you a sense of the typical steps involved. Chapter 7 also includes an ethical decision-making model that attempts to address diversity-related concerns throughout the process.

Corey, Corey, and Callanan's model (2003) begins with the first step of clearly identifying the problem. They then suggest the counselor identify all the potential issues involved. The third step is to review relevant ethical guidelines, such as the ACA Code of Ethics. The next step is to obtain consultation from other professionals or appropriate organizations. Then the counselor considers the potential consequences of various actions to determine the best course of action. The counselor then relies on the information gathered so far in the decision-making process to choose what appears to be the best course of action.

Welfel's model (1998) begins with the counselor developing ethical sensitivity. At this point the counselor is expected to understand the complex nature of ethical situations as they may occur in practice. Then the counselor defines the dilemma and options, and next refers to professional standards. The counselor is then expected to look into the matter further by reading research and other scholarly works regarding ethics. Next, the counselor should apply ethical principles to the situation and consult with others. The last three steps are to deliberate and decide, inform the counselor's supervisor and take action, and then reflect upon the experience.

These models significantly overlap, suggesting that a somewhat generic model of ethical decision making would, at the least, require the counselor to (1) begin with an understanding of ethical principles and behavior; (2) thoroughly investigate and understand the ethical issue in question; (3) seek consultation and education from the ethical codes, consultants, professional organizations, and relevant others; (4) formulate possible courses of action; (5) anticipate potential outcomes of these actions; (6) choose the best apparent action; (7) inform supervisors and consultants; (8) take action; and (9) evaluate the outcomes. Throughout this process, the counselor ideally would be informed and supported by consultants and/or supervisors. When responding to ethical concerns, community counselors are encouraged to ensure that they are never operating in isolation. Being able to rely on the informed expertise of others can help alleviate the stress of confronting ethical dilemmas, reduce the counselor's blind spots, and help ensure that all aspects of a situation have been assessed.

The "what if" questions and ethical dilemmas that arise in counseling can seem to go on forever. Ideally, ethical decision-making models, along with consultation from supervisors and peers, will help you navigate these types of situations. As we've mentioned, there is no way to adequately predict the outcome—or even all of the interrelated issues—that may be involved in any ethical dilemma. In addition, we must factor into our equation the importance of legal considerations affecting community counseling practice.

LEGAL ISSUES FOR COMMUNITY COUNSELING PRACTICE

We will resist the temptation to present any lawyer jokes here and state instead that a competent attorney may very well be a counselor's best friend. In fact, if you are planning to open a private practice, you would be well advised

EXPERIENTIAL LEARNING

The following case examples are taken from counselors' actual experiences. Consider what you would do in each situation, using one of the ethical decision-making models described earlier. Read the ACA's or a related organization's code of ethics prior to responding to the case studies.

1. I was assigned a new client—a ten-year-old boy—for play therapy. He had experienced multiple stressors. His baseball coach died, the little boy witnessed a car accident in which his dad was injured, and his uncle in the military had recently been sent to Iraq. After the car accident the boy started sleeping in the living room in front of the TV instead of in his own room. Mom was concerned that he was more upset than he appeared. I met with him once and was impressed with his resilience. He talked little about stress, other than to say he felt more comfortable sleeping in front of the TV. He said it was "less scary." I wondered about a diagnosis of Adjustment Disorder. During the second session I planned to assess for other criteria for the disorder, but the little boy reported that he was sleeping in his own room again. He also reported doing okay in other aspects of his life. I gave him a diagnosis of no diagnosis. I saw him two more times for "supportive" counseling and then we

terminated. Mom, the little boy, and I agreed that termination felt appropriate.

A month later I was contacted by an attorney for the little boy's family. His parents had sued the driver of the car who hit Dad, and they wanted the driver to pay for their son's "pain and suffering" as a result of witnessing the accident. After ensuring that all appropriate release of information forms had been signed by the little boy's parents, I explained to the attorney that there was no diagnosis. Mom then called me and asked if I'd help them out by giving their son a diagnosis. The family needs the money, she said, and after all, can I as the counselor actually prove that the little boy is really okay?

2. I see clients in a rural area, and I often do home visits. Several of my clients have mentioned their dealings with a local man who operates as an unofficial loan officer. This man, Mr. Nelson, has a local business and is well known for "helping out" people in need. However, I discovered that his help is a type of "loan shark" business. He charges inordinate amounts of interest, and I started to suspect that in a couple of cases Mr. Nelson has actually negotiated sexual favors in return for making loans. He seems to be preying on these clients'

(continued)

(Experiential Learning, continued)

poverty and their inability to get financial and other support from institutional sources. In fact, the banks and social service agencies have many times let these clients down, so most of these clients feel they have no other choice but to go to Mr. Nelson. What, if anything, should I do?

3. Maggie and Jeff, like all couples struggling to get past one partner's infidelity, were having a rough time. When Jeff guiltily revealed that he had a "fling" with an old high-school sweetheart, Maggie wasn't sure she wanted to stay in the marriage. I spent many sessions helping them to process the feelings of anger and betrayal, as well as helping them explore what underlying relational dynamics potentially contributed to Jeff's deceit. Maggie held the moral high ground, and she knew it. Jeff was appropriately contrite. He worked hard to assure her that it would never happen again, and he seemed sincere in his remorse. Maggie expressed no intention of dissolving the marriage, but I could also see that she had little inclination of ever letting Jeff make it right. She was hurt, and she was going to make him work hard to redeem himself.

One night I went to a local club. As I took a seat at a dimly lit table, I saw Maggie a few tables away. She was talking and laughing animatedly with a male friend. I have always felt a little uncomfortable when I bump into a client unexpectedly in a social situation, especially if the client isn't aware of my presence. Maggie must not have seen me because, much to my surprise, she put her arm around the neck of the man, leaned over and kissed him. It was much more than a friendly kiss. As she leaned into him, her other hand came to rest on the man's inner thigh just above the knee. I picked up my jacket, thinking I would discretely exit, when she turned her head and saw me rising from the table. She did a double take, and a look of panic spread over her features. Maggie quickly leaned away from the man, and settled back into her seat. She looked up at me, again making eye contact, clearly embarrassed. She then turned away and pretended to be interested in the band, which had just started to tune up on the small stage. Since she had already seen me, I stayed for the band's first set. I thought as I left, "Well, at least she will have a lot to say in our next session."

Wrong.

Maggie didn't mention seeing me at the club. It was as if the whole incident never occurred! The sessions continued as they had before, with her expressing her disappointment in Jeff, and questioning whether she could ever trust him again. Now it felt like a secret that Maggie and I were sharing. I noticed that she

(continued)

(Experiential Learning, continued)

began making sure that she was never alone with me in the room. Clearly, she didn't want me addressing this issue directly with her. I felt increasingly uncomfortable that I possessed knowledge obtained outside the session, and that she apparently had no intention of bringing it up. Each week I saw Jeff trying his best to appease Maggie, and to win her forgiveness, and each week Maggie ignored the event at the club. It was not a good feeling, and I knew that I had to do something.

4. I was a new counselor working with a thirteen-year-old girl with a history of sexual abuse, cutting, attempted suicide, and an eating disorder that by her parents' report had been successfully treated. After a few weeks we had established a good relationship and she began to trust me more with issues that she was dealing with. As she talked to me she made it clear that she did not want me to talk to her mother about the things she disclosed because her mother had not handled things very well in the past.

She was scared that she would "get in trouble" if her mother heard that she was hurting herself again. Her mother had her own issues of severe depression and was not emotionally available to the client. As we continued to meet, the client began making statements suggesting that she was struggling with an eating disorder again. When she told me that she was only eating enough to get through the day without fainting and that she had limited her diet to crackers and vanilla cokes I really began to worry. However, I knew this client could be very manipulative and often made statements just to get attention. I felt ethically responsible to get help for the client but the eating disorder clinic did not take a client under the age of fourteen without parental permission. I tried to persuade the client to tell her mother and helped to educate her about the danger she was doing to her body. She refused to talk with her parents, and often reminded me that I was supposed to be on her side.

to ensure you have access to solid legal assistance. Often, legal interpretation varies only slightly, and the best course of action for counselors facing legal issues is clear. Realize, however, that counselors can be sued, even if they feel they have been acting ethically and professionally. Some of the best practices you can undertake are to document your work, ensure you have been acting ethically in all counseling relationships, and always seek consultation and supervision if you are uncertain of the best course of action.

Legal issues are also relevant for the counseling profession in general, for it is through court cases that counselors have been recognized as professionals.

In 1960, a judge ruled that a counselor with a doctoral degree could not be held to the same standard as other mental health professionals because counselors were teachers (Swanson, 1983). However, in 1971 counselors were recognized as providing personal counseling in addition to education and vocational guidance. Thus, the legal system helped legitimate the profession. When this occurred, counselors were essentially held to a specific standard—that of a profession—and their relationships with their clients became subject to legal as well as professional guidelines.

In the most basic sense, laws affect community counseling by regulating counselor *credentialing*. Counselor credentialing ranges from licensure, the most specific form of credential, which suggests minimum education and experience levels; to certification, which implies a counselor has documented educational experience; to registry, which simply lists information about counselors. The level of credential offered in any state affects the counselor's scope of practice and is therefore of fundamental importance for community counselors.

As counselors are deemed members of a legally recognized profession, they then are held to professional obligations such as adhering to *standards of practice*. Counselors who fail to live up to the standards of practice and who hurt their clients in some way may be found legally negligible and charged with malpractice. According to Anderson (1996) and Vacc and Loesch (2000), malpractice charges may be brought against community counselors for

- Making faulty diagnoses
- Failing to adequately respond to client threats of suicide
- Practicing outside one's level of competence
- Breaching confidentiality
- Failing to protect clients
- Promising to cure
- Failing to follow appropriate standards of practice
- Failing to provide informed consent
- Intentionally harming clients

As we've said, legal interpretations change and vary. The list above is not inclusive of all instances in which a counselor may be charged with malpractice. Therefore, community counselors are encouraged to purchase professional liability insurance during their training program and to keep their insurance current during their practice. Insurance companies that provide this type of coverage are usually more than happy to provide consultation for their policyholders. In addition, insurance companies such as the Healthcare Providers Service Organization, which is endorsed by the ACA, provide publications for counselors who use their services. These publications include topics such as "Lessons from Court" and "In Legal Trouble, Now What?" (HPSO Risk Advisor, 2005). These companies can provide vital assistance to those who need immediate information and guidance regarding legal questions. We also recommend that you ensure that your agency has appropriate legal consultation available. Simply knowing and practicing within your ethical guidelines is not enough to adequately defend yourself if you get called to court.

Counselors in Court

Occasionally, community counselors are asked or subpoenaed to appear in court in order to discuss some aspect of a client's case. Even though the client may have given permission for the counselor to release information regarding the client's case, the counselor does not necessarily have to show up in court. State laws vary, so counselors are encouraged to seek legal assistance and anticipate the outcome of their potential testimony prior to testifying.

In some cases, community counselors have successfully avoided court testimony by discussing the potential outcome of their testimony with the client. For example, imagine a situation in which a client is seeking sole custody of a child during a divorce proceeding. The client has been coming to counseling faithfully for three months and has shown significant improvement in her ability to manage her anger over her spouse's infidelity. She has stopped drinking to excess and is less prone to what she describes as "sobbing and raging." The client now asks the counselor to speak on her behalf in court. If the counselor agrees, he is legally obligated to speak truthfully about the client's current condition. Thus, if asked to detail her presenting concerns, including her past and current condition, the counselor would have to respond with the truth. In the hands of a skillful attorney, the counselor's testimony could actually hurt the client's pursuit of joint custody, much less sole custody. Thus, counselors are also encouraged to consider how testifying may affect their relationship with the clients.

In other cases counselors are called to testify regarding their understanding of a client's abusive treatment of a child or elderly person, or to present the effects of abuse on a client. The counselor in this case may be less likely to try to avoid giving testimony, believing that testifying regarding the client's behavior, or perhaps on behalf of an abused client, is consistent with ethical obligations to do no harm and to protect the welfare of vulnerable people. However, she or he is still encouraged to be aware of the potential breach that may occur in the counselor-client relationship. Sometimes these relationships can be healed over time; other times the breach is irreparable.

Community counselors may also assume the role of expert witness. These counselors have sufficient expertise to make them valuable to the court in the legal process. For instance, some community counselors have multifaceted, in-depth knowledge regarding immigrants' issues, child abuse, substance abuse, or attachment concerns. These counselors may then be called upon to share their understanding and knowledge. They are considered to be working for the court during their testimony (Swenson, 1997).

The community counselor's interaction with the legal system may often feel anxiety-provoking and even frightening. Counselors are therefore encouraged to ensure that they never act in response to a legal request without first seeking legal consultation. Counselors' and clients' legal rights vary from state to state, and in some cases counselors have more legal rights than they know.

ETHICAL AND LEGAL ISSUES IN PRACTICE

Several fundamental issues are broad enough in scope to encompass both legal and ethical considerations in practice. We present these topics here in order to provide a basic foundation of ethical/legal awareness for community counselors. We begin with the Basic Four: Confidentiality, Informed Consent, Professional Competence, and Dual Relationships (Saccuzzoo, 1997), and go on to address agency policies and suggestions for avoiding ethical/legal problems.

Confidentiality

Confidentiality is, without a doubt, a vital ingredient of the counseling relationship (Swenson, 1997). Confidentiality, in most cases, is the client's right to privacy, and it is our responsibility as helpers to protect the client's rights. In most clinical situations, clients need to know that the information they share with a professional will stay with the professional unless clients give their permission to release it. Without this protection, many clients will be reluctant to share anything that may be sensitive or intimate in nature.

Clients' rights to confidentiality include the right to choose who will and who will not have access to their records and information about their treatment. Therefore, written permission by our clients must be obtained in order to share information about them with our supervisors, teachers, consultants, and classmates. Further, before counselors release any client information directly to others, such as physicians, social workers, or insurance companies, counselors first request clients' written permission.

In some cases, client records may be protected from being shared in court without the client's permission, meaning that the client's records may not be divulged to anyone involved in the court proceeding, including attorneys and judges. This protection is addressed by the legal concept of privileged communication, which parallels and limits the ethical concept of confidentiality.

The Supreme Court case *Jaffee* v. *Redmond* (1996) determined that information a client shared with a social worker was privileged. However, the concept of privilege varies among states, so the idea of confidentiality protection via privileged communication is not a given (Glosoff, Herlihy, & Spence, 2000).

Further, in an effort to protect clients' confidentiality, counselors are obligated not to discuss their clients with others. This prohibition often feels especially daunting for counselors who are in positions that do not provide ongoing supervision and consultation. The need to process our work can feel overwhelming at times, so it is natural for counselors to feel the need to ventilate and explore their reactions to clients. Our suggestion for any community counselor is to find and maintain appropriate supervision and consultative relationships, and keep work matters at work. By avoiding talking about your clients with your friends and family, you will be acting ethically and legally, safeguarding your professional boundaries, and protecting your personal relationships.

There are also several important exceptions to confidentiality that clients need to be informed of prior to beginning their counseling relationship. Ensuring that clients understand these exceptions is an important aspect of informed consent, which is discussed later in this chapter. A blanket statement regarding exceptions to confidentiality could sound something like this:

> Everything you say in here will be kept confidential by me with these exceptions: If I suspect child abuse or elder abuse (in some states), I am obligated to report this to appropriate agencies. If I seriously believe you may hurt yourself or someone else, I am obligated to intervene to protect your and others' welfare. If you give me permission, I will release relevant information about your case to your insurance company or other professionals, such as your physician. I would only release this information with your signed permission. In addition, if your records are court ordered I'm obligated to respond to the court, in that I may be forced to at least acknowledge that you are my client. In some cases a court may require me to divulge information about you as a client. It's important for you to know that I would inform you prior to releasing information about you. In fact, I would include you as much as possible in that process. Let's talk about these exceptions and see what questions you might have about them.

This blanket statement covers several key areas. First, counselors are usually labeled *mandated reporters,* which means they are expected to report suspected instances of child abuse, and in some states, abuse of elderly people and people with disabilities. When reporting such abuse, community counselors usually contact Child Protective Services or the Children's

Services Division of the Department of Social Services. Some states also have Elderly Social Services and Disability Protection Services. Take time now to find out the laws regarding reporting in the state where you will practice. Some states, for instance, require a verbal report within seventy-two hours and a follow-up written report to be filed as well. Any time you make a report, we encourage you to attend to the counseling relationship throughout the process. Include your client, whenever possible, in making the report. You should also consult with a supervisor or appropriate consultant and document your actions.

Another critical limitation of confidentiality occurs whenever the client threatens to harm him- or herself. In these cases, community counselors may find that they need to contact the police or begin proceedings for involuntary hospitalization. The exception to confidentiality was formalized in the case of *Tarasoff* v. *Board of Regents of the University of California* (1976). In the *Tarasoff* case, the client told his therapist at the University of California at Berkeley that he planned to kill his former girlfriend. The therapist told campus police. The police talked to the client, who claimed that he had no intention of killing his former girlfriend. He was released, and two months later he killed the woman. A case was successfully brought against the university for failing to notify the victim, and the California Supreme Court ruled that the therapist has a "duty to protect" that is more important than the client's right to confidentiality. Duty to protect, which is now also known as a "duty to warn," has been expanded in some states to include the requirement that counselors must warn any identifiable or even possible victims of violence as well as people whose property has been threatened (Remley & Herlihy, 2001). Again, we suggest you find out now your state's interpretation of counselors' duty to warn.

Counselors are also ethically and legally obligated to break confidentiality when responding to clients' threats to harm themselves. Assessing suicide risk will become an important helping skill, and one of the best instruments for this task is the SAD PERSONS Scale (SAD), developed by Patterson, Dohn, Bird, and Patterson (1983). Tools such as this will guide you in your counseling practice and the need to protect your client. Some community counselors aren't overly intimidated by the idea of counseling a potentially suicidal client. That's what part of their training is about, and they understand their obligation to thoroughly assess and then work with their clients. What may be more challenging, however, is the idea of creating a no-harm contract, contacting family members to solicit their support in watching over the client, or calling the police or emergency room for assistance. We suggest you use your counseling professors, supervisors, and professional consultants to help you as you make these difficult decisions. Practice role-plays in which you must respond to client threats to harm themselves or others, and attend to what feels most challenging to you throughout these processes. We provide more information regarding responding to client suicidality in Chapter 6.

Other potential limits to confidentiality involve insurance inquiries. In the current culture of managed care, insurance companies will often inquire about, and in some instances require, certain information on clients in order to provide benefits and payments. Keep in mind that although you may be required to provide this information, you should always have clear guidelines for communicating any disclosures to clients. Clients should know in advance who is receiving information about them. Further, counselors are encouraged to always provide the minimum amount of information requested, and, when appropriate, to resist attempts, including court attempts, to require counselors to share confidential information (Glosoff, Herlihy, & Spence, 2000).

Several safeguards for protecting client confidentiality are provided by Public Law 104–191, the Health Insurance Portability and Accountability Act (HIPAA) of 1996. As we mentioned in Chapter 2, HIPAA provides very specific guidelines regarding how client records and information are handled. Although many community counselors initially groaned at the thought of responding to this Act, in fact many of the HIPAA guidelines are basic good practice. Community counselors are expected now, for instance, to ensure that they don't just walk away from a computer with a client's information showing on the screen. Clients' folders are expected to be safeguarded as much as possible, and those who legally request client information now receive only the minimal amount of information required. Thus, counselors are expected to share only relevant aspects of a client's file when required to do so, rather than simply turning over the entire folder. Most agencies provide training on HIPAA compliance for their new employees. We recommend you view the regulations at the United States Department of Health and Human Services site at **www.hhs.gov.**

Informed Consent

All of the above mentioned exceptions to confidentiality, as well as an explanation of confidentiality itself, should be covered with the client through the process of obtaining informed consent. Any time clients enter a counseling relationship they are entitled to know exactly what they're getting into. Knowing the expectations and parameters of the relationship is what will enable clients to make reasoned decisions regarding their own treatment. Providing an informed consent document to the client, and then carefully going through that document, is therefore one of the first steps in creating a therapeutic alliance. As you explain expectations and respond to the client's questions, you are exhibiting your style and approach to your client. You are showing that you view the client as a valued partner and decision maker, and you are empowering the client to ask questions regarding the course of her treatment. You are also meeting your ethical and legal obligations to ensure that the client is giving consent for treatment and that you are fully disclosing all necessary information.

According to the ACA Code of Ethics (2005), informed consent includes letting clients know: (1) the purposes and techniques of treatments, including limitations and risks; (2) the implications of diagnoses; (3) information about tests they may receive; and (4) fee and billing arrangements. Clients also have the right to understand their confidentiality rights and the exceptions to confidentiality. They are entitled to information about their records and to be involved in the planning of their treatment. They have the right to refuse services and to understand the potential implications of refusing services. Further, clients must be offered the freedom to choose whether to enter into counseling and with whom. In those cases in which clients are not free to choose, such as when court ordered, those limitations should be clearly explained to them. Community counselors are also advised to provide information about their qualifications as a helper and to ensure that they are communicating with their clients in ways that are developmentally and culturally appropriate. The ACA Code of Ethics stresses the fact that obtaining and ensuring truly informed consent is an ongoing process in the counseling relationship.

The Professional Disclosure Statement is one way to provide a significant amount of information to clients in one document. Such statements not only provide information about the counselor, but they can form one aspect of the process of gaining informed consent. An example of a Professional Disclosure Statement is provided in the accompanying box. These statements should be tailored to the community counselor's unique agency, for some agencies have very specific requirements regarding issues such as taping client sessions, fees for cancellations, and emergency procedures.

Professional Competence

No matter how much you may want to help your clients, you must remember to practice within the scope of your professional training and experience. All community counselors must recognize the limitations of their abilities as helpers and must get comfortable asking for help when it is needed. You will never know everything there is to know about professional counseling practice, nor will you become a master therapist in all theories and techniques of counseling. You are not expected to know everything while you are still in training; you will be expected to work within your level of training and the limitations of your experience under the guidance of your professors and - supervisors.

Competence can include several facets of practice, including your commitment to represent yourself truthfully, to practice only within your level of

Sample Professional Disclosure Statement

Welcome to the ABC Counseling Agency, a comprehensive community agency providing a variety of counseling services to individuals and their families. The counselors at ABC provide a wide range of outpatient services including individual, child, couples, and family counseling. We also offer group therapy and certain types of psychological testing. All counselors in the agency are licensed mental health providers or counselors in training who receive careful supervision from licensed mental health professionals.

Confidentiality

As a client at ABC, you are entitled to confidentiality regarding your counseling sessions. The contents of your sessions will be held in strictest confidence and will not be revealed to any person or agency except under the following circumstances:

1. If you, as client or legal guardian/parent, give written permission to release the information. Such releases may include your permission for me to share information with physicians and other mental health professionals.

2. If you or your child reveals information which, in your counselor's judgment, indicates that you or your child intends to harm self or someone else.

3. If you or your child reveals information that indicates the existence of past or present child abuse. We are required to disclose this information as required by our state's Child Abuse and Neglect Law.

4. If an appropriate court order is received by the ABC Agency.

5. If your child is involved in a medical emergency while here at the agency, information may be given to medical personnel.

Professional Qualifications

I am a Licensed Professional Counselor in the state of _____. I obtained my M.S. Degree in counseling in 1985 and have received ongoing professional development and training annually ever since. I am a National Board Certified Counselor and a member of the American Counseling Association. I regularly work with children, adolescents, adults, and families regarding issues such as depression, anxiety, substance abuse, relationship concerns, and career concerns. I occasionally use psychometric tests in my practice. I will do so only after fully explaining the purpose of such tests, and then only with your consent. I use primarily a humanistic/existential approach to counseling, which

(continued)

(Sample Professional Disclosure Statement, continued)

means in part that I respect your inherent integrity and autonomy and rely on your willingness to engage fully in the counseling process.

Concerns and Complaints

If at any time you have questions or concerns regarding our work together, I request that you let me know right away. Unless there are any limitations on your freedom to choose to work with me, you have the right to end our relationship at any time. I can usually provide a number of referral options for you. If you are unable to resolve any complaints with me, you are also encouraged to contact our state licensing board at (address, phone number and/or website). Complaints may be made online or in writing.

Agency Policies and Procedures

The ABC Agency complies with all HIPAA regulations. A separate copy of your rights under HIPAA will be provided to you. You have a right to access your counseling records and to know to whom your information may be released.

Our fees are _____ for individual, _____ for group, and _____ for family sessions. We also bill for telephone and emergency consultations at the rate of _____ per half hour. Fees are expected to be paid at the end of every session. In the absence of a clear emergency, if you fail to notify us twenty-four hours in advance of a missed appointment, you will be charged for that missed session. The ABC Agency reserves the right to take legal measures to collect delinquent accounts, including the use of collection agencies. If legal action becomes necessary to collect payment, you may be responsible for all attorney and court fees involved in collection.

If you would like us to complete paperwork so that you may be reimbursed by your insurance company, we will be happy to do so. We encourage you to ensure that our services are covered by your insurance company.

Emergency Procedures

In the case of a mental health emergency you may contact the ABC Agency at _____ during regular agency hours of Monday through Friday, 7:30 A.M. to 6:00 P.M. If a mental health emergency occurs before or after agency hours, leave a message with our answering service. The on-call counselor will return your call as soon as possible. If you prefer, you are encouraged to seek immediate assistance at the Emergency Room of the closest hospital.

Conclusion

Initiating a counseling relationship is often the first step toward making meaningful changes in one's life. I look forward to our work together. Please let me know if you have questions about this document. If you fully

(continued)

(Sample Professional Disclosure Statement, continued)

understand and agree to these expectations, please sign below. I will keep one copy of this document in your file and provide one copy for you to keep.

I have read and understand the above and consent to services for myself and/or my child or family at the ABC Counseling Agency.

_____   _____
Signature of Client or Parent/Legal Guardian   *Date*

_____   _____
Signature of Counselor   *Date*

This form expires one year from the date of signatures.

EXPERIENTIAL LEARNING

1. Develop your own professional disclosure statement, being as specific as possible while attempting to authentically portray yourself as a counselor.

2. Share your disclosure statement with your peers for feedback and suggestions.

training, to seek ongoing professional development, and to seek help in resolving personal concerns that could impair your ability to provide effective counseling services (Robinson Kurpius & Gross, 1996). Further, according to Remley and Herlihy (2001), counselor competence exists on a continuum. Counselors may be considered minimally competent if they have met their licensure requirements, but, ideally, counselors continue working to expand their competence.

For instance, consider a licensed counselor who has several years' experience working with children and families. She takes on a new client who presents with depressive symptoms and what may be an eating disorder. The counselor has worked with depressed clients before in her family work, but she has not yet had a client with both depressive and eating disorder symptoms. The counselor begins to work with the client much as she has with her clients in the past. She relies on supportive therapy and encourages the client to monitor her food intake. She uses no formal screening devices to assess the level of depression or to investigate the eating disorder. Is this counselor performing competently? If the counselor fails to mention the potential helpfulness of medications for depression, perhaps not. If she does not understand the potentially serious implications of an eating disorder that is largely being left untreated, then perhaps not. When encountering new client situations, community counselors should consider what would be an accepted standard of care for their clients, and ensure they are providing that standard of care (Granello & Witmer, 1998). Counselors can be found legally liable for failing to provide the best appropriate treatment for their clients (King & Anderson, 2004).

Clearly, one of the best ways for counselors to practice competently is to make sure they are aware of recent developments regarding diagnosis and treatment, and to seek further professional training commensurate with their level of education and experience. It is acceptable for community counselors to limit their practice to a certain type of client or a range of client concerns, but failing to stay current regarding the best methods of treatment for that population and those concerns is not acceptable.

Many people also expect that competent counselors fully understand and abide by their professional code of ethics. As we've mentioned, ethical codes such as ACA's cover a wide range of counselor behaviors. Therefore, in this interpretation of competence, counselors who fail to keep accurate and timely records, who fail to develop multicultural competence, or who fail to understand and acknowledge their own limitations are not providing competent practice.

Dual Relationships

Gerald Corey (1996) defines dual relationships as occurring "whenever counselors assume two (or more) roles simultaneously or sequentially with a client" (p. 71). Section A.5 of the ACA Code of Ethics reminds us that counselors are expected to be aware of their power to influence clients, and to avoid exploiting their clients or using client dependency for their own gain. The ultimate goal in avoiding dual relationships is to prevent harming the client. How can a counselor being in two roles with a client at the same time hurt the client? The assumption is that when a counselor and client have formed a therapeutic relationship, any additional roles that either one may assume will confound that relationship. The additional roles may interfere with counselor objectivity, impose irrelevant or distracting issues, or complicate the imbalance of power that already exists in counseling relationships. For instance, if a community counselor provided counseling services for her son's teacher, how might the therapeutic relationship be affected if the teacher unfairly gave the counselor's son a bad grade? At the least, the teacher's behavior would likely be a distraction to the counselor. Furthermore, if the counseling relationship wasn't progressing well, the teacher could conceivably act out his frustration with the counselor on the counselor's son, which could frustrate the counselor, which could affect treatment even further, and so it goes, on and on, if not addressed directly, until the relationship becomes increasingly unprofessional, stressful, and potentially harmful.

Dual relationships can get even messier. When the topic of dual relationships arises, many people automatically think of counselors having sex with their clients. Indeed, engaging in a sexual relationship with a client is never permitted. Such relationships can involve, at the least, exploitation, abuse of trust, abuse of power, and lack of objectivity. The ACA Code of Ethics states that counselors should not have sexual or romantic relationships with clients within a minimum of a five-year period following termination of the counseling relationship. We strongly recommend that counselors work to keep their professional and personal lives separate.

Dual relationships usually generate interest among graduate students, because students often feel they are in many dual, and sometimes conflicting, roles. Students are peers in the classroom and may be friends outside of class, but they are usually required to counsel each other in peer counseling sessions for class assignments. Does this mean that you, or your training program, are acting unethically when you engage in peer counseling sessions? Not necessarily. Ideally, in training situations the dual roles are discussed in advance and negotiated with the assistance of faculty and supervisors. Similarly, you may not be able to avoid dual relationships when you begin your practice as a community counselor (Welfel, 2002). Living in a small town, for instance, means that you may indeed end up counseling your son or daughter's teacher. Or, if you assist in responding to crises in your community, you may be called on to provide assistance to people as close as your next door neighbors. Furthermore, the ACA Code of Ethics states that some counselor-client nonprofessional interaction may actually be beneficial for the client, such as visiting a client's ill family member in the hospital, or mutual membership in a professional organization. However, even in these cases, if a current or former client is harmed by the interaction, the counselor is responsible for attempting to "remedy" such harm (ACA, 2005, A.5.d.)

If a dual relationship cannot be avoided or is perceived to be potentially beneficial, the ACA Code recommends that counselors gain client consent and clarify issues such as the nature of the counseling relationship, the rationale for the interaction, and the anticipated consequences of the interaction. These procedures will help ensure that counselors are less likely to exploit the relationship or fail to retain objectivity. We must always remember that it is our client's *right* to be protected and it is our *responsibility* to do so for them. While hoping to help our clients, above all, we seek to do them no harm.

Therefore, it is best to set appropriate boundaries with your clients in advance so that they understand the nature of your relationship. Explain that in order to protect their confidentiality, if you bump into your clients at the grocery store, for instance, you will not introduce yourself publicly as their counselor or engage in conversation with them about personal matters. This is often very difficult in small communities where you may regularly find yourself in a social circle with a client. Set the boundaries clearly with your client, and do so early in the counseling relationship. If you are uncertain whether a relationship may be bordering on the inappropriate, consult with a fellow counselor or your supervisor for clarification. Counselors who eventually find themselves in ethical dilemmas often practice in isolation and have allowed their ethical sensitivity to become dull.

AGENCY POLICIES

Each community agency will have its own set of standards, rules, and operating procedures. It is important that you spend the time necessary to read the policy manual of the agency or organization where you are training and/or working. Be sure to meet with your supervisor if you need some clarification or have questions regarding the policies and procedures. Agencies will hold you accountable to their standards of practice whether or not you have read and understood the policies. Keep in mind, also, that interpretation of policy, and even law, varies. In one local county, for instance, counselors have been informed by an agency's attorney that they must inform parents if minor clients are pregnant and considering abortion. In the neighboring county, counselors were informed by their agency's attorney that the determination to inform parents would vary depending on the situation. Although we can't anticipate all of the policies that you will encounter, you are likely to face agency-specific policies regarding informed consent procedures; HIPAA compliance; emergency procedures, including documentation and follow-up; record-keeping, including adhering to a specific style, format, and deadlines; information sharing limitations; and procedures for using technology appropriately. Be prepared to follow closely the guidelines of practice set forth by your agency or organization. If the guidelines seem inappropriate or incomplete, ask for clarification.

DOING GOOD

This section could also be entitled "staying out of trouble," but we'd rather take an aspirational approach and assume that community counselors are committed to expanding their levels of competence to reach toward better levels of service. We therefore provide the following brief list of suggestions for maintaining ethical and legal practice.

- Read and understand the ACA Code of Ethics and Standards of Practice, as well as other ethical codes that pertain to your work setting.
- Be meticulous in ensuring that every aspect of your practice adheres to these codes.
- Understand the legal expectations regarding counseling in your state.
- Understand your agency's policies. Ask if you don't understand what is expected of you.
- Develop and maintain ongoing supervision and consultation relationships with peers who you know are competent, ethical practitioners.
- Keep accurate, timely records of your counseling sessions. Document any concerns, including how you responded to those concerns and the outcomes of your actions.
- Follow up immediately on any concerns you have regarding child abuse or neglect, client suicidality, or threats to harm others. Document your actions in your client's case notes.
- Ensure that your clients know what to expect of you and the counseling relationship.
- Seek ongoing professional development to ensure your practice is relevant, appropriate, and adheres to accepted standards of practice.

Finally, perhaps one of the most effective ways to make sure you act ethically is to work now to attend to issues you have that may make you vulnerable as a practitioner. Under what circumstances might you make questionable ethical decisions? If you think, *Never! I know I'll always act ethically,* you may be fooling yourself. Certainly some counselors who find themselves in ethical trouble do so because they are impaired. They're abusing drugs or alcohol, or they've failed to seek help for their mental health and physical needs. We can hypothesize that some counselors end up in trouble because they misunderstood or misinterpreted policies and laws. Others, however, are competent mental health professionals who lose their perspective. See "Bill's Soft Spot" for how one counselor's issues interfered with his work. How can you ensure you know yourself sufficiently to realize when you might be approaching the slippery slope of unethical behavior or losing your professional perspective?

CONCLUDING THOUGHTS

In this chapter we have provided you with an overview of ethical principles, codes, and decision-making models as well as common ethical and legal concerns you might face as a community counselor. This is just a starting point for

Bill's Soft Spot

"Maybe you need to bring in a co-therapist," remarked my supervisor. He was right, but I didn't like hearing him say it. I felt inadequate as a counselor, a bona fide failure. I was still in graduate school, and I had just started working with couples and families under the care and direction of a mature and experienced supervisor. He had noticed my tendency to align myself almost immediately with the wife/mother, even when it made no therapeutic sense to do so. As a matter of fact, occasionally I had done so in a way that blocked the couple or family's ability to get better. My own issues were getting in the way—countertransference to be sure. I perceived the families before me through the lens of my own family dynamics. The wife/mother always appeared to me as a victim, just as my bipolar mother had seemed. The husband/father always seemed to be the initiator of the problems and pain, similar to the way I viewed my dad. This is the way I perceived my own family, but it was an unfair and unjust comparison and unhelpful for others.

So, I had to see that I wasn't helping, and that I was potentially harming these couples and families. I was not providing best practice nor was I following the ethical principles of benefi-cence and nonmaleficence. I wanted to help these couples and families, and I certainly didn't want to cause any harm, so I had to adjust my perspective and change my approach. I started inviting a female co-therapist to join me for sessions with couples and families. This kept me honest in my work and provided the needed therapeutic balance. It became a standard practice for me to either bring in a female co-therapist, or at least consult with one on my couple and family cases. Taking this course of action helped me become a better counselor.

Questions for Reflection

1. We all have "soft spots." Parts of ourselves seem mysterious and unknown, and we glimpse those parts when we're weak, angry or tired. Based on your experiences, what do you suspect are soft spots for you? If you can't think of any, ask your friends and family what they think your soft spots might be.

2. Explore those soft spots, and consider how they might affect your competence as a counselor. What action can you take now to decrease the likelihood that you will lose your perspective as a counselor?

understanding ethical and legal issues in counseling. We want to encourage you to keep learning and growing in this vital aspect of counseling practice. We also want to urge you to avoid practicing in isolation. In our experience, the counseling professionals who have struggled most with ethical situations are those who've tried to go it alone. As a community counselor, you will inevitably face some ethical dilemmas. It comes with the territory. Practicing ethically and legally as a community counselor protects both your client and you. Remember, legal and ethical decision making requires knowledge as well as "virtues such as character, integrity, and moral courage" (Welfel, 1998, p. 9).

RECOMMENDED RESOURCES

In addition to the ACA Code of Ethics and Standards of Practice (always available at **www.counseling.org**) the ACA Ethical Standards Casebook (Herlihy & Corey, 1996) contains many examples of ethical issues and a wide variety of ethical case studies. This book is an excellent tool for personal reflection and classroom discussions. Each ethical situation addresses a particular standard of the ACA Code of Ethics.

Several comprehensive books regarding ethical practice and counseling are available. We recommend:

Corey, G., Corey, M.S., & Callanan, P. (2003). *Issues and ethics in the helping professions* (6th ed.). Pacific Grove, CA: Brooks/Cole.

Remley, T. P., & Herlihy, B. (2001). *Ethical, legal, and professional issues in counseling.* Upper Saddle River, NJ: Merrill/Prentice Hall.

Finally, we recommend that you review the counselor licensure regulations for your state. Most states have these regulations available online.

Other Resources

The Kite Runner by Khaled Hosseini is a compelling and often disturbing book that touches on the broad issue of moral decision making. *And the Band Played On: Politics, People, and the AIDS Epidemic* by Randy Shilts provides a fascinating documentation of the beginnings of the spread of AIDS in the United States and reveals the complexity of ethical considerations facing numerous health professionals.

Unfortunately, many, many movies are available that reveal unethical practice by helping professionals. *The Prince of Tides* and *Final Analysis* are two examples. Although you can definitely learn from the instances provided in these movies, you may be better served to look for ethical themes and practices in films such as *Brubaker*, *The Insider*, and *The Verdict.* These movies reveal how wrenching and life-changing our ethical decisions can be.

REFERENCES

American Counseling Association. (2005). *ACA Code of Ethics.* Retrieved August 22, 2005 from **www.counseling.org/Content/NavigationMenu/ RESOURCES/ETHICS/ACA_Code_of_Ethics.htm.**

American Counseling Association. (1995). *ACA Standards of Practice.* Retrieved July 15, 2005 from **www.counseling.org/Content/NavigationMenu/ RESOURCES/ETHICS/ACA_Standards_Ref.htm.**

American Mental Health Counselors Association. (2000). *Code of Ethics of the American Mental Health Counselors Association*. Retrieved July 15, 2005 from **www.amhc.org/code/.**

Anderson, B. S. (1996). *The counselor and the law* (4th ed.). Alexandria, VA: American Counseling Association.

Corey, G. (1996). *Theory and Practice of Counseling and Psychotherapy* (5th ed.). Pacific Grove, CA: Brooks/Cole.

Corey, G., Corey, M. S., & Callanan, P. (2003). *Issues and ethics in the helping professions* (6th ed.). Pacific Grove, CA: Brooks/Cole.

Cottone, R. R., & Claus, R. E. (2000). Ethical decision-making models: A review of the literature. *Journal of Counseling and Development, 78,* 279.

Glosoff, H. L., Herlihy, B., & Spence, E. B. (2000). Privileged communication in the counselor-client relationship. *Journal of Counseling and Development, 78,* 454–462.

Granello, P. F., & Witmer, J. M. (1998). Standards of care: Potential implications for the counseling profession. *Journal of Counseling and Development, 76,* 371–380.

Herlihy, B., & Corey, C. (1996). *ACA ethical standards casebook* (5th ed.). Alexandria, VA: American Counseling Association.

Healthcare Providers Service Organization. (2005). *HPSO risk adviser*. [Brochure]. Hatboro, PA: Author.

Health Insurance Portability and Accountability Act. (1996). Retrieved July 15, 2005, from **http://www.apse.hhs.gov/adminsimp/pl104101.htm.**

Insurance Institute for Highway Safety. (2005). *Child restraint, belt laws*. Retrieved July 13, 2005, from **http://www.iihs.org/safety_facts/state_laws/restrain.htm.**

King, J. H., & Anderson, S. M. (2004). Therapeutic implications of pharmacotherapy: Current trends and ethical issues. *Journal of Counseling and Development, 82,* 329–336.

Kitchener, K. S. (1984). Intuition, critical evaluation, and ethical principles: The foundation for ethical decisions in counseling psychology. *The Counseling Psychologist, 12,* 43–55.

Kottler, J. (2000). *Doing good: Passion and commitment for helping others*. Philadelphia: Brunner-Routledge.

Moursund, J., & Kenny, M. C. (2002). *The process of counseling and therapy* (4th ed.). Upper Saddle River, NJ: Prentice Hall.

National Board for Certified Counselors. (2005). *Code of Ethics*. Retrieved July 15, 2005, from **http://www.nbcc.org/ethics2.**

Patterson, W., Dohn, H., Bird, J., & Patterson, G. (1983). Evaluation of suicidal patients. *Psychosomatics, 24*(4), 343–349.

Pedersen, P. B. (1997). The cultural context of the American Counseling Association code of ethics. *Journal of Counseling and Development, 76*, 23–28.

Remley, T. P. (1985). The law and ethical practices in elementary and middle schools. *Elementary School Guidance and Counseling, 19*, 181–189.

Remley, T. P., & Herlihy, B. (2001). *Ethical, legal, and professional issues in counseling.* Upper Saddle River, NJ: Merrill/Prentice Hall.

Robinson Kurpius, S. E., & Gross, D. R. (1996). Professional ethics and the mental health counselor. In W. J. Weikel & A. J. Palmo (Eds.), *Foundations of mental health counseling* (pp. 353–377). Springfield, IL: Charles Thomas.

Saccuzzo, D. (1997). Law and psychology. *California Law Review, 34*(115), 1–37.

Swanson, C. D. (1983b). The law and the counselor. In J. A. Brown & R. H. Pate, Jr. (Eds.), *Being a counselor* (pp. 26–46). Monterey, CA: Brooks/Cole.

Swenson, L. C. (1997). *Psychology and the law for the helping professions.* Pacific Grove, CA: Brooks/Cole.

Vacc, N. A., & Loesch, L. (2000). *Professional orientation to counseling* (3rd ed.). Philadelphia: Brunner-Routledge.

Van Hoose, W. H., & Kottler, J. (1985). *Ethical and legal issues in counseling and psychotherapy* (2nd ed.). San Francisco: Jossey-Bass.

Welfel, E. R. (1998). *Ethics in counseling and psychotherapy.* Pacific Grove, CA: Brooks/Cole.

Welfel, E. R. (2002). *Ethics in counseling and psychotherapy: Standards, research, and emerging issues* (2nd ed.). Pacific Grove, CA: Brooks/Cole.

Chapter 4

Exploring the Counselor Within: The Facilitative Self

Know thyself.

Socrates

This above all: to thine own self be true. And it must follow, as the night the day, Thou canst not then be false to any man.

Shakespeare

You can't tell the dancer from the dance.

William Butler Yeats

GOALS

Reading and exploring the ideas in this chapter will help you:

- Appreciate the importance of your self-awareness in becoming a successful community counselor
- Gain an understanding of how you can become a facilitative self

OVERVIEW

This chapter presents information on counselor characteristics and behaviors that influence the helping process. Above all else, you are your most important counseling tool. Therefore, in addition to learning the theories and techniques of counseling, you must strive to better understand yourself and commit yourself to being authentic with your clients. No counseling technique is successful unless it is used by someone who is a facilitative self. A facilitative self is one that is open to the experience of others, unencumbered by one's own concerns and limitations, and therefore able to let the other's genuine needs and experiences emerge in the relationship. The paradox is that you help another to become truer to him- or herself by becoming more of yourself. In this chapter, you will become acquainted with the concept of self, learn how central your own self-awareness is to any successful counseling, and participate in experiential learning activities to explore yourself. We believe that, regardless of the counselor's theoretical orientation, exploration of the self is imperative for effective community counseling work.

NATE'S DEFINING MOMENT: Cleaning Up

Nate is currently a counselor educator and practitioner with over twenty years of experience. A full professor and licensed counselor, Nate is known nationally for his advocacy, preventive work, and crisis response interventions. He seems born to the profession. According to Nate, however, he found his niche only after a defining moment that permanently altered his view of his potential life's work. He relates his story below.

"I was expecting the blood, but not the skull fragments and bits of gray matter. The body, of course, was gone. However, what remained were all the small remnants that could not be gathered quickly together. My first reaction also surprised me. For some reason, I had worried that I might feel shocked or disgusted by the scene. Instead, I had a feeling of unreality, as if I were in a bizarre dream where nothing was where it was supposed to be. Blood should be hidden away in veins and arteries, but here it was splattered on the wall. A skull should be under the skin and intact, but it was shattered into gritty shards everywhere. And the brain should be something neatly contained within a head, but here it was strewn all over as if it were water flung about by a soaked dog.

"The scatter pattern that the wreckage formed on the wall looked to me like the watermelon that I had once dropped on the patio at home. It had the form of a cartoon drawing of an explosion—countless sharp spires of red extending far away from the point of impact. Strangely, the complexity and detail of the design gave the shape a sense of movement, elegance and grace.

"I was a college student home for the summer vacation. That night, I had been having dinner with my girlfriend, Janice, and her family when we began to hear sirens. The wailing grew louder, until several emergency vehicles pulled into the driveway of a house across the street. A woman was on the porch; she waved frantically to the rescue workers, screaming, 'My husband's dead! He blew his head off with a shotgun!'

"Janice's parents rushed to offer support to the woman and brought her into their home while the emergency medical technicians quickly determined that there was nothing that they could do but gather the remains into the ambulance and leave. It was then that I wanted to be useful. Janice's brother Terry and I volunteered to clean up the basement recreation room, the scene of the suicide.

"Armed with rubber gloves, sponges, mops, buckets and disinfectant, Terry and I gathered together the disassembled pieces of what used to be a man. Although I had been considering the counseling profession for a long time, this experience was my defining moment. I decided then and there that I wanted to do whatever I could to prevent this tragedy from happening again."

Questions for Reflection

1. What were your reactions as you read the story of this defining moment? What do these reactions suggest about your feelings regarding suicide, violence, and your own ability to respond to crisis?

2. It's impossible to accurately predict how we will behave in situations such as the one presented above, but consider how you might react if you were in Nate's shoes. What would be your specific strengths in such a situation? What would be your specific weaknesses?

WHAT IS A SELF?

Stephen Priest (1991) has given one of the best answers we have found to the question, "What is a self?" The answer is succinct, clear, and just as confusing as the self itself:

> an individual that is conscious of the individual
> that it is . . . [and] conscious that it is the
> individual that it is conscious of. That is what
> a self is, whatever it is (p. 221).

How's that for an explanation? Understanding the self can be difficult because, as Levin (1992) pointed out, our sense of self is at once the most obvious, and the most fleeting, experience we have. "The self to which we think we are so close eludes definition and, indeed, becomes more elusive as we attempt to grasp it" (p. 1). While self-knowledge always remains somewhat elusive, its attainment can be improved with practice. There is good reason to believe that only mature adults can achieve a fully developed sense of self; before adulthood, only a partial sense of self exists. A baby, for example, knows that the foot she is able to put into her mouth is not for eating, because it is part of herself. But the baby has little self-understanding. Small children can achieve a rudimentary level of self-consciousness, but only later does it become possible for them to begin to think about their own feelings and behaviors, as well as their impact on other people.

Parents of children who are preteens know how difficult it is to get them to be concerned with combing their hair, wearing matching socks, or to keep them from putting on smelly clothes that they pull out of the hamper. But, at some point, a miracle happens! Almost overnight, children become aware of how they appear to others. They then become preoccupied with how others view them. Long hours are spent grooming and studying themselves in the mirror. They have developed what has been called the "imagined audience," the notion that other people have nothing better to do than to observe their every action and either praise or criticize them. The child now has an "exposed self" (Lewis, 1995).

Yet even earlier, when the child is a toddler, another milestone on the way to the exposed self can be seen. In children, recognition of self can be part of the child's repertoire between the ages of eighteen and twenty-four months. In an ingenious experiment developed by Gordon Gallup during the 1970s, children were placed in front of a large mirror with a dab of red rouge surreptitiously placed on their foreheads. Children under the age of eighteen months generally showed a response that indicated no recognition of self. They talked to and even played with the "baby in the mirror" as though it were another child. Sometimes, they would look behind the mirror, just as monkeys do when they see their image in a mirror. The children seemed to display no recognition that the "baby" was their own image, and they took no notice of the rouge on their foreheads. But sometime after the age of eighteen months, the children showed a recognition response. They stared into the mirror, noticed the rouge spot, and then touched their own foreheads. Now they knew that the person in the mirror was themselves and that there was rouge on their foreheads.

Most developmental psychologists mark this discovery as the child's budding self-reflection, and the beginnings of the ability to develop self-esteem—for better or worse. At this stage, the child becomes aware that he or she is an object for self and others to scrutinize. The interesting emotional reaction that many children show at this instant of "rouge-recognition" is the blushing of embarrassment.

BECOMING WHO YOU ARE

So how do we move from this rudimentary level of self-awareness to the keen level of attunement expected of master counselors? In order for you to become attuned to your client's emotions, you must continually strive to become fully who you are. In this way, you tune your instrument to receive your client as fully as possible. You must also work to clear up any of your own issues that might get in the way of this attunement. This process has been compared to the work of a nineteenth-century photographer. In those days, cameras captured their images on photographic plates made of glass. If the plate became smudged with fingerprints or debris prior to its use, then the smudge turned up in the picture. But if the photographer kept a clean plate, then the photos were clear images. Likewise, your work as a counselor is to bring a "clean plate" to your encounter with your client.

Arthur Deikman (1999) pointed out that the encounter between a medical doctor and patient is very different from that between counselor and client. The physician uses scientific techniques in an impersonal manner; the counselor connects with the client through participatory knowing, in which the relationship is collaborative through connection. In a counseling relationship, you constantly tune into yourself, as well as the client. The objective stance of the physician exists in marked contrast to the "emotional communication" that takes place between you and your client. In emotional communication we "understand another's emotion by experiencing a similar feeling . . . such subjectivity, the essence of art, is antithetical to rational science" (pp. 30–31). This is a never-ending process for all of us in the profession (Martz, 2001). Unless we are fully ourselves, we cannot be fully with our clients. The ancient admonition of Socrates to "Know thyself" remains good advice in the twenty-first century. As Midgley (1999) put it, "We cannot really understand other people unless we make some serious effort to understand ourselves as well" (p. 85).

When you are true to yourself, you are then able to be *empathic* with your client. We discuss empathy in more detail later, but for now realize that when you are empathic you are able to temporarily bracket your own self-experience and enter your client's inner world of thoughts, feelings, and fantasies (Martz, 2001). You walk around in the client's world as if it were your own, but you never lose the realization that that world belongs to your client. You are a respectful and inquisitive observer, joining with the client to fully understand as much as possible what he experiences. Through listening, understanding, and validating the client's self-expression you communicate to the client that he has been received in the way that he intended.

Many would agree that effective counselors—regardless of their theoretical orientation—are also able to be *authentic* and *congruent* with their clients. To be authentic means you must be the person you are. You don't assume a façade, act out a role, or hide your true essence as a person. You are congruent when your behavior with your client matches what you are actually feeling or sensing at the time. Thus, if you find your client confusing, you acknowledge your confusion. If you find yourself becoming annoyed with a client, you respond to the annoyance rather than ignore it. These qualities

Chalemane's "Baggage"

Chalemane was worried about her relationship. In particular, she was *very* upset about a blowup that had occurred the night before. As she was waiting for her 10:00 A.M. client, she was thinking to herself about how her life had become so complicated. Her partner Bethany had accused her of still having feelings for her ex-husband and had left their apartment in a jealous rage the night before.

After a sleepless night, Chalemane was tempted to call in sick the next morning, but she just couldn't do it. She knew that she was fortunate to have her job as a community outreach counselor, and she felt she owed it to her clients to be available when they needed her.

Chalemane gritted her teeth and resolved to concentrate on her work. She looked at the clock and saw that she still had a few minutes before her appointment, so she decided to call Bethany at work and make a date for a late lunch. The telephone rang twice at her ex-husband's office before Chalemane realized what she had done.

After hanging up abruptly, she tried to compose herself as she walked down the hall to meet her client. Chalemane felt the need to go to the bathroom and splash cold water on her face, but she was running late and decided to tough it out.

After about ten minutes into the session, Chalemane realized that her client had stopped talking and was looking at her expectantly. "Well, should I or shouldn't I? I think he meant it, don't you?" the client asked.

Chalemane had no clue what her client was talking about, who "he" was, and what he "meant."

Questions for Reflection

1. What steps could you take to avoid putting yourself in Chalemane's position in session?

2. If you did lose your focus during a session, how would you handle it?

3. How do you think this lapse would affect your relationship with the client?

---

combine to create a transparence on the part of the counselor that some people refer to as facilitative genuineness (Rogers, 1961).

On the face of it, this doesn't seem so hard. After all, you are the person you are. So how could you have a problem knowing, and being, yourself? In actuality, knowing and being your true self can be incredibly difficult. During your training to become a counselor, you will find that comprehending concepts and practicing techniques will be much easier than exploring yourself and understanding others. Consider the case of Chalemane, for instance, in "Chalemane's 'Baggage.'" Unlike your undergraduate education, in which you could keep the curriculum at a distance, becoming a counselor is a journey that involves becoming more fully who you are. You must be yourself.

THE HUMAN DILEMMA

We humans think of ourselves as both an "I" and a "me." "I" is the center, the observer, the ground of being, while "me" is the object of our perception, our identity, and the part of us we motivate and evaluate. Rollo May (1967) has said that the "human dilemma" is our capacity to experience ourselves as both subject and object at the same time. That I can say something about myself, or about me, is the essence of the human dilemma.

Carl Rogers (1961) stated that the human dilemma is a paradox with which we need to live. Truly, "me" is always tinged with the quality of thingness, but "I" never is. "Me" seems to be a part of my body. But the "I" that I am is not the same as my body or the "me" that I observe. "I" always maintains an elusive quality. Whenever I turn back to locate my "I," it instantly turns into "me" and "I" jumps into the center of my consciousness. It feels a bit like being in a carnival sideshow house of mirrors—reflections of reflections can seem to go on forever, but there is only one real, true, and original "I." So how can you explore your "I"? For that matter, why should you?

Owning Yourself

R. D. Laing, in his 1969 classic *The Divided Self,* created for us a vivid picture of the implications for having a secure base in life. When someone feels fundamentally secure, the person can go "out into the world and meet others: a world and others experienced as equally real, alive, whole, and continuous" (p. 39). Rogers (1959) would consider such a person as "fully functioning." On the other hand, according to Laing (1969), the insecure person experiences the self as "disowned," lacking consistency and cohesiveness, feeling insubstantial and uncertain that she or he is good and valuable (p. 42).

Because we were all raised more or less under *conditions of worth,* (Rogers, 1959) we may have, then, denied some aspect of ourselves that our parents, teachers, and other significant evaluators considered unworthy. When people begin to act in accordance with the conditional regard of others, they come to prize some aspects of themselves that are valued by others and to mistrust other aspects of self. In these situations, "we allow ourselves to become only part of who we really are. . . . Such falsification of ourselves and our experience is . . . a natural, though tragic, development" (Prochaska & Norcross, 1994, pp. 131–132).

Nathaniel Branden (1971) wrote extensively regarding this phenomenon of self-alienation, which he called "the problem of *the disowned self*" (p. 3, emphasis in original). This condition of self-estrangement affects us all; it is not only about those with diagnosable personality disorders. Victor Frankl (1959) described this "existential vacuum" as characterized by boredom, apathy,

EXPERIENTIAL LEARNING

Join with two classmates to form a small discussion group. Talk about a time that each of you made a Faustian Bargain by "selling out" in some way in order to be accepted or successful with others. Be sure to include in your own story a description of what it felt like afterwards when you realized that you had not been true to yourself.

cynicism, and lack of direction. There is a feeling of emptiness poetically described by Sissy Spacek's character in the movie *Badlands:* It is "that 'blah' feeling. Like when you're sitting in the bathtub, and all the water's run out."

We are all estranged from ourselves to some degree. At those times when we lose touch with the sense of being that goes with living life fully alive, we experience what Seinfeld (1991) called "the empty core." We lose the subjective sense of existing—the conscious experience of *what it is like to be* (Nagel, 1986). At these times, we may be engaged in stultifying daily routines, mindless diversions, and occupations. We may be making important decisions dispassionately and monitoring our behaviors so that we manage our impression according to social expectations. We are not truly alive.

Because all this leads to a feeling of insecurity, we can find ourselves trying to manage the sensations that accompany it by ignoring them or closing ourselves off to this awareness. But by reducing our conscious experience of these feelings of insecurity, we also reduce our feelings of enthusiasm and joy for living. We become slaves to external pressures and demands.

If we give in to those people who insist that we become someone other than who we really are, we let them take ownership of us. If we continually trim ourselves to fit others, we'll have nothing left of ourselves. This is the experiential truth of the Faustian Bargain, in which Faustus made a deal with the Devil, achieved success and riches, but lost his soul in the process. In order to gain the esteem of some people, we sell out.

The disowned part of the self is always waiting to be reclaimed. And when this happens, whether it's through participating in counseling, resolving a crisis, or keeping a journal, the person feels whole and experiences life as vivid. In his book *The Discovery of Being,* May (1983) offered a portrayal of such a breakthrough experience reported by one of his clients in psychotherapy. Reclaiming one's self is like "receiving the deed to my house. It is the experience of my own aliveness" (p. 99). Fundamentally, once you *find* yourself, you *own* yourself.

After reading this section, you may believe that in order to be a successful community counselor, you must first attain complete security and self-understanding. But most of us have only achieved a self-awareness that is "good enough," and we usually can recognize a small glimmer of our insecurity in the dark corners and recesses of our selves. Furthermore, when we are in circumstances in which our self-esteem is on the line, we feel this insecurity intensely.

Your training program will require you to practice your skills in front of other students, on videotape, or while being observed through a one-way mirror. At these times, you're likely to feel insecure. You may find yourself so focused on what you are going to say next that you hardly hear what your client is saying. Over time, and with practice and supervision, you will begin to allow the real you to be present and emerge as you work with your clients.

Several key areas are fundamental in enhancing your ability to wrestle with the Human Dilemma. We present below the topics of self-disclosure, trusting one's intuition, empathic accuracy, and countertransference as particularly relevant for counselor training. Focusing on these areas will enable you to maintain your facilitative self and ensure that you continue to grow as a person and community counselor.

SELF-DISCLOSURE

It is likely that during your training program you will be asked to disclose personal information about yourself. Perhaps you will become a client for another counselor trainee, or be required to write and turn in a personal journal, or become involved in a process group in which you are invited to "get real." What possible relationship can this sort of self-disclosure have to your becoming a successful counselor?

Becoming a counselor involves much more than simply learning theories and developing skills. You must work to become more fully who you are as a person. In doing so, you will come to a greater level of self-understanding and learn to recognize when your buttons are being pushed by your clients. You will learn to recognize more vividly the values that you hold and the prejudices that you harbor. You will be able to finish some of your "old business" and become a more authentic human being. And you will, in the process, achieve more success in helping your clients to become more authentic.

Sidney Jourard began conducting research into the benefits of self-disclosure as far back as the 1950s. In *The Transparent Self* (1971), he stated that people who are comfortable with self-disclosure tend to be mentally healthy. We counselors ask that our clients disclose personal information to us, but the therapeutic value of revealing oneself to another human being is

EXPERIENTIAL LEARNING

Many people keep a private diary or journal of their day-to-day lives. In it, they may record important events, articulate their innermost thoughts, and give voice to their deepest feelings. For a week, keep a "public diary" by recording the significant self-disclosures you make to others. Reflect on the experience.

1. With whom did you share?

2. What were the common themes of your self-disclosures?

3. How did it feel to reveal yourself to someone?

often overlooked because we tend to focus more on the content of what is disclosed. Jourard's assertion was that self-disclosure *itself* is curative. Jourard provocatively asked whether perhaps people needed counseling because they had not yet disclosed themselves to others who were important in their lives. His response to this rhetorical question was that people need to self-disclose in order to get better, and that all of us would be better off if we allowed ourselves to be known as who we truly are and gave up hiding behind our roles. If self-disclosure leads to greater mental health, shouldn't you seek more opportunities to talk authentically about yourself?

Self-Exposure and Shame

Why would we resist letting others see us fully? Why do we more often present our fake persona, rather than our true person? Perhaps we do so because allowing ourselves to be fully revealed feels like being undressed, and it brings with it the terror of shame—the feeling that others will see into our core and find us lacking.

Where did we get such an idea? It seems to come to all of us naturally in the process of growing up. As we have mentioned before, there is a moment in early childhood when we first realize that others are evaluating us. From that time on, we begin to feel exposed to their scrutiny. We begin to despise aspects of ourselves that we consider to be unacceptable to significant others. And, sure enough, others seem eager to give us feedback regarding those unacceptable parts of ourselves. We cringe, for example, to remember times when we were labeled "bad girls" or "bad boys" because something we were doing at that moment didn't sit well with our caretakers.

At these times, we confront our conditions of worth. People send us the message that they will love us *if, and only if,* we look and behave in ways that they find agreeable. As a result, we come to feel that only those aspects of ourselves that can pass muster are worthy, and we hope to hide, or even kill off, the unacceptable parts. Shame embodies the terror that we will, in an unguarded moment, inadvertently reveal the "unacceptable" parts of our true selves, and then love and regard will again be withdrawn.

When those children in the Rouge Test finally realized that they saw themselves in the mirror, many of the children displayed what appeared to be embarrassment. Most developmental psychologists mark this discovery as the beginnings of the ability to not only develop self-esteem, but to develop shame as well. In order to experience shame, a person must be able to evaluate his or her own behavior or situation in terms of some external standard (Lewis, 1995). The failure to meet a standard results in shame because we have some level of objective self-awareness. Seeing oneself as physically unattractive, impoverished, or deformed in some way may produce shame. An unrequited smile or a situation in which one feels foolish can also create shame. Any circumstance in which people believe that they do not "measure up" may bring on embarrassment and the fear of being exposed.

In shame, a person experiences a heightened sense of self-consciousness. This type of self-perception is accompanied by the feeling of being small and helpless, and in this situation the person feels ineffective or inadequate. This is the humiliation experience in which people perceive a loss of control that brings about the desire to hide or disappear. The intense pain or discomfort may be accompanied by the feeling that we are no good or unworthy. We feel like a victim of the external standard and helpless to avoid condemnation.

Keep in mind, though, that shame is a self-attribution. It is an evaluation of the self that produces lowered self-esteem because of the belief that who one *is* is simply not good enough. Such evaluations are often first conveyed by others and then internalized as aspects of the self. Lewis (1995) suggested that negative self-attributions can even come from seemingly harmless teasing, which he compares to an engine for humiliation.

A display of disgust or contempt on the face of another person gives rise to feelings of shame. Withdrawal of love also creates a sense of failure, worthlessness, and shame. Anyone who has experienced any of these humiliations—and we all have—has known shame. Unchecked or unexamined shame has the potential to keep you from being fully present, authentic, and congruent with your clients. We all have it—what do you plan to do about yours?

The Imposter Phenomenon

You wanted to become a community counselor because you believed that you had the "right stuff." You were a good listener, you cared about others, and you were drawn to helping when you saw people in trouble. But when you began to take classes, you realized that there was a standard that counselors must meet. Initially, when that benchmark may have seemed beyond your grasp, perhaps your first reaction was to hide your lack of competence. As you recall those feelings of insecurity and inadequacy, you might remember that you tended to secretly believe that you were a fraud, and that sooner or later you would be found out and excommunicated from the ranks. There was a lot more to becoming a counselor than you had realized and you were not certain that you had what it takes. Perhaps those professors who accepted you into the program had made a serious mistake!

Such a belief is what Clance and Imes (1978) and Harvey and Katz (1985) called the "imposter phenomenon." Most people who achieve some level of success while at the same time wondering if they truly possess the requirements for the job, initially believe themselves to be frauds. The requisite level of performance seems out of reach and thus they feel a sense of shame. As a community counselor in training, you have probably occasionally felt this sense of being an imposter.

Swann (1996) pointed out that when we humans are in the midst of a negative self-evaluation, we cannot accept positive feedback from others. Nothing anyone can say will cheer us up. Therefore, when something good happens to us that we believe may be undeserved, our level of self-esteem can actually drop. We may then wish to withdraw from any activity in which we will face the evaluation of others. The famous comedian Groucho Marx once explained his reason for withdrawing his membership from the Hollywood chapter of the Friar's Club by declaring, "I just don't want to belong to any club that would have me as a member" (Swann, 1996, p. 18). Groucho avoided the humiliation of being found wanting by not participating.

Perhaps you have found yourself doing this as well. Or maybe your way of dealing with your imposter phenomenon is to hunker down and try to avoid situations that involve scrutiny. Either remedy will rob you of the opportunities you need to become a successful counselor. Unless you become open to feedback from others, and, better yet, begin to disclose your misgivings about yourself, your only choices are to hide out or leave the field. You cannot find refuge in adopting a "professional" persona that is not who you are.

Self-Disclosure as an Antidote to Shame

According to Jourard (1971), although being open and honest with others—and, as a result, with yourself—can be painful at times, "it is likely to be an effective preventative of both mental illness and certain kinds of physical sickness. Honesty can literally be a health insurance policy" (p. 133). Ironically, when you present yourself to others as you truly are, you will find yourself becoming more accepting of yourself. As a result, you can be more accepting of your clients. Remember that clients may initially be reluctant to let themselves be known. This unwillingness to share themselves inhibits their freedom when interacting with you. They may, at first, attempt to manipulate your perceptions of them. They may present as "the good client," "the helpless client," "the tough guy," or "the know-it-all."

Your job is to offer acceptance of who they are behind this façade so that they can be more self-disclosing. Once clients realize that you will not respond to them with scolding, shock, scorn, or moral indignation, they will feel encouraged by this lack of expected censure and will likely go on to reveal deeper and more honest views of themselves. You will then have created a condition that Carl Rogers (1961) termed unconditional positive regard. This condition is the antidote to the conditions of worth under which we have all suffered.

According to Jourard (1971), if counselors are genuinely themselves with their clients, they can then let their clients and themselves be who they truly are. There will then be no need, or at least less of a need, for clients to hide or deny their true feelings and desires. The result for the client, and very likely for the counselor as well, is growth. Similarly, Buber (1937) believed that the most facilitative and growth-producing relationship anyone can experience is the "I-Thou" relationship. This is an encounter between authentic human beings who both grow as a result of their time together. It is a relationship of mutual congruence. Carl Rogers (1961) asserted that congruence, which involves encountering another without a façade or defensive front, is fundamental for successful counseling. Buber contrasted this "I-Thou" type of relationship with an "I-It" relationship, in which we are treating the client as the object of our manipulations and treating ourselves as the professional, relying on our expertise and training rather than our *self* for understanding.

Of course, authenticity does not mean that you say anything and everything that comes to your mind. The ethical use of self-disclosure means that you reveal yourself to the client as this becomes important for the *client's* benefit. It is counterproductive when counselors self-disclose to clients because of the *counselor's* own need to discharge unresolved emotions or issues that do not pertain to the client's situation. While Jourard found in his research that people who self-disclose are better liked than those who are guarded, he also found that those who gratuitously self-disclose are shunned. If you have ever been trapped on an airplane next to someone who wants to tell you all the gory details of his or her life, you know that there is an optimal level of self-disclosure. Too much or too little self-disclosure makes for strained relationships.

Furthermore, inappropriate self-disclosure on the part of the counselor can be an annoying distraction, or worse, a jarring, fatal flaw. The counselor who spends time complaining about his work or colleagues, sharing gossip, or revealing intimate details of his life is wasting the client's time and breaching

EXPERIENTIAL LEARNING

Successful counselors have developed certain personal qualities that have helped them to be effective with clients. Take some time to look inside and see where you are right now on your journey toward becoming a facilitative self. When you're ready, complete the checklist below. Check "Y" for "Yes, I've definitely achieved this quality. Check "?" for "I'm not sure, but I think I'm making progress." And check "N" for "No, I have major work to do in this area."

1. Y _____ ? _____ N _____
   I admit my weaknesses without an overwhelming sense of shame.

2. Y _____ ? _____ N _____
   I am often spontaneous.

3. Y _____ ? _____ N _____
   I am strongly committed to helping other people.

4. Y _____ ? _____ N _____
   I consider myself a worthwhile person.

5. Y _____ ? _____ N _____
   I am endlessly fascinated by the behavior of people.

6. Y _____ ? _____ N _____
   I am eager to grow and change.

7. Y _____ ? _____ N _____
   I take time for myself in order to feel rejuvenated.

8. Y _____ ? _____ N _____
   I enjoy deep personal connections with a few other people.

9. Y _____ ? _____ N _____
   I try to find good in people, even when I don't approve of their behaviors.

10. Y _____ ? _____ N _____
    I try to behave ethically, even when I am not sure of what path to take.

11. Y _____ ? _____ N _____
    People seem to trust me.

12. Y _____ ? _____ N _____
    I can see situations from different angles.

13. Y _____ ? _____ N _____
    I often trust my "gut" feelings when making a decision.

14. Y _____ ? _____ N _____
    I know myself pretty well.

15. Y _____ ? _____ N _____
    I have a good sense of humor.

16. Y _____ ? _____ N _____
    I enjoy my own company.

17. Y _____ ? _____ N _____
    I am willing to take risks in relationships.

18. Y _____ ? _____ N _____
    I can listen without needing to have my say.

19. Y _____ ? _____ N _____
    I am generally a fairly calm person.

20. Y _____ ? _____ N _____
    I can see that I probably "fudged" a bit on some of my answers above.

Once you have finished this checklist, look over your answers for any patterns or common themes. What areas are more fully developed than others? What areas require significant work?

the expectations of a professional relationship. In all cases, counselors must consider their professional role and the intention behind self-disclosure.

In the final analysis, optimal self-disclosure reduces feelings of shame, while increasing a sense of confidence that who we are is okay. Armed with this confidence in ourselves, we tend to interact more comfortably with others. Without such confidence, counselors tend to hide behind a professional role and establish "I-It" relationships with clients. Unfortunately, this robs both the client *and* the counselor of what could have been achieved in their work together.

Outside the client/counselor relationship, it is important for you to be with significant others with whom you can self-disclose without fear of negative consequences. Find other counselors who understand what you are going through and who will serve as consultants and confidants. So long as you keep attempting to share who you truly are, and don't succumb to hiding to avoid shame, you will be able to allow your clients to realize their own authentic selves. You will not simply be a person who possesses theories and skills; you will be facilitative by your very presence.

Remember that all of us, including the counselors who have written this book, are continually in the position of not being as good now as we can be in the future. We are engaged in a lifelong process, and there should be no shame in it so long as we are striving to be better. The best we can do is to commit to transcending where we are now. And as *we* get better, our clients will get better, too.

TRUSTING YOUR INTUITION

As indicated in the items of the checklist, often counselors find themselves in ambiguous situations where the right thing to do is unclear. There is no recipe book for successful counseling. At such times, you must be willing to trust your "gut" feelings or intuitions. Of course, it is wise to seek consultation regarding your clients and learn as much as you can from supervisors, research, and workshops. Nevertheless, you will regularly find yourself in situations without an external beacon for direction, and you will have to rely on your inner sense. But exactly what are intuitions and where do they come from?

One of the more interesting treatments of the nature of intuition is Goldberg's (1983) analysis of what he called the "faces of intuition." Goldberg asserted that when intuition shows itself, it can take many forms. *Discovery* intuition, for example, is the type of intuition often experienced as a flash of insight, during which the solution is laid bare, as if by a flash of lightning. People who experience such intuitions—or insights—report a strong sense of release at the moment of the "Eureka!" or "Aha!" This is not to say that all intuition must come as an orgasm of the mind. *Evaluation* intuition, on the other hand, is often experienced as an adjunct to rational decision making. Rational and quantitative evaluations can still leave us with uncertainty and ambiguity. In the end, it appears that whether we accept something as true will depend on how it feels in our gut. This type of intuition can also guide us in our creative expression and is probably also the intuition that is our conscience. Once we have internalized a sense of the rightness or wrongness of something, we are signaled by the evaluation function of our intuition when we must make a choice about our actions.

Operation intuition, according to Goldberg, is the "most subtle, almost spooky form of intuition . . . [which] guides us this way and that, sometimes with declarative force, sometimes with gentle grace" (p. 54). In this form of intuition, we are drawn to certain actions, sometimes in spite of ourselves, because of what feels like the call of necessity or destiny. Sometimes we find ourselves compelled by a goal, or simply impelled by a need to move. At those moments, we are usually at a loss to explain why. We simply know, albeit vaguely, that what we do now has implications for our future—that we have been "called." Goldberg delineates other types of intuition, but for our purposes, it's relevant to focus on how intuition has influenced you so far, and how it might affect your work with clients, as it did with Enrique in "Jon's Revelation." At times, simply trusting oneself can help the client access more genuine emotions.

EMPATHIC ACCURACY

Your world is populated by others whom you presume to be like you. They are beings who walk, talk, and bear a categorical resemblance to yourself. In your own experience, you are a self, while everyone else is the "other" in your world. How then, is it possible for you to achieve empathic knowledge of others? How can you connect in an "I-Thou" manner, rather than remain in an "I-It" relationship with others? How do you avoid treating people as mere objects?

We automatically experience our own thoughts and feelings, but we do not have direct access to the subjective experience of another person. Philosophers call this "the problem of other minds," which we discuss in more detail in Chapter 6. In response to the problem of other minds, the question we must ask ourselves is how it is possible to relate to others as well as we do when we are mostly just guessing about what goes on in their personal worlds. Furthermore, some people seem to be quite adept at understanding these other minds, while other people seem hopelessly clueless in dealing with others. What accounts for this difference in ability? Ickes (1997) wrote that resolving this problem of understanding the minds of others "is likely the second greatest achievement of our species (the first being having achieved consciousness)" (pp. 1–2).

Jon's Revelation

It was early December, and Enrique was pleased that the semester would soon be ending. He was successfully completing his first semester of internship at the university counseling center, and he was ready for a break. During the semester Enrique had learned much about himself as a counselor. He, like many interns, had initially struggled with insecurity. He had therefore recently been gratified to feel within himself a growing sense of self-efficacy as a counselor. He was meeting for the first time with Jon, whom he knew had sought counseling for personal issues. He listened to Jon talk casually about going home for the winter break and observed as Jon laughed off his inability to sustain a steady relationship.

"I know my parents are going to ask me for the millionth time when I'm going to bring home a 'nice girl' for them to meet. I mean, I'm a senior. They're starting to wonder why I never really have an ongoing relationship." Jon paused, looked at Enrique, and then looked away. "But whatever. It's not a big deal." Jon looked at Enrique with a smile and shrugged. "I guess my main concern is just dealing with the stress of the end of the semester."

But what really brought you here? Enrique wondered. He felt himself grow quiet within. He focused intently on Jon, trying to feel his experience. He looked steadily at Jon, and after a few seconds said, "Yet, as you describe it, it seems like there's something unsatisfying, unfinished about all this."

"Well, I don't know," Jon stumbled over his words. "I just don't know if I'm ready . . ."

Enrique waited.

"I'm gay," said Jon. "I'm not sure I'm ready to talk about it. With my parents or with you."

"Okay," Enrique said. "You lead."

Questions for Reflection

1. What self-doubts and baggage might interfere with your receptiveness to yourself?

2. When are you best able to hear and respond to your own intuition? How can you enhance this ability in your work with clients?

One way to characterize this ability is to say that people who have it are empathically accurate in their understanding of others' subjective experience. According to Ickes (1997), empathic ability is a biologically inherited predisposition to apprehend the experience of another person. However, people, especially those who want to become counselors, *must* learn how to use this innately based communication capacity. Although we can practice and refine our empathic skill, empathy involves a kind of knowing that is beyond or beneath logic or analysis. This is a "wired-in" social ability that has evolved over the eons and that is the result of our being social animals.

As mentioned, *empathy* is our ability to sense and appraise the current condition of another person. Lazarus (1991) stated that there are two modes of this appraisal: one is "automatic, involuntary, and unconscious" and the other is "time-consuming, deliberate, volitional, and conscious" (p. 188). The first mode of appraisal is more of a feeling, sometimes called "emotional contagion." In contrast, the second is a kind of reasoning, usually referred to as "role-taking" or "perspective-taking."

Combining these modes of empathic appraisal makes for a more complete and accurate understanding of others. When we sense that another person is feeling such-and-such a way, we make this appraisal in the form of a "gut reaction." However, this does not necessarily mean that the other person *is* feeling that way, because empathy belongs to the observer and not the observed person. Empathic accuracy therefore occurs when our gut feeling matches the feeling of the other.

For both client and therapist this level of empathic encounter can be very powerful and moving; the client has the experience of being profoundly heard and confirmed. Emotional resonance and sensitivity are crucial to empathy. True empathy also includes the ability to see your client's unique perspective on things and to use the client's frames of reference for meaning making and understanding experience. Thus, the most helpful and responsive attitude of the counselor is one of *sustained empathic inquiry* as an investigative stance (Stolorow & Atwood, 1992).

In both animal and human studies, it has been shown that attachment difficulties in infancy and trauma in childhood can dull empathic accuracy. To the extent that you have suffered in your life, that is the level of preoccupation with your *self* that you must overcome in order to improve your empathic accuracy. Put bluntly, if you are still licking your wounds, you cannot give your full attention to others. Self-disclosure with intimate others, such as you might find in a personal counseling relationship, will help you work through such deprivation and injury, allowing you to devote more of your energies to empathy (Jourard, 1971). This is one reason why it is so important for counselors to do their own personal work. The admonition of Socrates to "Know thyself" is still good advice after 2,500 years.

COUNTERTRANSFERENCE

Inevitably, all people have sensitive areas of emotional injury that they have not fully explored—hidden and sequestered by protective layers. Sometimes these unresolved emotional injuries become activated in their present relations with others. Someone "touches a nerve" or sensitive issue that provokes a response that may seem out of proportion to the current situation.

Or perhaps the person finds himself responding very negatively toward some-one, but unable to identify why he experiences that person as so obnoxious. In other words, the ways in which we have been injured, frustrated, or disap-pointed in our past relations with others can affect how we perceive and respond to new relationships in the present.

This is particularly true if you have not yet fully explored and understood how past injuries or interpersonal problems with others have influenced you. Part of your journey of self-exploration will include becoming more aware of these areas of unresolved conflict. The less you are motivated by protective and defensive efforts designed to shield you from emotional pain, the more you will be able to engage others with full awareness of your authentic thoughts and feelings.

Playing out unresolved personal issues in your current encounters with other people is a human tendency that Freud (1924) called *transference*. In the therapeutic relationship, Freud observed that a client often acted as if the therapist were a sort of stand-in for another important person in the client's life. The client may express emotions toward (and assign motivations to) the therapist that rightly belong to that client's experience of someone else. Gaining insight into the origins and meaning of the client's transference con-stitutes one of the main goals of psychoanalytic therapy.

Although you're not intending to become a classic psychoanalyst, never-theless you will encounter transference in your clients. What's more, you will find that clients will evoke in you certain feelings and reactions that touch upon your own personal conflicts and unresolved issues. Freud called the counselor's reaction in this situation *countertransference*. He cautioned that it has the potential to derail a productive therapeutic relationship, because the counselor's own unresolved feelings and conflicts get in the way of the client's self-expression. In other words, the counselor may distort the client's behavior to conform to the counselor's expectations or biases.

Freud's concept is not a relic that is irrelevant to either counseling or interpersonal relationships in general. Most modern forms of counseling include some variant of the concepts of transference and countertransference. Now, however, many counselors believe that countertransference can be a source of insight for both the counselor and the client to be explored rather than simply avoided (Teyber, 2000). Countertransference can alert the counselor to his or her own weaknesses or unresolved conflicts. It can also provide telling informa-tion that can illuminate the essence of a client's problems. For instance, if a counselor feels bored by her client's tendency to tell long, rambling stories about his past, then the counselor may have some sense of how other people in the client's life feel about that client. This reaction of boredom, if shared judiciously and genuinely with the client, can help the counselor and client conceptualize the client's ongoing problems with interpersonal relationships.

You can probably think of times that stand out as examples of when you have had a strong transference reaction to someone. These situations may have been primarily about you, or primarily about that other person. The important point to remember is that self-awareness is a lens through which you see your relationship with your clients, and the finer the lens the clearer the image.

MAINTAINING YOUR FACILITATIVE SELF

Since *you* are your instrument in counseling, your ethical obligation is to maintain yourself in good working order. In this sense, the self of the counselor and the role of the counselor are two sides of the same coin. If you should become chronically anxious or depressed, physically ill, or burned out in your work, you will be less useful to your clients.

As you read in Chapter 2, the work of a community counselor is stressful. You will hear stories of people's agony that will sometimes leave you struggling to shake the images of their awful lives. Your clients may make demands on you that could only be met by a superhero. Even though you realize this, you will sometimes experience guilt for not being good enough. You will be disappointed that clients in whom you have invested a great deal of energy will backslide or choose not to change in the way you believe they should. Your clients' positive and negative transference will leave you emotionally defensive and confused. Sometimes the demands of routine paperwork will have you feeling buried and stultified. Denial of payment by insurance companies for services will frustrate and anger you. And because you are involved in relationships that are always focused on the needs of others, at times you will feel as though you have given all you can.

But the demands on you do not end when you part from your client and leave the counseling room. Community counselors also must function within a larger organizational system that can be both facilitative and frustrating. You will be involved with such activities as community outreach, crisis services, case management, and provision of emergency services. All of these important aspects of community counseling require high levels of coordination by many people working within an administrative structure. You will be challenged to understand how you fit in to such a system.

Can you use your self-knowledge to enhance your role as a "team player" while keeping your own values, ideas, and creativity? Can you contribute to productive change, but also be a cooperative counselor and adjust yourself to play by the rules that keep the system intact? Some adjustment will certainly be required of you to work productively with others to meet the needs not only of clients, but also of the institution in which you work. When you are underpaid and overworked it will be more difficult to maintain your

An elderly Cherokee Native American was teaching his grandchildren about life. He said to them, "A fight is going on inside me; it is a terrible fight and it is between two wolves. One wolf is evil—he is fear, rage, envy, shame, arrogance, self-pity, greed, lies, and suspicion.

"The other is good—he is joy, hope, compassion, serenity, humility, empathy, truth, and faith.

"This same fight is going on inside you, and inside every other person, too."

The children thought about this for a minute, and then one child asked his grandfather, "Which wolf will win?"

The old Cherokee simply replied, "The one I feed."

balance and to use yourself to understand your clients while meeting the demands of the agency. All of this can leave you feeling as if you were filled with thoughts and feelings that have nowhere to go. Your role as a counselor may feel at odds with your "self" as a counselor.

In some cultures, people with life problems go to the shaman for a cure. Since it is believed that some human difficulties are due to possession by evil spirits, the shaman's job is to perform an exorcism. The shaman asks the client to lie on the ground while ritual symbols are employed, along with certain incantations. Then the shaman lies head-to-head with the afflicted person and summons the evil spirit to exit through the skull of the client and enter the skull of the shaman. The shaman, having maintained excellent physical health and knowing certain cathartic procedures, wrestles with the evil spirit until at last the shaman is able to vomit out the offending spirit. After that, the shaman has to undergo a recovery period in order to return to a facilitative condition of mind and body.

Like the shaman, you will employ certain rituals and incantations with your client in the counseling room. You will summon the afflicting spirit to leave your client. It's not hard to imagine that sometimes you will feel poisoned by the struggle, requiring that you engage in some procedure to restore yourself to optimal physical and mental health. You may have heard the expression, "The job's not finished until the paperwork is done." In counseling, the job is not finished until you have re-tuned your instrument—and the instrument is you.

The Reality of Stress

Hans Selye (1976) was among the first to describe how psychological stress resulted in physical illness. He stated that distress (negative stress) and

EXPERIENTIAL LEARNING

Write down the top sources of stress in your life right now. In what ways are these sources of stress sabotaging your ability to achieve all that you want in your personal and professional life? How might counseling help you in dealing with these stressors more productively?

eustress (positive stress) were indistinguishable in terms of the body's reaction. When we experience conditions of stress, Selye said that we develop a "flight or fight" mechanism in our bodies that gets us ready to respond to a threat. Various chemical reactions are triggered, such as an increase of adrenaline, cortisol, and other hormones that ramp-up our ability to act quickly.

Perhaps in the days when we humans were in constant danger of being eaten by predators, this flight-fight mechanism was quite useful. Today, our physical well-being is less often threatened, but we undergo psychological stress on a regular basis. As a counselor, you will experience psychological stress more often than the average person. According to Selye, what happens in situations of chronic stress is that we tend to accommodate the stress and carry on. However, we can only ignore our bodies for so long. Eventually, a threshold is reached where the saturation of our bodies by stress chemicals causes a breakdown of our immune system and we either become physically ill or decline psychologically.

While none of us will ever be problem-free, it is our responsibility as counselors to always work to maintain "personal soundness" as we respond to the stress in our lives. You don't have to be a paragon of mental health in order to be a successful counselor. All of us have our personal hang-ups, periods of ups and downs, and unfulfilled potential. Your own counseling can help you stay in touch with yourself when the strains of everyday life begin to erode your confidence (McLeod, 1998). Working with troubled clients costs you a great deal of psychic energy and can result in residual confusion and burnout unless you continually process your experiences.

THE NEED FOR PERSONAL GROWTH

Truax and Mitchell (1971) reviewed over one hundred studies of counselor effectiveness and found that counseling techniques are useful only when the counselor's personality is inherently helpful. Others (Perez, 1979; Seligman,

1995) found the counselor's personality to be the most important criterion for effectiveness with clients. Like members of the clergy who follow their vocation, successful community counselors have somehow been called to their life's work and are ready to fully give themselves to it. The more willing you are to make such a commitment, the more likely you will be to experience joy and success in the work of helping others.

The journey that has brought you to this profession has taken many years. It is likely that negative experiences in your life have sensitized you to the misfortune of others and stimulated in you the desire to be helpful. Henry (1977) found that, as children, counselors often had experienced illness, loneliness, or bereavement. Counselors were likely to have endured more traumatic events, and their families of origin were often in turmoil. Not surprisingly, counselors were likely to have been clients themselves before entering their training. Such findings have led to the "wounded healer theory" (Guggenbuhl-Craig, 1971; Rippere & Williams, 1985), which suggests that the healer's history of misfortune or trauma confers the power to heal.

First-hand experiences of loss and suffering are certainly helpful in understanding what life might be like for clients. A counselor trainer of our acquaintance often says, "I wouldn't give you a nickel for a counselor who hasn't suffered." Such painful events in the counselor's life are, however, a two-edged sword. While they may aid in the establishment of empathy, they could also result in the counselor overidentifying with the client's pain. One thing you will need to check in yourself is how strong your "rescue fantasy" might be. A rescue fantasy is the urgent need to fix the client's situation and then to be appreciated for the extraordinary intervention.

You also need to explore your value system in order to become more aware of what pushes your buttons and what makes you uncomfortable. For example, you may have strong opinions regarding abortion, incest, infidelity, child abuse, alcohol, or drug use. It's okay for you to have these opinions, but it is important that you work on respecting and accepting clients, even when their opinions or behavior are different from your own. Often, your discomforts and prejudices may lie beyond your awareness. In such cases, you may communicate to your client, without realizing it, that talking about such subjects is out-of-bounds in the counseling relationship.

For example, when he was a graduate student, Jack once met with an admired professor, who later that day committed suicide. Being aware only of the feeling of guilt at having been the last person to see this man alive, Jack subsequently graduated and entered practice. Two years later, while discussing a particularly vexing case with a supervisor, Jack was asked if the client had talked of suicide. At that moment, Jack realized that none of his clients had ever spoken of suicide. Somehow, he had subliminally communicated to all his clients,

"Don't talk about suicide—it makes me uncomfortable." After that epiphany, Jack's clients often spoke of suicide. Like Jack, you may unconsciously hope that your clients do not bring up certain topics in counseling because they might make you feel threatened or helpless. Do you know what these topics are?

It is difficult to lift up bandages to look at old wounds, and even more difficult to go poking around when the wounds are not fully healed. But as you can see, those wounds that are still festering will invisibly influence your behavior toward others. Shoving painful life events down into a cellar of forgetting just makes you afraid to go downstairs to where your deepest, richest feelings may live. It is a natural human tendency to want to move on from painful life events. How you choose to move on becomes vitally important to whether you become an integrated and fully alive person, or whether you surround yourself in a shroud of insulating forgetfulness. As Freud observed, it is what we forget that we repeat.

The more you are distanced from your true self, the more likely you are to make fundamental mistakes in counseling. Misunderstanding a client's concern, pushing one's own values on the client, or even misdiagnosing a client can all be the results of counselors who are unaware of their own problems and concerns. For this reason, we strongly encourage all counselors in training to receive their own counseling. Working as a client will help reduce the potential for strong countertransference reactions that could interfere with your own work with clients. Further, being a client allows you to experience the relationship from the client's perspective, which helps to foster an enhanced understanding of the challenges the client faces. You will be able to remember what your own counselor did that worked best for you and begin to incorporate those skills into your repertoire.

ETHICAL AND LEGAL ISSUES IN PRACTICE

One last reason to know yourself well in order to be an effective instrument of counseling involves your role as an ethical decision maker. It is easy to read and understand the ethical guidelines about what is appropriate or not in counseling relationships. However, counselors often find themselves in situations where there is no cut-and-dried rule, and they discover that they must interpret an overarching "principle." In other words, they must draw on their expertise, judgment, and self-knowledge to determine a course of action that serves their client's best interests. Counselors must feel confident that the important decisions that they make are not influenced by their own unresolved issues or unexamined biases.

The legal implications of your work as a facilitative self are similar to ethical considerations, in that any time your selfhood interferes with your ability to effectively treat your client, you may be at risk for sanction or legal action. Perhaps the most blatant ethical and legal concerns that we see arising from the counselor's misuse of self are those occasions in which counselors engage in inappropriate relationships with clients. Having sex with clients is never appropriate. Engaging in unnecessary dual relationships is discouraged, as is any counselor-client relationship in which the client can be misled or hurt. As we mentioned in Chapter 3, community counselors know the expectations of ethical and legal behavior; yet every year counselors are charged with inappropriate behavior. Why?

Explanations vary, but our general sense is that counselors have let their personal desires override their professional judgment (Smith & Fitzpatrick, 1995). Counselors who have not attempted to fully explore themselves, who hide from their own shaming experiences, or who fail to attend to their ongoing emotional, physical, and spiritual needs seem most at risk for engaging in inappropriate behavior. Thus, we again assert the need for counselors to receive their own counseling and consultation throughout their careers (Smith & Fitzpatrick, 1995). Our blind spots can be debilitating unless we continually take action to address them.

CONCLUDING THOUGHTS

You are the instrument of counseling. Your *self* (your *youness,* your *being*) is the tool through which counseling occurs. Understanding who you are and who you are becoming, and then allowing yourself to be fully you, are unending tasks for all counselors. We conclude this chapter with the encouragement that you heighten your self-investigation during your training program. Write, reflect, seek counseling, and consult with your peers and professors. Now is the best time for you to figure out who you are and to understand how you will use who you are when you work with others.

RECOMMENDED RESOURCES

In order to get in touch with the elusive idea of one's self, consider reading some of the texts we've mentioned in this chapter, such as:

Jourard, S. M. (1971). *The transparent self*. New York: D. Van Nostrand.

Laing, R. D. (1969). *The divided self.* New York: Pantheon Books.

Levin, J. D. (1992). *Theories of the self.* Washington, DC: Hemisphere.

You may also be interested in literature on attachment and object relations.

Bowlby, J. (1969/1982). *Attachment.* New York: Basic.

Buckley, P. (Ed.). (1986). *Essential papers on object relations.* New York: New York University Press.

Other Resources

Frida, A Biography of Frida Kahlo, a dynamic book by Hayden Herrera, paints a picture of one woman's life, revealing how she comes to terms with herself, her loved ones, and her life. The book *A Lesson Before Dying* by Ernest J. Gaines also presents a very compelling view of two men's explorations of their own self-hoods.

Cast Away is an intriguing movie that allows us to see how one man deals with his sense of himself as he responds to enforced solitude. *Being John Malkovich* provides a quirky look at what it's like when someone literally gets inside someone else's head, while figuring out what's going on for himself at the same time. For an intriguing glimpse into the personal growth of a moviemaker, watch *Sherman's March* by Ross McElwee, and then watch his later videos *Time Indefinite* and *Six O'Clock News.* You'll see how he matures and develops into a more authentic, complex, and interesting self.

REFERENCES

Branden, N. (1971). *The disowned self.* Los Angeles: Nash Publishing.

Buber, M. (1937). *I and thou.* New York: Scribners.

Clance, P. R., & Imes, S. A. (1978). The imposter phenomenon in high achieving women: Dynamics and therapeutic intervention. *Psychotherapy: Theory, Research and Practice, 15,* 241–247.

Deikman, A. J. (1999). "I" = awareness. In S. Callagher & J. Shear (Eds.), *Models of the self* (pp. 421–427). Charlottesville, VA: Imprint Academic.

Frankl, V. (1959). *Man's search for meaning.* New York: Simon & Schuster.

Freud, S. (1924). *A general introduction to psychoanalysis.* New York: Washington Square Press.

Goldberg, P. (1983). *Understanding intuition and applying it in everyday life.* New York: Tarcher/Penguin.

Guggenbuhl-Craig, A. (1971). *Power in the helping professions.* Dallas: Spring.

Harvey, J. C., & Katz, C. (1985). *If I'm so successful why do I feel like a fake?: The imposter phenomenon.* New York: St. Martin's Press.

Henry, W. E. (1977). Personal and social identities of psychotherapists. In A. S. Gurman & A. M. Razin (Eds.), *Effective psychotherapy: A handbook of research* (pp. 47–62). Oxford: Pergamon.

Ickes, W. (1997). *Empathic accuracy*. New York: Guilford Press.

Jourard, S. M. (1971). *The transparent self*. New York: D. Van Nostrand.

Laing, R. D. (1969). *The divided self*. New York: Pantheon Books.

Lazarus, R. S. (1991). *Emotion and adaptation*. New York: Oxford University Press.

Levin, J. D. (1992). *Theories of the self*. Washington, DC: Hemisphere.

Lewis, M. (1995). *Shame: The exposed self*. New York: Free Press.

Martz, E. (2001). Expressing counselor empathy through the use of possible selves. *Journal of Employment Counseling, 38,* 128–133.

May, R. (1967). *Psychology and the human dilemma*. Princeton, N.J.: D. Van Nostrand.

May, R. (1983). *The discovery of being: Writings in existential psychology*. New York: W. W. Norton.

McLeod, J. (1998). *An introduction to counselling* (2nd ed.). Buckingham, UK: Open University Press.

Midgley, M. (1999). Being scientific about our selves. *Journal of Consciousness Studies, 6,* 4, pp. 85–98.

Nagel, T. (1986). *The view from nowhere*. Oxford: Oxford University Press.

Perez, J. F. (1979). *Family counseling: Theory and practice*. New York: D. Van Nostrand.

Priest, S. (1991). *Theories of the mind*. Boston: Houghton Mifflin.

Prochaska, J. O., & Norcross, J. C. (1994). *Systems of psychotherapy: A transtheoretical analysis* (3rd ed.). Pacific Grove, CA: Brooks/Cole.

Rippere, V., & Williams, R. (1985). *Wounded healers: Mental health workers' experiences of depression*. New York: Wiley.

Rogers, C. R. (1959). A theory of therapy, personality, and interpersonal relationships as developed in the client-centered framework. In S. Kock (Ed.), *Psychology: A study of a science* (pp. 184–214). New York: McGraw-Hill.

Rogers, C. R. (1961). *On becoming a person*. Boston: Houghton Mifflin.

Seinfeld, J. (1991). *The empty core: An object relations approach to psychotherapy of the schizoid personality*. Northvale, NJ: Jason Aronson.

Seligman, M. E. P. (1995). The effectiveness of psychotherapy: The *Consumer Reports* Study. *American Psychologist, 50,* 965–974.

Selye, H. (1976). *The stress of life*. New York: McGraw-Hill.

Smith, D., & Fitzpatrick, M. (1995). Patient-therapist boundary issues: An integrative review of theory and research. *Professional Psychology: Research and Practice, 26,* 499–506.

Stolorow, R. D., & Atwood, G. E. (1992). *Contexts of being.* New Jersey: The Analytic Press.

Swann, W. B. (1996). *Self-traps: The elusive quest for higher self-esteem.* New York: W. H. Freeman.

Teyber, E. (2000). *Interpersonal process in psychotherapy: A relational approach* (4th ed.). Belmont, CA: Brooks/Cole.

Truax, C. B., & Mitchell, K. M. (1971). Research on certain therapist interpersonal skills in relation to process and outcome. In A. E. Bergin & S. Garfield (Eds.), *Handbook of psychotherapy and behavior change* (pp. 299–344). New York: Wiley.

Chapter 5

Experiencing Counseling: Concepts, Dynamics, and Change

People are changed, not by intellectual convictions or ethical urgings, but by transformed imaginations.

Madonna Kolbenschlag

GOALS

Reading and exploring the ideas in this chapter will help you:

- Envision the process of a counseling relationship from beginning to end
- Understand the contract that exists between counselor and client
- Assist your clients in achieving meaningful change
- Develop techniques that are commonly used in counseling, such as immediacy, reflection, and confrontation
- Successfully terminate with clients

OVERVIEW

This chapter presents information on essential interviewing and helping skills as well as an overview of the fundamental aspects of the therapeutic relationship. From establishing the relationship to terminating, successful counseling goes through a generally predictable process. As the counselor, you begin by communicating that you are willing to listen to, understand, and validate your client's story. You then establish a contract for your work together. After that, you influence change in your client through the use of such techniques as role-play, interpretation, guided imagery, reflection, and confrontation. You will master a variety of approaches and therapy methods. You will also have to develop strategies for working with difficult or resistant clients.

However, the quality of the relationship between you and your client is paramount, no matter what techniques you use. As you learned in Chapter 1, whether your approach to counseling is cognitive-behavioral, psychodynamic, humanistic, or constructivist, the process is far more likely to be successful when you have achieved a positive therapeutic alliance with your client (Wampold, 2001). Throughout your time together, you both travel on a path that is intended to lead to the client achieving important personal goals and you having a profound learning experience. According to Yalom (2002), you must first allow your clients to matter to you, "to let them enter your mind, influence you, change you—and not . . . conceal this from them" (pp. 26–27). If this "mattering" takes place, the relationship between you and your client will likely end with both of your lives enhanced.

JACK'S DEFINING MOMENT: The Escape

Jack is a counselor and counselor educator who has spent much of his professional career studying the therapeutic relationship. For years he has been awed by the healing potential in counseling and has spent a considerable amount of time exploring what makes counseling work. As a result, Jack has developed the capacity to be particularly responsive to clients' experiences and needs. In his case, the genesis of his unique counseling strengths was created by the substantial pain he experienced as a child.

When he was a boy, Jack hated his parents. No, maybe he just hated being around them when they fought. Sometimes their arguments escalated into physical fights, and Jack's father wouldn't stop hitting until his mother succumbed. Once, when he was about twelve, Jack made the mistake of trying to protect his mother and his father began striking him. After that, Jack didn't try to intervene in any of their conflicts, no matter how serious. Instead, he locked himself in his room or left the house if he could—although he would often be slapped around for taking these actions without permission. There was always a reason given for the "discipline," as his father called it, but it really didn't matter. His father's moods and how much he drank depended on what kind of a day he had at work, or how his favorite ball team had fared that weekend, or what real or imagined criticism he heard in his wife's comments.

The abuse continued over the years, and Jack became more and more reclusive. His favorite retreat was behind the garage, where an old car seat was propped up against the wall. Overhead, a single dim outdoor bulb provided just enough illumination to read by and to keep a squadron of moths occupied. While this weed-infested portion of the backyard was an eyesore by day, at night it was a sanctuary for Jack. He taught himself to become so deeply engrossed in his reading that he screened out the sounds coming from the house.

One hot and humid night in August, Jack's father crept around the side of the garage and slapped Jack hard on the head. Without thinking, Jack leapt to his feet and twisted around to face his attacker. He glared at his father, who was only inches away from his face. Jack had just turned fifteen and was now a shade over 6 feet tall; he'd added 20 pounds of muscle since his last run-in with his father. Dodging a backhanded slap, Jack landed a blow to his father's rib cage. All of his father's breath escaped in a rush and he fell to the ground as limp as a rag doll. Jack had a violent image of himself beating and kicking his father, but resisted the impulse, turned his back, and began to walk away. He paused only long enough to say, "The next time you touch *any* of us, I'll do it again."

Several weeks later, Jack finally decided to get things off his chest and talk to a counselor. Like the dam that finally broke, it all came pouring out in a torrent—his father's drinking and the constant abuse. Burning with shame, and trembling with the effort of getting it all out, Jack looked at his counselor. The man shook his head sadly and asked, "Jack do you go to church?"

Surprised, Jack uttered a barely audible reply, "Yes, well I have . . . but not much lately."

"Do you know what the Fifth Commandment is?"

"No, I'm sorry I don't remember"

"Well, it's to honor thy father and mother, and I think that's where you need to start."

Jack was stunned. Was this how counseling was supposed to work?

Questions for Reflection

1. If you had been the counselor, what would you have said to Jack after hearing his story?

2. Jack went on to become a successful community counselor. In what ways do you think he may have used this experience in his own journey toward becoming a counselor?

3. What have been your own sufferings that you can use as an empathic bridge to clients?

THE COMMUNITY COUNSELOR'S TASK

As a community counselor, you play a unique and important role. Often you are the helper of last resort, because the person in need may have exhausted many other methods of addressing her or his difficulties. The new client brings a fragile hope that the counseling process can provide something new and different to help improve the situation. Your task is to be ready to face these challenges and to use them therapeutically.

The variety of client problems you will encounter is truly remarkable. You have the opportunity to work with persons who are coming from all walks of life—different family, socioeconomic, and ethnic backgrounds. They are facing all stages of development, from toddlers to the aging. And they are seeking a wide range of goals, from maintaining sobriety to resolving a personal crisis.

This diversity of client characteristics and experiences will challenge you to be flexible and to tailor your counseling activities to suit the specific requirements of each client. However, the process of counseling involves some core constructs that inform all counseling-related activities. In other words, although each client will be different and have unique concerns, the process you will go through together is fundamentally similar. You will be successful in helping your client once you are able to:

- Make sense of yourself
- Make sense of the client
- Understand the relationship between you and the client
- Use the therapeutic relationship effectively
- Help clients change

Once you possess a good understanding of these fundamental processes of counseling, then you can develop your skills and apply them to a wide variety of counseling settings and situations.

UNDERSTANDING WHERE YOU AND YOUR CLIENT "COME FROM"

Each person "comes from" someplace unique. That is, each of us grew up in a particular family, culture, and environment that was a "psychological space" in which we formed as a person. We are often unaware of just how profoundly our early environment, relationships, and experiences have influenced our personalities, our way of seeing the world, and how we experience ourselves and others. To be a successful counselor, you need to understand these influences and how they have affected you.

In our families and communities, we unconsciously learned what sorts of self-experiences and self-expressions were permitted. We also learned what emotions and thoughts were welcomed and valued, or squelched and forbidden. We also formed a picture of ourselves from the points of view of those around us that vastly influenced our self-image. In other words, each of us grew a particular "self" while steeped in this interpersonal world.

As you learned in Chapter 4, becoming a successful counselor requires that you accept as your first task the project of understanding as thoroughly as possible what values you hold, what image you have of yourself, and what behaviors in others trigger automatic responses in you. Ideally, you have changed your "self" in order to help others change. Having traveled this terrain of personal growth, you will be in a better position to help others take the journey of personal development. Perhaps this process of self-understanding is one of the reasons you found the helping professions attractive in the first place. You are not only fascinated with what makes others tick, but also interested in discovering more of your own inner dynamics.

Beginning counselors often think that counseling merely involves acquiring a set of skills to help people solve their problems. Good practitioners know, however, that successful resolution takes place when clients explore their inner world of thoughts, feelings, hopes, and possibilities. Only then can clients achieve true and meaningful change. How can you ask someone to embark on this process unless you are willing to do the same hard work of self-examination and cultivation of greater awareness? Your own self-understanding is the corollary process that makes it possible to help clients achieve their potential. Only when you explore the dimensions of your own inner world will you be able to effectively help others take a similar journey. Making sense of yourself is fundamental to helping others understand themselves and is potentially your best training experience.

Origins of Self-Experience

Apart from the organically based psychopathologies, the problems for which most clients seek counseling are interpersonal and social in nature (Teyber, 2000). At the core of these interpersonally based problems is a disruption in the person's ability to achieve an integrated and coherent sense of self (Kohut, 1971). The quality of early emotional contact with others is a critical factor in the developmental processes that contributes to an integrated and coherent sense of self. It is especially vital that other people provide the growing person with a validating empathic emotional connection. Because family relationships are the first and most emotionally powerful social learning experiences, they serve as primary forces shaping people's perception of self and others. When early caregivers are empathically attuned, the child's emotional world is validated, and the child is able to "own" and embody his or her feelings (Kohut, 1977). Part of this developing ownership is the child's capacity to articulate and name ever more subtle emotional states. In other words, the child learns to have an emotional vocabulary and "range."

In this safe and accepting environment, the child achieves a growing sense of independence without losing connections with others. She or he then feels a sense of belonging and protection. An environment of emotional support and empathic attunement sets the stage for the child to negotiate critical developmental tasks. As the child grows, he or she is able to contain, modulate and express internal states, even when the caregiver is no longer present to lend support.

Children who haven't been given this accepting environment usually struggle to integrate a solid sense of themselves. Their options feel limited, and their range of behaviors seems restricted. Clients who fail to achieve an integrated sense of self tend to behave in self-defeating ways, have trouble expressing their emotions, and act defensively. It is not enough for you as a counselor to merely act as a technician, attempting to control or eliminate the client's problems. Rather, you must be able to address the underlying "self-experiences" that give the client's symptoms utility and meaning. Otherwise, you will not be able to make sense of the client's experience. When clients come to counseling in crisis, it is the counselor who must now provide a "containing" function—a safe, supportive environment—and lend the client the necessary support to preserve an intact sense of self.

Affect and Trauma

It is, of course, impossible to grow up and not endure some psychological knocks and bruises. Even with the most fortunate of children, the environment is not always responsive or empathically attuned to their needs. However, this does not automatically mean that everyone is doomed to a life of personal turmoil. Sometimes disruptions and struggles even enable the individual to find new areas of strength. As Donald Winnicott (1965) put it, we only need "good enough" nurturing to grow into stable and fully functioning adults.

However, for many children, the environment is unpredictable, oppressive, and even dangerous. When fundamental developmental needs are rarely met, the stage is set for chronic personal problems. Many clients presenting at community agencies have long-standing emotional difficulties that have become dispositional—a part of their personality. Since these conflicts may have their origins in early relationships, you can use the counseling relationship itself to resolve these conflicts. In other words, as a counselor you can provide your client with a new kind of relationship structured around positive, healthy interpersonal experiences. These experiences can serve as the building blocks that strengthen the self (Shapiro, 1995).

When frustrated developmental needs become the source of inner conflict and pain, a person always *does something* to prevent that pain from becoming overwhelming and disruptive. Most of the time, what a person does is healthy and adaptive; he or she makes a choice or change that addresses the core conflict. Sometimes, however, although the choice is adaptive in the short run, it ultimately undermines long-term well-being. The core conflict has not been addressed—the person's actions have served only to reduce the threat of overwhelming anxiety or pain. In this case, we usually call what the person does a "symptom."

A symptom is a way of preserving some core area of the self. Rollo May (1979) observed that a neurosis is not a *lack of adjustment,* an adjustment is *precisely what a neurosis is*—an effort to reestablish self-equilibrium. No wonder that clients are not eager to give up their symptoms or problematic behaviors when they have become so effective at preventing something worse from occurring.

Schemas

Another issue central to answering the question, "Where do you and your client come from?" involves the process of "making meaning" of experience. We are meaning-making creatures. We insist that the world must make sense to us, and we become anxious when encountering a situation with too much ambiguity. Piaget (1951) observed that each child is a little scientist, constantly figuring out the rules of how the world works. As we grow, we construct *schemas,* which are internal representations of the world, and these depictions are usually mostly accurate in predicting how things behave. Our culture contributes greatly to the internal "map" that we develop to give an overview of the physical, psychological, social, and spiritual terrains of our lives. This "map" lets us know not to step in front of a bus, that people are hurt when we betray their trust, and that we are finite and will one day die.

The problem is, as Gregory Bateson (1980) observed, the map in our heads is not the same as the "outside" territory. The categories of experience that serve as a person's internal map cannot be assumed to correspond to an "objective" or "real" world. In other words, we each live in a constructed world (Brunner, 1990).

This concept of a constructed world is perhaps best illustrated if we consider people in the midst of crisis. During these times people undergo disorienting shifts in their usually stable schemas. For instance, a woman whose husband has just died in a car accident might experience a traumatic crisis of meaning regarding the point of life and the validity of her religious beliefs. Ten months later she may have a very different view of her life. Our schema— our assumptions about ourselves, others, and the world—can be shattered in times of crisis (Janoff-Bulman, 1992). Although people assume that their organizing schemas represent the "real reality," in fact, they really possess only a "working model" that is continually under revision.

For most persons, the underlying categories and meaning-making templates that organize self-experience tend to be latent (Stolorow & Atwood, 1992). That is, our meaning making is not ordinarily the focus of our awareness. However, one of the primary goals of counseling is to help your client make these meaning-making templates overt. You help to create conditions in which clients can explore and understand the underlying organizing rules that give their experiences meaning. Clients are often startled when counseling helps to make their latent assumptions explicit. Self-defeating thoughts and behaviors appear in a new light when illuminated by the process of counseling. The client not only becomes more self-aware, but also discovers new alternatives and choices.

But there's a catch. As the counselor, *your* underlying schemas are also subjective—a constructed model that reflects a long history of experience, biases, and values. Why are your schemas any more "real" than the client's? They all represent a history of meaning-making events that solidify into a more or less unified model of experience. Some beginning counselors imagine that the client would be eager to substitute another perspective (the counselor's) for the client's "distorted" or defective view. However, this is rarely the case, and is certainly not desirable. Counselors are not in the business of converting people's fundamental beliefs or substituting their beliefs for the client's.

Instead, you must make a personal effort at self-exploration and ask, "How can using my schemas facilitate or hinder the discovery process of this client?" It is through mutual participation, through the interaction of your worlds, that your client's underlying organizing principles are revealed (Stolorow & Atwood, 1984). Clearly, you need to know how your own internal maps are drawn as well as understand your client's reality in order to help that client explore possibilities and achieve successful resolution.

Family Roles

When seeking to understand ourselves and our clients, we may also want to consider identity as shaped by family expectations. Researchers studying communication patterns in families have pointed out that often children are scripted into familial roles. Some of these roles include the responsible, good child, the problem or bad child, the hero child, or the mediator child (Teyber, 2000). These childhood roles reflect unspoken rules that govern the family. The roles are powerful identity shapers because children discover that when they perform these roles well, family stability increases. The problem is that long after leaving their families of origin, many adults are still so bound to these roles that they do not fulfill their potential. Children who have carried old role expectations and demands into adulthood often find themselves repeating these role patterns in other significant relationships. Thus, it is essential that you examine the roles you played in your own family, especially because some adults wish to play out their old role of "family healer" by becoming counselors! Working out your own unresolved issues through your clients can only hinder the growth of both yourself and your client.

Exploring clients' original family roles and recognizing the remnants in current relationships is often a central part of increasing client self-awareness and promoting change. For example, the "good girl" finds that in marriage she is perfectionistic and compliant—unable to express anger, burdened with guilt, worried, and ultimately depressed. The person reenacting the mediator role often finds that he has no feelings or opinions of his own, but instead is eager to be conciliatory and pleasant, avoiding all conflict, at the expense of truly enjoying anything. The "bad boy" occasionally finds himself unconsciously defying all authority figures, disrupting relationships, cheating on his wife, and still acting out an old rebellion, even though he left the family years before.

Roles define how the family allows critical developmental tasks to be accomplished. *Must* the conforming boy follow in the footsteps of his attorney father and go to Harvard Law? *Must* the teenage daughter develop an eating disorder so that she can distract the family's attention from the guerilla war silently going on between her parents? How are these children allowed to individuate from the family and ultimately leave home?

Once learned, family roles, myths, rules, and relationships are hard to abandon and frequently persist across many generations (Bowen, 1978). One of the difficult tasks of counseling is for clients to come to grips with the good and the bad that happened in their families. Then, they can become more aware of how old agendas are playing out in current relationships where they don't belong.

STAGES OF COUNSELING

As a community counselor, what will you be giving your clients that they could not get from their friends or their parents? The answer to this question illuminates what a trained counselor does. Gerber (2003) suggested that there are four stages to a counselor's work with clients. He labeled these stages "ventilation, clarification, alteration, and accommodation" (p. 11).

Ventilation

In Gerber's first stage, *ventilation,* there is little difference between people speaking with a community counselor or telling their story to a bartender,

EXPERIENTIAL LEARNING

Draw a picture of your family-of-origin and label each member according to the role he or she played in your family dynamic. Make each figure relatively large or small, depending on the amount of power the person exerted on the other members of the family. (Remember that passive roles, such as chronic illness or depression, often are more powerful than obviously aggressive roles.)

1. What was your primary role?

2. What behaviors did you regularly exhibit in this role?

3. What remnants of your family role are still present in your current relationships?

friend, or minister. This does not mean that ventilation is an insignificant process. Sometimes, when people have intense feelings, they give expression to these emotions by talking, crying, or writing about them. During this process people get their issues "off their chests." What the person requires for this ventilation to be useful is another human being who will listen. Usually, after a good ventilation session, the person reports feeling better. But the issue or problem that has caused the person to be upset remains the same. "If nothing more is done, the emotions will build up again and a cycle of ventilation-build up . . . is created" (p. 11).

Metaphorically, ventilation alone is like a steam boiler releasing pressure or letting off steam while the fire under the boiler still rages. If nothing is done to resolve the real problems, then the person is locked in this cycle of always seeking a sympathetic ear. Clients will sometimes view the counseling session as a situation in which they do nothing but ventilate. They come to the counselor wanting to dump excess emotional energy by telling a new "war story" or elaborating on an old one. Even if clients leave believing that the session has been useful, the counselor has done little to help them alter their situation.

Clarification

Gerber suggested that beginning with the second stage, *clarification*, a skilled counselor becomes necessary. This is the point of departure between a counseling relationship and a friendship. In this stage, the counselor helps the client tease apart the elements of the recurring dynamics in the various situations that the client finds to be problematic. As the client's story becomes more specific and orderly in the telling, themes begin to emerge. The client starts to realize that circumstances that seemed to be separate occurrences are linked together by the person's manner of responding (Teyber, 2000). As the old saying goes, "Everywhere you go, there you are."

At this stage, clients begin to make important discoveries about themselves and their circumstances. They may begin to question the personal and cultural assumptions that undermine their own potential. They may start to appreciate their own strengths and the resources available to them in the community. They may recognize how they have internalized oppression. Armed with these new insights and perspectives, clients begin to envision new possibilities and realize that they can take responsibility for meaningful personal and social change in their lives.

Alteration

The *alteration* stage (Gerber, 2003) occurs when clients assert their desire to change in ways that might alter the circumstances of their lives. The sticking point at this stage, however, is that while clients may have insight into the personal and social dynamics that are problematic, this insight may not be sufficient for true and lasting change.

For example, think of a time when you may have been dieting and happened to see a delicious-looking piece of chocolate cake. You had insight into the fact that this piece of cake contained an enormous number of calories. You may even have told yourself that eating this cake will set your goal of achieving a desired weight back several days. But you might have rationalized eating the cake by telling yourself that you have had such a difficult day that you deserve this tempting morsel. Eating "comfort food" is something we all do occasionally when our spirits are low. Simply knowing that this is not the best way to solve our current problem is not a useful insight for us at such critical moments.

Furthermore, clients have, over a long period of time, developed a characteristic style of reacting. Even though they may possess the insight that their automatic thoughts and behaviors are not successful, they may believe they have no other tools in their repertoire. Even inadequate tools are better than no tools at all, so our clients stick with what they always do.

Having at least some way of reacting is a bit like comfort food. It feels familiar and reassuring, even if we know it is not good for us. As some would put it, "Better the devil you know than the devil you don't." At this alteration stage in the counseling process, clients therefore need a great deal of support. They know they must change, but change to what? It feels to them as though giving up their habitual but unsuccessful ways of reacting would be like stripping down to their underwear in public. They have no new clothes to put on. Counselor support at this stage is therefore vital.

Accommodation

Gerber's *accommodation* stage begins when the client has attempted a change, is meeting with some success, and is getting used to thinking and behaving in new ways. This is often referred to as the "working through" phase of the process. Now the client is collecting a new set of tools or acquiring a new wardrobe. Gerber stated that people in this stage have begun to thaw out their previously frozen ways of responding to situations in their lives. "Unfreezing has to do with becoming aware of what pattern is causing the problem" (p. 12).

As clients increasingly practice new ways of responding, their situations can remain problematic, but they begin to realize that there are other ways of dealing with interpersonal and social issues. The client, in effect, becomes more creative and flexible. Abraham Maslow (1968) once said that when the only tool you have is a hammer, then everything begins to look like a nail. As clients move through the accommodation stage, they develop an entire toolbox, and situations begin to appear less singular and more manageable. On completion of this stage, clients are ready to go it alone in dealing with daily stresses, ongoing oppressive conditions, and other challenges of society.

THE THERAPEUTIC RELATIONSHIP

As they sit in the waiting room anticipating their first counseling appointment, many clients hope that behind that door they will be able to un-shoulder their heavy burden and leave it behind forever. As a counselor in training, you may be under the misguided impression that it's your job to fulfill that fantasy by taking up the burden and rescuing clients from their turmoil. Seasoned community counselors know that this is not only impossible, but also undesirable.

Like periods of happiness and fulfillment, suffering is an essential part of growth, change, and life. Suffering is one of the existential "givens" of life— a part of the human condition. The most that you can offer is to help your clients deal with their suffering honestly and productively, not neurotically and in a self-defeating fashion. But how does this occur? Your assumption must be that your clients can use counseling to discover and tap into their own personal strengths and resources to meet the painful vicissitudes of life. For clients, it often gets worse before it gets better. Or, in the common parlance: "No pain, no gain."

It is the *counseling relationship* that makes client change possible. But what does this mean? The counseling relationship is a type of human connection that is unlike any other available in ordinary life. As a counselor, you encounter your client solely in service to his or her growth and resolution.

In this sense, the relationship is not reciprocal. The client does not, as in all other relationships, need to take care of the "other side," worrying about how his or her words, feelings, or fantasies affect you.

The counseling relationship is a real, human relationship that rests on (1) a foundation of trust on the part of the client and (2) empathy and unconditional positive regard on the part of the counselor. You cannot hide behind a role or technique. The worlds of counselor and client come into contact with one another in a real encounter, which can be very powerful for *both* participants.

As a counselor in training, you may sometimes feel intimidated by these relational aspects of counseling. At times, you may rather "do something to," rather than "be someone with," the client. Strong emotions, disturbing revelations, sexual attractions, and confusing transferences are all potential parts of the counseling relationship. Therefore, you must be able to maintain your reference points while deeply engaging and participating in the inner world of the client. A strong and secure sense of self is necessary for you to remain unthreatened by this level of participation. Using your unique personality to stay grounded in the relationship gives greater power to your interventions and helps clients to achieve their counseling goals. Below we provide an overview of the fundamental elements of building therapeutic relationships, from an initial focus on recognizing strengths to the final stage of terminating the counseling relationship. As you read, keep in mind that you will be enacting these elements in your own unique way, building on your strengths and experiences to create counseling relationships that are genuine working alliances.

Recognizing Strengths

As we begin working with clients, our initial efforts to make sense of their concerns is essentially the process of conceptualization. We wonder about our clients' early self-experiences, we guess at their schema, and we hypothesize about family roles and relationships. As we do this, we gather relevant information and attempt to create a coherent picture of the client and his or her world. The more accurate and complete our picture, the more focused and potentially effective will be our interventions. We must, therefore, ensure that we include in our conceptualizations the recognition of our clients' strengths.

Community counselors are wellness-oriented. We focus on what is right, working, and strong for our clients in addition to acknowledging their obstacles, weaknesses, or illness. For some of our clients, we may be hard-pressed to find strength. In our university-based community counseling center, for instance, we often meet with clients who face multiple stressors. They're grappling with substance abuse. They've mistreated their children. They show characteristics of personality disturbances that interfere with their ability to function effectively with others. They struggle with poverty and lack of access to resources. As we work to conceptualize our clients—to make sense of them and their worlds—we sometimes initially feel despair.

As community counselors, though, we always ask, *Where is the client's strength? What is working for this person? What does she have going for her?* At times, the fact that the client showed up for counseling might be the only strength we can immediately identify. However, that ability to show up might be just what the client needs in order to make effective change in his or her life. Neglecting this resolve on the client's part fails to acknowledge that client's potential. Our job is to ensure that as we conceptualize we never sell our clients short. Building on our clients' strengths is the foundation for creating a therapeutic relationship with them.

Listening, Understanding, and Validating

As we look for clients' strengths, we realize there is no generic or one-size-fits-all method of counseling. As a counselor you may be reflecting someone's emotions, inviting the client to explore goals, or bearing witness to someone's traumatic experience. All successful counseling involves creating a condition of acceptance and caring in which the client feels safe. This is an active process— you do not simply listen passively. You must continually communicate that you are listening. Presbury, Echterling, and McKee (2002) suggested that you do this by offering the "LUV triangle": Listen, Understand, and Validate.

Listen. What does it mean to listen so that the client understands that you are paying full and deep attention? According to Egan (2002), it helps to have an open body posture, maintain appropriate eye contact (appropriate based on your client and her or his culture), and present a calm, attentive physical presence. This helps to ensure that you are presenting your authentic, congruent, *facilitative* self to your client. Doing so will enable you to better focus on your client rather than yourself.

Understand. How will the client know that you understand what is being said? There are a variety of specific strategies that you can use to communicate your understanding. You can paraphrase what your client is saying and check your understanding by stating what your client means and asking for verification. You can also state, or "reflect," the feelings you hear the client expressing, or the feeling you sense under the surface. It also helps if you can nonverbally match your client's mood and the pace of his or her communication, and use words, phrases, and expressions that are similar to the client's.

Validate. What can you do in order to convey your willingness to validate the client? There are a number of simple behaviors you can use to communicate that you support and respect the client. For instance, you may offer minimal encouragers ("um-hmm," "I see," and "yes, go on"), nodding affirmatively now and then as your client speaks. Counselors also should refrain from conveying skepticism, doubt, or the desire to debate with the client. Of course, you do not ask questions which may indicate that you are repudiating your client's presentation of his or her experiences, or behave in any way that suggests you are devaluing the person. Instead, by validating, you are indicating, in every way you can, your openness and willingness to believe what the client is telling you.

This simple use of the LUV triangle serves to establish a relationship and a condition in which the client will feel that you are someone who cares and can be trusted. It is most important that you approach the client in this manner from the beginning. However, when you experience your client resisting the work as your relationship progresses, you will find that returning to the LUV triangle will serve to reestablish your working relationship.

The Contract

After you've used the LUV triangle to connect with your client and see that your client is responding to your willingness to help, you can begin establishing a contract for your work together. This contract is based on what your client wants from counseling. However, this will not always be clear at the beginning. Moursund and Kenny (2002) stated that it is not unusual for clients to be unsure about what has brought them for counseling. Some may begin counseling by presenting a problem that's safe, instead of the issue about which they feel shame and embarrassment; "only later, when you have passed the test of trustworthiness, will they dare reveal what they are really concerned about" (p. 22).

A contract is an agreement between two people in which each promises to perform in some way that the other person finds acceptable. As a counselor, you are promising to perform a service for the client in return for the client's collaboration. The client promises to cooperate in return for your continued work. The contract ultimately is based on the client's goals for counseling. As the client's goals become clearer, the contract may be renegotiated. The important thing is that both parties must agree. For example, if the client wishes to establish a contract that you will work to change someone who is not in the room, you cannot accept. On the other hand, you may think that your client needs to work on anger, but the client does not agree. In either case, you have no contract.

Contracting for well-formed goals is an ongoing process. Much of the time, when asked what they want from counseling, clients will say that they want something in their life, or in themselves, to go away. Examples of this might be, "I want my husband to quit controlling my life," or "I wish I wasn't

doormat with other people." You will find that attempting to get a con-
⎯⎯or a goal that expresses the presence of something—rather than the absence of something—is more workable (De Jong & Berg, 1998). For example,
alternative goal statements to the above might be, "I would like to have a better relationship with my husband," or "I would like to get better at saying 'no'
to people." When the presence of something is the goal, you can more easily
gauge progress toward the goal.

In general, well-formed goals have the following aspects:

- They are the presence, rather than the absence, of something.

- They are based on something the client can do, rather than a hoped-for
  change in others' behavior.

- They are simple enough that they can be accomplished.

- They are stated in such a way as to be measurable by either an observable change in behavior or a scaled self-report. (For example, "I now feel
  I'm at a 3, and I would like to get to at least a 7.")

- They reflect work that is important to the client.

As your work with your client progresses, you may at times lose track of
whether you still have a contract. In many cases, new information is presented, the client's goals and motivations shift, and the focus of sessions becomes less clear. At those times, you can remind the client of your original
agreement and ask whether their initial goals have changed. This way, you
remain on course.

An Internal Focus

After establishing a contract for your work together, one of the primary tasks
of the counselor is to encourage the client to assume an attitude of self-
examination. This process involves helping clients gain the skills to look
within themselves and to explore the inner world of thoughts, emotions,
fantasies, and conflicts. You may have been drawn to the counseling profession because you are interested in self-exploration and thrive in a process of
continual reflection. You have likely spent considerable amounts of time
wondering about your motivations and desires, perhaps experimenting with
your own processes of personal change. However, the search to uncover and
understand internal drives is not universal. You may not appreciate just how
difficult looking inward can be for some clients.

One reason this inward-looking process can be so difficult is that clients are
often responding to events that are inflicted upon them. Poverty, oppression,
racism, lack of access to resources, lack of education, and isolation are real and
mighty factors that can genuinely disrupt your clients' lives. Furthermore, some
people find self-exploration inconsistent with their traditions and upbringing.

Often, these clients do not initially or voluntarily seek counseling. They may, however, come to counseling feeling they have no other options.

When clients are dealing with environmental or external concerns that seem out of control, you can help them cultivate self-reflective awareness. By exploring themselves in counseling, clients can discover their personal strengths and resources. As we hear clients give voice to their experiences of disenfranchisement and marginality, we can help them reconnect with their own worth and appreciate their own potential. One particular technique you can use to help clients maintain an internal focus is to emphasize the *immediacy* of their self-experience.

Immediacy

Real life happens in the present. The past has already gone. The future has not yet happened. It is precisely the present moment in which people feel their feelings, make their decisions, and experience their existence. For this reason, it is essential for you to work in the "here and now" with your clients (Yalom, 2002).

Clients do not resolve their problems merely by exploring the past, gaining insights into the source of their problems, or acquiring new skills. Clients change by experiencing something new in their encounter with you in the counseling relationship. First, they practice on you, and then they try their new behaviors with other relationships and in other situations in the real world "out there."

Working in the here and now means that you help clients focus on what is happening within themselves as they relate to you. You can facilitate this awareness of what is happening in the present moment by using *process comments*. Process comments are observations that make explicit what is happening in the interaction between you and your client. Working in the process reveals the obvious in a way that other social relationships forbid. For instance, you would not ordinarily observe out loud to someone at a party that although she is smiling and putting on a brave face, this didn't seem to fit with the experience she is communicating at that moment. However, in counseling, you might share with a client, "Judging by the scowl on your face, you seem to be angry at my suggestion that maybe you are disappointed with your father, as well as your boss." With another client, you may say, "Every time you talk about your daughter, your words seem to convey a sense of shame." Such observations are not considered good manners in social situations.

In counseling, therefore, the normal social conventions do not apply—in fact, they tend to get in the way. As a beginning counselor, you may find yourself struggling with this difference between the kind of communication that takes place in social vs. counseling situations. You probably have been well socialized to not be "rude," "intrusive," or "impolite." But when you are engaged in *actively* listening to your clients, this conversation is unlike any other available to the client. You actively listen by abandoning these social conventions and sticking to the client's expressions and experience. You temporarily "bracket" your own thoughts, feelings, and associations in order to make space for the client's. You use language that *mirrors* or *reflects* the client's expressions in such a way that the client feels truly heard and understood. Therefore, no topic is off-limits in counseling. As a facilitative counselor attempting to build a strong therapeutic relationship, you will use immediacy to acknowledge not only your client's socially acceptable feelings and thoughts—you'll also recognize and explore what the client may perceive to be unacceptable, disgusting, or forbidden.

More than anything, your active listening fosters the empathic climate that permits clients to focus their attention internally and feel a sense of safety and trust. When you use process comments to facilitate clients' self-expression, they become more aware of their own immediate internal and relational processes. Carl Rogers (1969) observed that when people feel truly heard and understood, they become more aware of what is happening within themselves.

Promoting Self-Awareness

As clients learn to develop or maintain an internal focus, they can become ready to actively explore their thoughts, feelings, and actions, connecting their "inner world" with their presenting concerns. Even those clients who are actively resistant to self-reflection can be encouraged to explore how their thoughts and feelings affect their daily functioning. However, making a major change in our lives is challenging, even when we're highly motivated. Helping clients change requires counselor interventions that move beyond actively listening.

Your immediacy invites your client to look inward. But when attending to the inner world becomes confusing, painful, or anxiety producing, your client sometimes looks to you to help make sense of experience in a new way. Interventions like *interpretation* and *confrontation* aim at intentionally disrupting old patterns. These interventions operate by addressing aspects of client self-experience that are denied, disowned, repressed, or in some way not fully realized or available to the client.

Interpretation, or Sharing Hypotheses

An interpretation goes beyond simply calling attention to the client's behavior. When you interpret, you provide your hypothesis for what might be happening. For instance, the counselor may say, "I heard you say that you are really sad about losing your job, but I sense that you are also angry at your boss for giving you a negative evaluation. It seems difficult for you to express that side of your feelings." Such interpretations emerge from what is currently happening as you help to expand the client's awareness.

As you come to better understand your client, you begin to form a better picture of habitual patterns, conflicts, and needs. You gradually grasp the repetitive nature of the client's difficulties and begin to understand how the client may have become stuck in these problems. As this picture of the client's inner world becomes more elaborated, you may choose to share your specific impressions. This sharing may take the form of helping the client make sense of experience in a new way. It may involve offering an alternate version of the client's story or narrative, one that includes your impressions and experience of the client *in the relationship itself.*

Sigmund Freud (in Gay, 1989) considered interpretation to be *the* intervention that produces therapeutic change. Contemporary methods of counseling expand the use of interpretation to bring to light ways in which the client habitually structures his or her experience. In this sense, interpretation may be used to further understand how the client's values, attitudes, assumptions, and thought processes shape his or her world. Interpretation is no longer assumed to only address "repressed" material, but is used to help the client take a different view of his or her own meaning making and cognitive architecture.

As we said earlier regarding schemas, each of us structures our world by principles that we believe reflect an external reality. These values, assumptions, and beliefs are not ordinarily the focus of our awareness. Your task is to help the client make these organizing frames of reference more available to the client's deliberate scrutiny. Interpretations serve as alternate hypotheses to the client's normal ways of making sense of themselves, others, and their world. Hamlet's famous line that "nothing is good or bad but that thinking makes it so," captures something of the subjective nature of self-experience. Interpretation is one of your most potent tools for helping clients to look within and to build the capacity for greater self-awareness, a central goal of all counseling.

Confrontation

Another intervention that helps promote client self-awareness is confrontation. For the client, confrontation is often experienced as surprising and therefore initially disconcerting. When you confront the client, you call attention to discrepant or distorted aspects of the person's story or self-experience. For instance, a counselor might say to the client, "You said earlier that you really resented your sister for all the attention she demands, and then you just explained how you offered to throw her a party. I'm wondering how those two things go together." This type of confrontation calls attention to a discrepancy in the client's telling of the story.

At another time, a counselor may observe, "You are describing how awful and emotional it has been these first few weeks after the divorce, but as you talk about it with me you seem unemotional, describing it as if it happened to someone else." This type of confrontation points out an incongruity between what the client is saying and the nonverbal accompaniment to the statement. Confrontation can help clients get in touch with ambivalent or conflicted feelings and thoughts and become more aware of unacknowledged parts of their inner world. Confrontations can create an opportunity for new and alternate ways of being to take hold in the client's repertoire. If a client *always* feels soothed, and is never anxious or upset in counseling, then deep therapeutic change is probably not occurring.

As a beginning counselor, you may be reluctant to use interpretation and confrontation. Perhaps you believe that confronting a client is punishment or criticism. But confrontation does not imply a lack of empathy. In fact, confronting a client can show a depth of understanding and resonance that the client experiences as highly confirming. The client feels that you really *see* the entire person—not just the superficial persona. Furthermore, if interpretations and confrontations are performed lovingly, the client gets the feeling that you are willing to accept all aspects of his or her inner life, even those the client despises. Interpretations and confrontations, though they may be difficult for the client, are another expression of your empathy.

Another reason that you may be reluctant to interpret or confront is that you do not wish to upset or distress your clients. Not only might a client not like or approve of you, but you may want to see yourself as supportive and easing the client's suffering, not increasing the pain. Your own anxiety is aroused if you feel responsible for the client's unwelcome thoughts or distress. If you are struggling with these issues, you need to take a close look at *yourself,* and wonder how you may be inhibiting the client's full range of emotions. The truth is that the self-knowledge and productive change clients discover in counseling is often hard won and emotionally painful. Both you and your client must be up to the task.

At this point we should remind you that no intervention will be successful if the counseling relationship itself is not marked by your respect for and understanding of the client. Your use of immediacy, your sharing of hypotheses or interpretations, and your confrontations will be meaningless to a client who does not trust you. It may be tempting to rely on techniques to convince ourselves that we are "doing something" in our sessions. We may even feel we're showing our clients the light! What counselors do best, however, is to help clients see their own light. Successful counseling, counseling in which

EXPERIENTIAL LEARNING

Find an agreeable fellow counselor-in-training who will serve as a client for you. Ask the person to talk about something that is of persistent concern in that person's life. As you notice discrepancies, distortions, or incongruities in the telling of the story, call attention to these. Notice how you feel at those moments when you are confronting. Any reluctance on your part to be honest with your client means that you have issues that might get in the way of your development as a counselor.

1. What issues may contribute to your reluctance?

2. How will you work on these issues?

clients are genuinely changed, rests on a collaborative, trusting connection between counselor and client.

Knowing When to Stop

In a very real sense, bringing counseling to a successful end begins with the first session. The question "How do you know when to stop?" can only be answered when you and your client have kept in mind the original purpose of your being together. If you have established a reasonably articulated contract and revisited it from time to time, then it should be clear to both of you when you have sufficiently achieved the client's goals. Approximating the goal brings with it the signal that termination is imminent. The Cheshire Cat's advice to Alice when she visited Wonderland was, "Keep going till you get there . . . then stop." Good advice.

Of course, stopping your work with a client should not be an abrupt event. Obviously, both of you have been aware from the beginning that a time will come when your sessions together will end. Despite this knowledge, you must prepare for termination. Nobody, including an experienced counselor, is really good at goodbyes. Saying goodbye in counseling leaves both people with ambivalent feelings. Goodyear (1981) stated that termination is a "loss experience" in which people can relive their prior goodbyes, but also an "index of success." According to Boyer and Hoffman (1993), at termination the counselor is likely to feel pride and regret at the same time.

One way we have found that helps us to determine when the appropriate time for termination is approaching is to scale the client's concerns. Early on in your relationship you can ask, "On a scale of 1 to 10, with 1 being that this problem is the worst it has ever been, and 10 being that it has completely vanished, where are you right now?" After the client has given you a number, you then can ask (presumptively), "When our work together has been enough of a success to let you know that you can carry on without coming here, what will your number be then?" Whatever number the client gives you will be the measure of when you are nearing termination. As you begin to suspect that the ending time is coming near, you can say, "I remember that you said when you got to a (the number previously named by the client), that you felt you could carry on without me. Where are you now?"

This method helps to make concrete the progress that has been made during the counseling sessions, as well as indicate to the client that the concerns of living are never completely solved . . . nobody gets to a 10 in life. Further, if the number that the client currently reports is lower than the desired number, you can ask, "How much more work do you think we will have to do in order for you to arrive at your 'taking it on your own' number?" By responding to this question, your client is predicting success by a certain point in time. This prediction can then become a self-fulfilling prophecy and a predicted end point.

Teyber (2000) suggested that when clients report that they are consistently feeling better and are responding more adaptively to conflict situations, they are indicating they have worked through many of their concerns. They have rehearsed new behaviors with you so that they can now operate more independently. In addition, when the client can respond to you "in new, more direct, egalitarian, and reality-based ways that do not enact their old interpersonal coping styles or maladaptive relational patterns" (Teyber, 2000, p. 296), this is a good indication that termination is near. Also, when clients report that others are giving them positive feedback on their behavior or their perceived attitude or mood, this is a clue that the old repetitive patterns that got them into interpersonal difficulty have eased or been altered.

Avoiding Client or Counselor Flight

Research suggests that the modal number of sessions for any type of therapy is one (Talmon, 1990). Clients very often fail to return for the second session. When they do return for multiple sessions, still they tend to expect that they will not be in counseling for a long period of time. Lambert, Shapiro, and Bergin (1986) stated that 75 percent of the clients who benefit from therapy do so within the first six months, and that the major positive impact of therapy takes place in the first six to eight sessions. Garfield (1978) concluded that in both private practice and community mental health centers, the average duration of therapy was five to eight sessions, regardless of the theoretical orientation of the therapist.

Because short-term counseling tends to be the norm, the community counselor might want to think of each session as if it were the only one, staying fully engaged with the client. Such an attitude not only promotes a sense of "happening" in each meeting, but also, paradoxically, makes it more likely that the client will return for the next session. The short-term nature of most community agency counseling makes it especially important that the counselor keep an eye on the initial goals that were set with the client and on the emerging goals that crystallize out of the developing therapeutic dialogue. When all you have is eight or ten sessions, you must make each one count. Some agencies allow for longer-term work with clients, but when brief approaches are the norm due to agency requirements and resources, the imperative to terminate may come too soon for both client and therapist.

In the medical model, termination comes only after a cure has been achieved. At such a point, the patient is dismissed. This model of ending psychotherapy casts the therapist as the surgeon who excises malignant issues from the client's consciousness. If the client seeks help after termination, either the therapy has been a failure or the person has a new illness. There's also a possibility that the individual may have experienced a "flight into health," a rather sudden—but false—experience of improvement, which may have caused the premature termination of therapy in the first place.

The conventional wisdom suggests that when such a flight into health occurs, the counselor should persuade the client that the time is not yet right to end the therapy. In fact, some therapists would predict doom for these clients, leaving the impression that there was a ticking bomb in their psyche that would eventually bring them back to therapy (Presbury, Echterling, & McKee, 2002). Conversely, counselors who do brief work expect to terminate with clients as soon as possible. When they suspect that their clients are experiencing a flight into health, they suggest that the treatment of choice is "Keep them flying." In this case, if counselors acknowledge their clients' progress, discuss the potential for relapse, and remind their clients of available resources, they can support the client's sense of self-efficacy and empowerment. To insist that every client's early termination is a flight into health that will be unproductive in the long term is to deny the client's autonomy and strength.

It is true, however, that sometimes counselor-client relationships end prematurely, before the client has achieved all that could be achieved. Sometimes this happens because the client is threatened by the process or misunderstands how the counseling relationship is to develop. For example, clients more than occasionally arrive believing that the counselor will quickly assess their concerns and give sage advice that will instantly alleviate their problems. After all, TV therapists such as Dr. Phil accomplish their work within one hour of programming by giving glib, entertaining, and "expert advice."

On the other hand, sudden client termination is a moment for you to take an introspective inventory to see what part you may have played in the client's failure to return. Sometimes counselors collude with clients to prematurely end their sessions. This often takes place out of the counselor's awareness. The counselor may experience discomfort with a particular client and feel that the client is "not ready for counseling," and so will subliminally suggest that the client not return. The counselor may experience a personality clash, a strong cultural difference, or a client concern that is overwhelming (Hackney & Cormier, 2001).

For example, if you suspect that a client might attempt suicide, has an issue that is beyond your competence, or is struggling with a condition such as borderline personality disorder, you may feel alarmed and incompetent. We all wish to avoid situations that make us feel inadequate. When you find yourself experiencing any of the above feelings, you should attempt to understand what is stressing you so that you do not communicate your reluctance to your client. All counselors occasionally have clients that they cannot work with or who would create such stress as to render the counselor ineffective. In such cases, a referral is indicated, but you should also accept such incidents as a "heads up" that you might have some personal issues that need work.

We also know that minorities are underrepresented in the counseling profession and that minority clients are more likely to terminate counseling after one session (Sue & Sue, 2003). Although there are many reasons why clients may come to one session and never return, you need to consider how competent you are to work with clients who are culturally different from yourself. How adept will you be at building and maintaining a therapeutic relationship with clients who are strikingly different from you? "Mei, Misunderstood" presents one student's experience with a counselor's multicultural incompetence.

Dealing with Client Reluctance to Terminate

Assuming that you and your client have worked well together and are nearing termination, you may find your client reluctant to end the relationship. On the one hand, termination is cause for celebration. After all, your client has successfully achieved the goals for counseling. However, because you and your client have developed an intimate and meaningful relationship, it may be difficult for both of you to let go. For your client, this may have been the first time that anyone has devoted unwavering attention to him or her. Feeling helped by you, your client may be unsure as to whether he or she can go it alone. In addition, your client could have feelings of abandonment or of being set adrift in a sea of trouble. Endings often can be ambiguous (Teyber, 2000), and you should anticipate and attempt to clarify this ambiguity. Finally, the client will often feel unfinished. He or she may believe that all concerns must be addressed and resolved before counseling can stop.

Sometimes clients feel angry or depressed when talk of termination becomes the focus. They may, however, keep silent because of their fear that

Mei, Misunderstood

Mei was a counseling graduate student who had moved to the U.S. from China. She decided to seek counseling at the university counseling center in order to address some of the personal issues that she suspected might interfere with her own counseling competence. She knew that her experience as a Chinese woman would affect how she related to her clients. When asked at intake about her presenting concern, Mei replied that she was interested in working on her adjustment to U.S. society.

At her first counseling session, her counselor met her with enthusiasm. "I'm so happy to meet you," the counselor said. "I see you're from China. One thing I know about immigration experiences is that they can be traumatic. Tell me about your stress reactions. I'm very familiar with PTSD and its treatment."

Mei stared at the counselor. Her immigration experience had included a long plane trip, a couple of in-flight movies, and some average airplane food. *What in the hell is she talking about?* Mei thought. *Does she think all Asian people are alike?* Mei felt embarrassed, angry, and yet vaguely sorry for the counselor. Mei completed the session and never returned.

In some ways, Mei was fortunate. She was not in distress. She was savvy and psychologically minded. She could write off her counselor's incompetence as the counselor's problem, not her own. Most of our clients, however, are going to be more in need of our assistance than Mei. They expect us to be able to understand them and help them.

Questions for Reflection

1. How might your assumptions about your clients help or hurt your initial work with them?

2. Do you think Mei's counselor could have repaired the therapeutic relationship with Mei? If so, how?

---

they are not being a "good client" and that you might be disappointed in them for having misgivings. They may believe you think they are stronger than they really are.

You can open a discussion of client reluctance by saying, "When people have accomplished the goals that they have set for themselves and it's time to stop counseling, even though they feel confident and able to carry on, they might also, at the same time, have some negative feelings about stopping. I wonder if there is any of that going on with you." With such a statement, you can validate these concerns and invite your client to openly address these issues (Presbury, Echterling, & McKee, 2002).

The depth of the relationship that you have established will likely determine how easy or difficult termination will be. A relatively impersonal "professional" relationship, such as when you work with an accountant or a real estate agent, is easy to terminate. A "therapeutic" relationship is deeper than this and implies that you and your client have experienced something together that others would not fully understand. This type of relationship is more difficult to give up, because it is very special. Beyond this, therapeutic relationships often bring transference (and perhaps countertransference) distortions into the work. At times, during your sessions, your client may regard you as a punitive or nurturing parent, a rejecting or beckoning lover, or a judgmental or accepting authority figure. You will have worked through these transferences and arrived at a more realistic relationship by the time for termination, but you and your client will have been through an arduous journey together, and ending it will be a significant event. Someone has said that during the process of a therapeutic relationship, first you are your clients' mother, then you are their father, then you are their friend, and then they are gone.

While termination is often difficult, it may not be the agonizing event that has been suggested in the psychoanalytic literature (Hackney & Cormier, 2001). Quintana (1993) reviewed results of several termination studies (Mann, 1973; Marx & Gelso, 1987; Quintana & Holahan, 1992; Ward, 1984) and found that most clients accept termination as the culmination of a process and an indication that they have achieved their goals. Quintana concluded that these studies "suggest that only a small minority of clients experience a psychological crisis over the end of therapy, and the crisis seems to focus on the disappointing level of client outcome rather than specifically on loss" (p. 427).

If, in your preparation for termination, you have helped the client consolidate his or her gains and bring personal resources into awareness, the client should feel reasonably confident and ready to end counseling. But remember that termination may be an awkward experience for both you and your client and should be prepared for throughout the counseling relationship.

COMMUNITY COUNSELORS AS FLEXIBLE PRACTITIONERS

The community counselor working in an agency is like a jack-of-all-trades, and he or she must be flexible in the mode of intervention. As mentioned, community agencies most often encourage relatively brief models. This is because resources are usually limited, client loads tend to be high, and the goals of counseling are to address specific problems that interfere with basic life functioning. However, sometimes clients may stay for longer periods if the agency allows and if resources permit. The counselor will need to learn to adjust the counseling relationship to reflect the limitations and possibilities available.

In addition to short and longer term types of intervention, the community counselor must also develop the necessary skills to respond to a crisis.

Community agencies offer crisis counseling in response to a wide variety of situations. Perhaps a natural disaster, a school shooting, a terrorist event, an automobile accident, or a fire generates the crisis. Community counselors often don't have the luxury of sitting in their offices and waiting for clients to come to them, but must go out to meet those in need where they are struggling with huge challenges. Again, the therapeutic relationship, that constant in providing effective interventions, must conform and adapt to the circumstances that characterize the life situation of any given client.

Another facet of community agency work tends to resemble the functions of social work. You will work with all levels of community systems as you provide outreach, referral, and case management services. Often the persons and families that rely on the community agency counselor are from the lower strata of the socioeconomic scale. These clients often need help with basic life needs before they can engage in the kind of therapeutic work that would give them a greater quality of life and more success in interpersonal relationships. If you recall Abraham Maslow's hierarchy of needs, the most basic needs for proper food, clothing, and shelter must be met before the person can progress to pursuing higher level needs such as self-actualization.

As a community counselor, you will advocate for your clients, connecting them with important social services and resources to meet their fundamental requirements before any real counseling can happen. The story is told of a young Jesuit missionary who enthusiastically traveled to his new territory. Despite his eloquent speeches, he could not achieve a single convert, even though he poetically promised the fruits of earth and heaven would come to any who would believe. Finally one of the village elders approached him and began to tell him stories. The old man spoke for hours, well past the young missionary's lunchtime. Finally, when his aching stomach took precedence over his desire to be polite, the missionary said, "I'm interested in what you have to say but I must eat before I can pay attention." The village elder looked him in the eye and said, "Yes, we are also interested in the fruits of earth and heaven when we listen to you. Could we likewise start with the fruits of earth first?"

Community counselors also work with clients who are mandated by an outside institution to receive services. Court-ordered clients may present with issues involving truancy, child custody or neglect, sexual deviance, spousal abuse, violence against property, substance abuse, or any of a wide range of problems that have resulted in legal trouble. These clients often do not want to meet with a counselor. They are forced to attend a certain number of sessions to satisfy court requirements, and they show up feeling resentful and resistant to any help the counselor wishes to provide. These mandated clients are some of the most difficult the community agency counselor will face, and they frequently present with issues that the counselor finds unsavory or repugnant. Sometimes creating a supportive and therapeutic relationship will be a challenge for both client and counselor as the counselor works to resolve strong reactions to the client's behaviors. However, as we have said often, the sustained empathy of the counselor may evoke a desire in even very resistant clients to participate in a real therapeutic relationship. Indeed, because the strong resistance of some clients represents a history of injuries, disappointments, and traumas, this resistance is often the best proof that the client needs what the counselor has to offer.

The community counselor, then, must be flexible and skilled in many different types of interventions and services. And if the preceding were not enough to convince you, you should know that the counselor will also find that working with managed care, documenting and exchanging information, and handling the "logistics" of cases will draw on another skill set that is entirely different from your empathic and analytic abilities. Did we mention that to work effectively as a community counselor it helps to have super powers?

ETHICAL AND LEGAL ISSUES IN PRACTICE

Profound, therapeutic relationships rest on the counselor's vigilance in working ethically and legally. As we've said, the counseling relationship is unique; its force is powerful and transformative. The only way to ensure that the power of the relationship is used productively is for counselors to constantly safeguard their clients' rights. Thus, dual relationships, especially those that are exploitive, are always a concern in professional practice. In addition, the fundamental needs to protect client confidentiality and respect clients' dignity and worth must be ongoing facets of the counseling relationship.

From a legal standpoint, the same issues apply. Counselors who misuse their client's trust, fail to keep their promises, or harm their clients are at risk for being charged with malpractice. Furthermore, there remains for many laypeople, and in fact for many counselors, a sense of mystery regarding the counseling process. Therefore, counselors who abuse their clients' trust project a negative, confusing, and potentially very damaging message to the public. We can all be tainted and negatively affected by the unethical and illegal practice of a few practitioners.

We rely on our legislators and policymakers to protect our practice rights, so any time we breach our own professional obligations and ignore regulations and laws that affect our practice, we undermine our own profession. Our encouragement is that as you delve deeper into the mysteries and potential of therapeutic relationships you always be cognizant of the very pragmatic ethical and legal boundaries around your practice.

CONCLUDING THOUGHTS

This chapter has provided an overview of the counseling process. You will undoubtedly co-create this process many times, and in many ways, with your clients. We encourage you to take advantage of your training experience to fully explore your beliefs about how counseling works and how counselors function. Identify and clarify your theoretical leanings. Begin or renew your own counseling. And, when given the opportunity to observe a counseling session or work as a counselor, take it! Practice will answer many of your questions and help you address many of your concerns.

RECOMMENDED RESOURCES

Several texts have been written on counseling skills and the counseling relationship. We recommend the following:

Egan, G. (2002). *The skilled helper* (5th ed.). Pacific Grove, CA: Brooks/Cole.

Gerber, S. K. (2003). *Responsive therapy: A systematic approach to counseling skills*. Boston: Houghton Mifflin.

Moursund, J., & Kenny, M. (2002). *The process of counseling and therapy* (4th ed.). Upper Saddle River, NJ: Prentice Hall.

Teyber, E. (2000). *Interpersonal process in psychotherapy: A relational approach* (4th ed.). Pacific Grove, CA: Brooks/Cole.

Other Resources

The Gift of Therapy by Irvin Yalom is a wonderful gift to give yourself. Yalom openly acknowledges the mistakes he has made, the lessons he has learned, and the joys that he has experienced over his long career as a therapist.

Most of the movies that portray the process of counseling and therapy are dreadfully inaccurate even if they are entertaining. *Analyze This, Tin Cup,* and *What About Bob?* are several examples. However, there are many excellent movies that focus on the rich and complex process of becoming more authentic and real in relationships. For example, *Amelie,* a delightful movie directed by Jean-Pierre Jeunet, is a whimsical reflection on the mysterious ways that people encounter and affect one another. Another powerful example is *Dead Man Walking,* in which a dedicated nun's relationship to a man on death row displays many parallels to counseling.

REFERENCES

Bateson, G. (1980). *Mind and nature: A necessary unity.* New York: Bantam.

Bowen, M. (1978). *Family therapy in clinical practice.* New York: Aronson.

Boyer, S. P., & Hoffman, M. A. (1993). Counselor affective reactions to termination: Impact of counselor loss history and perceived client sensitivity to
loss. *Journal of Counseling Psychology, 40,* 271–277.

Brunner, J. (1990). *Acts of meaning.* Boston: Harvard University Press.

De Jong, P., & Berg, I. K. (1998). *Interviewing for solutions.* Pacific Grove, CA:
Brooks/Cole.

Egan, G. (2002). *The skilled helper* (5th ed.). Pacific Grove, CA: Brooks/Cole.

Garfield, S. L. (1978). Research on client variables in psychotherapy. In S. L.
Garfield & A. E. Bergin (Eds.), *Handbook of psychotherapy and behavior
change* (2nd ed.) (pp. 190–228). New York: Wiley.

Gay, P. (Ed.). (1989). *The Freud reader.* New York: Norton.

Gerber, S. K. (2003). *Responsive therapy: A systematic approach to counseling
skills.* Boston: Houghton Mifflin.

Goodyear, R. L. (1981). Termination as a loss experience for the counselor.
Personnel and Guidance Journal, 59, 347–350.

Hackney, H. L., & Cormier, L. S. (2001). *The professional counselor: A process
guide to helping.* Boston: Allyn & Bacon.

Janoff-Bulman, R. (1992). *Shattered assumptions: Towards a new psychology
of trauma.* New York: Free Press.

Kohut, H. (1971). *The analysis of self.* New York: International Universities Press.

Kohut, H. (1977). *The restoration of self.* New York: International Universities
Press.

Kolbenschlag, M. (1988). *Lost in the Land of Oz: The search for identity and
community in American life.* San Francisco: Harper & Row.

Lambert, M. J., Shapiro, D. A., & Bergin, A. E. (1986). The effectiveness of
psychotherapy. In S. L. Garfield & A. E. Bergin (Eds.), *Handbook
of psychotherapy and behavior change* (3rd ed.) (pp. 157–211).
New York: Wiley.

Mann, J. (1973). *Time-limited psychotherapy.* Cambridge, MA: Harvard University Press.

Marx, J. A., & Gelso, C. J. (1987). Termination of individual counseling in a university counseling center. *Journal of Counseling Psychology, 34,* 3–9.

Maslow, A. H. (1968). *Toward a science of being* (2nd ed.). Princeton, NJ:
D. Van Nostrand.

May, R. (1979). *Psychology and the human dilemma.* New York: W. W. Norton.

Moursund, J., & Kenny, M. C. (2002). *The process of counseling and therapy*
(4th ed.). Upper Saddle River, NJ: Prentice Hall.

Piaget, J. (1951). *The child's conception of the world.* New York: Humanities
Press.

Presbury, J. H., Echterling, L. G., & McKee, J. E. (2002). *Ideas and tools for brief counseling*. Upper Saddle River, NJ: Merrill/Prentice Hall.

Quintana, S. M. (1993). Expanded and updated conceptualization of termination: Implications for short-term individual psychotherapy. *Professional Psychology, 24,* 426–432.

Quintana, S. M., & Holahan, W. (1992). Termination in short-term counseling: Comparison of successful and unsuccessful cases. *Journal of Counseling Psychology, 39,* 299–305.

Rogers, C. R. (1969). *Freedom to learn.* Columbus, OH: Merrill.

Shapiro, S. (1995). *Talking with patients: A self psychological view of creative intuition and analytic discipline.* New Jersey: Jason Aronson.

Stolorow, R., & Atwood, G. (1984). *Structures of subjectivity: Explorations in psychoanalytic phenomenology.* New Jersey: Analytic Press.

Stolorow, R., & Atwood, G. (1992). *Contexts of being: The intersubjective foundations of psychological life.* New Jersey: Analytic Press.

Sue, D. W., & Sue, D. (2003). *Counseling the culturally different: Theory and practice* (4th ed.). New York: Wiley.

Talmon, M. (1990). *Single session therapy.* San Francisco: Jossey-Bass.

Teyber, E. (2000). *Interpersonal process in psychotherapy: A relational approach* (4th ed.). Pacific Grove, CA: Brooks/Cole.

Wampold, B. E. (2001). *The great psychotherapy debate: Models, methods, and findings.* Mahwah, NJ: Erlbaum.

Ward, D. E. (1984). Termination of individual counseling: Concepts and strategies. *Journal of Counseling and Development, 63,* 21–25.

Winnicott, D. (1965). *The maturational process and the facilitative environment.* New York: International Universities Press.

Yalom, I. D. (2002). *The gift of therapy.* New York: Harper Collins.

Chapter 6

Conceptualizing Clients: Individual Assessment

The secret of knowledge is knowing the names of things.

Confucius

The data we learned *about* the patient may have been accurate and well worth learning. But the point, rather, is that the grasping of the being of the other person occurs on a different level from our knowledge of the specific thing about him.

Rollo May

GOALS

Reading and exploring the ideas in this chapter will help you:

- Understand the basics of using tests in counseling
- Integrate assessment material into client conceptualization
- Assess and respond to suicidal clients
- Understand ethical issues associated with assessment in counseling

---

OVERVIEW

This chapter presents information on basic concepts of individual assessment, including evaluation of varied client populations. Any time you are in contact with other people, you are continually assessing their moment-to-moment behavior and predicting what will happen next in your interaction with them. Since behaviors are all we can ever observe (we cannot see mental processes), we must then interpret these behaviors in order to imagine what is going on in people's minds. In a very real sense, we are all "mind-readers"

(Baron-Cohen, 1996). The minds of others exist in our own minds; the minds we are "reading" are works of fiction that we ourselves have authored. Our map of their mental territory is never the territory itself.

Now that we have offered this disclaimer, we will proceed to suggest ways in which you might be able to more accurately approximate the processes and structures of other minds. As you attempt to make sense of other people in counseling settings, you will always be making maps and using these maps to understand how your clients have strayed from their desired destinations and how you might help them back on the path to fulfillment in their lives. Your mapmaking tools will consist of (1) clinical interviews in which you note certain client behaviors that seem to indicate their unique style and their problem areas; (2) client self-reports in which they reveal to you their version of their inner-workings and their relationships; (3) standardized assessment instruments that place the client in certain categories relative to others; (4) reports from third parties (family, friends, physicians, courts, etc.) as to the person's behaviors; and (5) your own life experience and acquired knowledge of how people work.

LORI'S DEFINING MOMENT: Alicia's Story, True or False?

Lori is a seasoned community counselor. She has worked in community agencies for seven years and now has supervising as well as counseling responsibilities. She is adept at formal and informal assessment procedures, and her caseload usually includes several referrals for assessment-related services. When she first started working, however, Lori found even the most informal type of assessment to be daunting. Her recollections of a particularly challenging moment are below.

"Initially I felt very prepared for my first job as a community agency counselor. I had done well in school and taken advantage of numerous opportunities in practicum and internship to work with a fairly diverse caseload. The first week of my new job, though, I was reeling. I had what felt like way too many clients and way too little supervision. I faced my biggest hurdle when I met for the first time with Alicia. Alicia was twenty-four years old. She had been placed in foster care when she was three and had moved around the country for several years. Now she lived in a homeless shelter, had a two-year-old daughter, and had recently been arrested for possessing methamphetamine and for neglecting her child. She had been encouraged to seek counseling by her court-appointed attorney.

"I knew a little about Alicia's story before I first met with her, so I was ready to face a challenge. I wondered if she would be belligerent, angry, or simply unwilling to talk. I wondered about the child neglect charge and, if it was true, whether it was related to her drug usage or to additional pathology. I started organizing in my mind the questions I would ask and the potential direction I would take toward assessing her motivation for change.

"When Alicia came in, I was surprised to find that she was quiet, deferential, and respectful. She appeared fatigued and confused. After I introduced myself, Alicia began sobbing, saying she didn't understand the charges against her, she was confused about the child neglect charge, and she felt like killing herself. She said she had a learning disability and wondered if she had signed papers she shouldn't have signed. Her depression and hopelessness seemed acute, so I was very concerned about her suicide threat. I began to feel increasingly anxious, wondering if Alicia's charges had been in error. Could she have been a victim of a series of misunderstandings? I continued to listen to and question Alicia, with a growing sense that she had been wronged by 'the system.' She stated that the drugs in her bag weren't hers. She suspected they were put in her bag by an acquaintance. She insisted that she had never understood the child neglect charges. 'I've always been stupid,' she said, 'I know that. But that doesn't mean they can threaten to lock me up and take away my kid.'

"When the session ended I quickly found my supervisor. After filling him in on my impression of Alicia's story, he was quite dismayed with my assessment of this client. He sincerely believed that Alicia had pretended to be not only innocent, but also ignorant, in order to convince me that she had been falsely accused. He said she was setting me up to testify on her behalf in court, and if nothing else, to help her get prescription drugs that she could either use herself or sell. I felt like an idiot, but I also felt incredibly unprepared for this work."

Questions for Reflection

1. If you were Alicia's counselor, what issues would you want to address first in your assessment of her?

2. How would you determine whether or not Alicia was telling the truth?

3. How might Alicia's background, including her level of intelligence and/or lack of adequate education influence her, your diagnosis, and your work with her?

MAKING SENSE OF ASSESSMENT IN COMMUNITY COUNSELING

How will you begin the work of mapping other people's minds? Assessments vary in type and kind depending on what information is being sought about the client. The purpose of an assessment is to gain detailed information, usually through some structured interview or testing protocol, so that the counselor can provide effective interventions that are relevant and specific to the client's concerns (Whiston, 2000). The goal and techniques of assessment vary according to the client's initial presentation. In general, though, information gained through assessment allows the counselor to begin to develop a core understanding of the client's issues, measure the scope and severity of a client's concerns, develop a relevant treatment plan, and focus on the client's capabilities (Young, 2001).

One assessment method that you may employ is a structured intake interview, perhaps with the goal of making a diagnosis of the client's problems. Other assessment devices can specifically target concerns regarding the client's intellectual functioning, achievement, personality, or aptitude. Often clients come to community agencies in crisis, and an assessment must attempt to gauge a client's suicidal potential or propensity to harm another. In some instances, you may be part of a larger team, perhaps involving schools or legal systems, which is involved in helping the client. Specific assessments can help structure these collaborative efforts and provide information on which to base important decisions (Young, 2001).

Assessment is also a type of intervention. By involving the client in decision making during the assessment process, counselors can help clients explore their own understanding of their concerns. The mere act of focusing on one aspect of a client's experience, such as emphasizing the client's depression or substance abuse, invites the client into dialogue regarding her or his opinion of the severity of and prognosis for the concern. Further, such conversations invite clients to share their opinions about critical topics such as: How does this problem (concern, issue) affect them on a daily basis? How does the client define improvement or a lessening of the problem? What does the client think regarding the etiology of the problem? What does the client want to know about his or her problem? What does the client want from counseling in general? These assessment-oriented questions, and others like them, can empower the client to feel immediately involved in the progress of his or her own counseling.

Before You Begin to Assess

Client assessment is an ongoing process. In order to be most effective, this process requires the counselor to be systematic and thoughtful in her approach. The process of clinical decision making is best informed by a comprehensive approach to assessment, which includes several steps (Hood & Johnson, 2002).

1. Figure out exactly what you hope to accomplish in the assessment, and be sure to involve the client in making these determinations.

2. Plan to use multiple methods of assessment. One test, or a basic mental status exam, is likely to be insufficient to adequately inform diagnosis and treatment plans, especially if the client has overlapping concerns.

3. Consider the unique experience and context of the client when choosing assessment techniques. Which particular assessment or test will be appropriate for this client, given her background, culture, and educational level? Are the clinical issues presented by the client complicated by, or perhaps caused by, environmental factors such as poverty? If so, the purpose of the assessment may shift from one based on exploring pathology to an approach designed to measure and build upon resilience.

4. Maintain a tentative approach in assessment (Hood & Johnson, 2002), seeking to emphasize clients' strengths while realizing that no assessment process is perfect.

5. Share information with the client about the assessment process to ensure that the client is given as much agency as possible in her own treatment.

We realize that many counselors prefer the one-on-one diagnostic interview to the use of standardized assessment instruments, and we present aspects of that part of the conceptualization process in this chapter. We begin, though, with a discussion of testing as a formal assessment procedure in order to ensure that we do not understate the importance of these types of interventions in community counseling.

TESTING AS ASSESSMENT: THE CRITICAL DIMENSION

Community counselors often display great ambivalence regarding the use of tests in their work with clients. We counselors deal with the most intangible aspect of human beings—their mental life. Since mental life has no weight, length, height, or other measurable aspects, some people claim that attempting to measure such things as intelligence, interest, ability, and personality is a useless project. But E. L. Thorndike, one of the pioneers of mental testing, stated early on that if something exists at all, then it exists in some amount

(Aiken, 1988). It follows that if something exists in some amount, it can be measured. When working with a client like Alicia, for example, the counselor is likely to find that she or he must use a diagnostic procedure that includes not only an intake interview with mental status exam but formal assessment procedures as well. Simply talking with Alicia is unlikely to provide sufficient information for the counselor to create a thorough, accurate conceptualization of her.

Tests are everywhere. Open the Sunday supplement to your newspaper, and you might find tests that claim to measure whether you have a good marriage, if you are truly happy, or how much sex appeal you possess. You may also find that the homepage of your Internet service provider will occasionally offer a test for you to take in order to determine your intelligence or an inventory you can self-administer to seek a compatible mate. And, of course, you have been tested on your achievement in school for many years. Since you are a "test-wise" person, your intuition should tell you that most of these popular tests are bogus, meaningless, and ill-constructed. Part of your job as a counselor and a user of tests is to be able to recognize useful, informative, well-normed, and well-constructed tests when you see them. To that end, we will offer you a crash course in measurement theory. This minicourse will be enhanced when you take courses in Psychometrics and Assessment, Research Methods, and Statistics during your training program.

As a community counselor, your role will entail conducting assessments and interpreting appraisals of individuals. Psychological and educational test data can provide objective and reliable information to help you make choices in counseling, vocational guidance, selection, diagnosis, classification, placement, and screening. You need to know assessment principles and practices in order to be successful in a profession in which you will make many crucial decisions about people based on test score results.

In assessing an individual or a group, you start with a *construct,* a particular type of concept used to explain behavior. Since constructs are abstract notions—intelligence is one example—you need to operationally define them by looking at specific *variables,* measuring these variables, and then drawing conclusions based on some established criteria. To be able to assess a variable, you *measure* it by relying on some agreed upon rule set for assigning numbers or values to quantify the existence of some level of the attribute. For example, if you consider the ability to solve a math problem a variable involved in intelligence, you might decide that the speed at which people come up with the answer to a math problem is an intelligence variable. In other words, the amount of time people will need to solve the problem will *vary* depending on how intelligent they are. Smarter people take less time, while people who are less intelligent require more time. Time, then, becomes the *measure* of intelligence in this case.

Reliability and Validity

You may be unconvinced that speed of problem solving is a measure of intelligence, and perhaps your skepticism is warranted. We would have to establish the *validity* of such a measure before accepting it, but prior to this step, we would need to know that our testing procedure is *reliable*. Reliability refers to the test's consistency and stability. That is, all other things being equal and constant, if you took multiple measures of a variable with a test, would you always get the same result? We might check our reliability by giving people the same math problem, or a similar one, two weeks later and comparing their times from the first to the second administration. But what if everyone we were measuring took vastly different times to solve the problem during our test-retest trials? In other words, their results seemed completely random. With this result, we might suspect that our measure is not reliable. No test is perfectly reliable. Reliability is usually expressed as a coefficient of correlation. For example, what is the numerical relationship of the first test administration to the second one? Doing the math, we might find that the correlation between these two testing sessions is .20, not reliable enough to go to the next level and check for validity.

On the other hand, say that we found our results to produce a *reliability coefficient* of .90. We could then say that our measure looks very reliable, but what are we actually measuring? This is the question of validity: Does the procedure measure what we think it measures? One path to answering this question might be to compare the speed of problem solving with some outside measure, say, each person's grade point average in college. If we found that there was a high correlation between the speed with which people solved our math problems and their GPA, and if GPA is correlated to intelligence, then we might begin to think that we have a valid measure. If in this case people who were slower on our problem-solving measure had GPAs that averaged around 1.8, and those who were fastest had GPAs approaching 4.0, we might conclude that we are actually measuring *intelligence*.

Different types of tests are used for different purposes; it is important that the test be valid for the judgment or inference we seek to make. For example, achievement tests measure one's performance on a sample of questions intended to represent a certain subject matter. With such tests, *content validity*—demonstrated by showing how well the items on the test sample the greater class or subject matter—is especially important. A mathematics test, for example, should not include test items asking you to conjugate verbs. An item about the Battle of Hastings in 1066 would not be part of the proper content for a test of your achievement in a music theory class.

Some tests are used to predict an individual's future standing or performance, or to estimate an individual's present standing on one construct based on his or her performance on a related construct. The GREs that you took to get into graduate school are an example of this use of tests. What is important with these types of tests is their *criterion-related validity,* which is demonstrated by comparing the test scores with one or more measures of the criterion. We have found that students in counseling programs vary to a great degree as to the scores they achieved on the GRE. Getting extremely high scores on this test does not seem to predict one's success in such training. In fact, there seems to be a curvilinear relationship between GRE scores and good counselors. Very low GREs seem to predict lack of counseling ability and lower grades in graduate school, but very high GREs sometimes also predict a lower achievement of counseling skills than those people who score somewhere in the middle range. What this appears to suggest is that there are criteria that are more important than GRE scores in predicting counseling success and that whatever is being measured by GREs may be more predictive of success in other academic fields.

Finally, some tests are used to infer the degree to which an individual possesses some trait or quality that is assumed to be reflected in the test performance. Intelligence tests are prime examples of this, as are many personality tests. Here, we are especially interested in *construct validity.* Let's say you have a measure of state anxiety. For your test to have construct validity, we would expect scores to increase in situations designed to provoke anxiety and decrease in more calming, relaxing situations. Thus, the test performs according to the theory of the construct. Also, a test that has good construct validity would be expected to relate highly with other measures of the same construct. For example, an individual's performance on a new intelligence test should relate positively to his or her performance on other established intelligence tests. For example, someone who scores in the moderate mentally retarded range on the Wechsler Adult Intelligence Scale would be expected to score in the same range on the Stanford-Binet Intelligence Scale.

Standard Error

Now, let's go back to the idea of reliability and talk some about test scores. A psychological test is a standard procedure designed to obtain a sample of behavior from a specified set of measurable behaviors. The information provided by tests, in contrast to natural observation, is unique in that it is explicit, quantitative, and reproducible (Nunnally, 1978). But as we have pointed out, assessment is not an exact science. There is error involved. Thus, for all the reasons discussed previously regarding reliability, one's performance on a particular test may vary from administration to administration.

All of this variation is known as the *standard error of measurement.* Needless to say, some instruments, by their nature, lend themselves better to

EXPERIENTIAL LEARNING

Try this experiment. On a blackboard or a large sheet of paper, carefully draw a line 45.25 inches long. Now, have ten other individuals use a yardstick and measure the line to the nearest quarter inch. Record all the answers. Did they all get exactly 45.25 inches? You probably have results varying around it, such as 45 or 45.5 inches.

achieving higher levels of reliability. For example, thermometers and watches are much more reliable instruments than measures of intelligence, depression, and self-esteem. As you are looking at the manual of a standardized test, you will usually find the standard error reported as a number. For example, if you see that the standard error on the Wechsler scales of intelligence is 5, this means that if you administered the test to an individual a thousand times (which would be tedious indeed), there is a roughly 68 percent likelihood that their true score on the test could vary 5 points on either side of the score he or she achieved on the single administration (Anastasi & Urbina, 1997). The 68 percent likelihood is derived from the fact that in a normal curve 68 percent of the data should be within one standard deviation of the mean. (We discuss this in more detail in the next section.) Thus, an obtained score of 100 might come up as 95 or 105 next time they were administered the test. (Things can get more complicated than this, but for the sake of conveying the concept of standard error, this addresses the basic idea.)

We are primarily concerned with two basic types of errors in psychological measurement: *systematic* or constant error and *random* error. Systematic error occurs when there is a known bias in the test. For example, a test of intelligence whose items are representative of only one culture would be systematically biased against individuals from other cultures. Great care is taken in test construction to avoid systematic bias, but it is still something for you to investigate before making decisions regarding the assessment of your client. Before you use any assessment instrument, you should ensure that it is appropriate for use with your particular client's age, reading level, preferred language, and culture.

More common are the random errors. The more reliable the test, i.e., the higher the coefficient of reliability, the less likely there is to be random error. Sources of error may be subject-related (the person had a bad cold that day), situation-related (the room in which the test was taken had poor lighting or was too hot), or test-related (there are some built-in problems with the test). Fortunately, we usually have a very good estimate of E, the error. For groups, the estimate is the reliability coefficient and, for individuals, the estimate is the *standard error of measurement*. Theoretically, if one were to take the same test, say the GRE, over and over again, one would amass a distribution of scores that would approximate a normal curve with the true score (T) as the mean and variation of other scores around this mean reflective of the standard error of measurement. That is, the higher the reliability, the lower the standard error of measurement; and the tighter the grouping of scores around the mean, considered to be the true score.

Standard Deviation and Normal Distribution

Consider the case of George. George was in his first semester in college. He had been an "A" student all through high school, and much was expected of him. Having taken his first exam and receiving his score, George sent his mother an e-mail telling her that he had gotten a 75 on this exam. His mother was appalled! Everyone knows that a 75 is not a very good score, or is it? George wrote back and said that while there were 100 items on the test and he only got 75 of them correct, there were also 100 students in the class, scores ranged from 45 to 75, and he had received the highest score of anyone in the class.

So, what do we know about George's performance on the test? First of all, we know that the professor may not have constructed a very good test, since the level of difficulty was too great. But aside from that, how do we make sense of a score of 75, or 65, or 55 under such circumstances? One way would be to take all the achieved scores, add them together, and divide by 100 (the number of students in the class). We would then know the *mean* score and we could go on from there to determine the *standard deviation* (SD) of the achieved scores. The SD would give us information as to how the scores were distributed. Students often call this procedure "curving" the results. While we suspect that George's score is a very good one, we could learn more from this procedure about the way in which scores were arrayed, making our interpretation more meaningful. For example, if 99 students achieved a score of 75 on the test, and only one got a 45, George's score is less impressive. On the other hand, if the scores were normally distributed, George achieved an outstanding score, provided the instructor considers this to be a norm-referenced test, meaning that test-takers' scores are compared against each other. We provide more information on norm versus criterion-referenced tests below.

Statisticians assume that a bell-shaped distribution is a natural phenomenon. For example, if you line up a group of men according to their height, you will find that there will be many more of them whose height ranges from 5 feet 9 inches to 6 feet one inch than there will be those who stand 5 feet 4 inches or 6 feet 10 inches tall. If you have a large enough group, it is likely that if you arrange the men by height, they will form that bell-shaped pattern in their height range. So it is with scores on intelligence tests. Approximately 68 percent of all people will score between 85 and 115 on the Wechsler scales, while only 14 percent will score between 70 and 84, and another 14 percent will score between 116 and 130. The remaining 4 percent will be equally divided between those who score below 69 or above 131. This is what is called a *normal distribution*.

There are two major ways to interpret scores from tests. The first, *criterion-referenced,* requires that an individual's performance on the test be compared to some previously established standard of performance. An example would be requiring a mastery level of 70 percent on an assessment of math skills—either the individual meets the criterion or not; and the individual's performance is only interpreted in relation to this criterion, not the performance of others. You may encounter this type of situation when you take a counselor licensure or certification exam. If George's test (above) was a criterion-referenced one, and a 70 percent mastery level was expected, he passed, but we might not consider his performance to be excellent. If, on the other hand, his test was *norm-referenced* based on the one hundred students who took the exam, and the distribution of scores was a bell curve, George did very well. He will need to explain this to his mother.

This second type of interpretation of test scores is based on that normal distribution curve. Most psychological tests employ a *norm-referenced* approach to interpret an individual's score by comparing it to how others have performed on the test. On published tests, normative groups are determined prior to standardization of a test to reflect the population for which the test may be appropriately used. Thus, an adult measure of personality should include a normative group reflective of the current adult population—covering variables such as gender, age, race, geographic location, socioeconomic status, and cultural/ethnic backgrounds. You would not expect to find teenagers in this normative group given the purpose of the test. The performance of this normative sample constitutes the *norms* for the particular test. These norms depict "average" performance of the normative group. Some of the more commonly used methods for expressing norm-referenced scores include percentiles, standard scores, and transformed standard scores.

Percentiles indicate the percentage of individuals in the normative group who are at or below a particular score. Thus, if you scored at the 50th percentile on a test, this would mean that 50 percent of the people in the norm group have scores equal to, or less than, your score.

Standard scores and *transformed standard scores* express the relative position of a score in a distribution in terms of standard deviation units from the mean. In other words, standard scores provide a way to look at your individual score in relation to the mean, or average score, of the norm group,

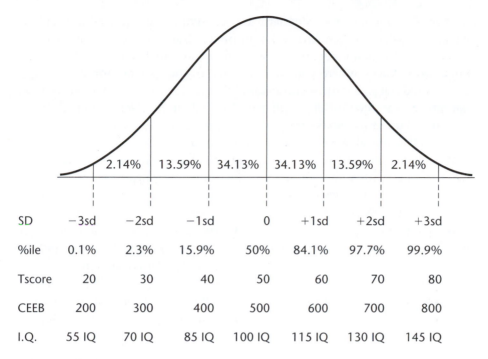

SD	−3sd	−2sd	−1sd	0	+1sd	+2sd	+3sd
%ile	0.1%	2.3%	15.9%	50%	84.1%	97.7%	99.9%
Tscore	20	30	40	50	60	70	80
CEEB	200	300	400	500	600	700	800
I.Q.	55 IQ	70 IQ	85 IQ	100 IQ	115 IQ	130 IQ	145 IQ

SD = Standard Deviation
%ile = Percentile Scores
Tscore = Standard Score (MMPI)
CEEB = College Entrance Exam Scores (SAT)
I.Q. = Derived Intelligence Quotient Scores (Wechsler and Stanford-Binet)

Figure 6.1   Normal Distribution Curve

taking into consideration a standard way of measuring the distance from your score to the mean (i.e., the standard deviation). This is useful in making comparisons for an individual across multiple standardized measures.

Above, in Figure 6.1, we have constructed a graphic of a normal distribution curve showing standard deviation, percentiles, T scores, College Entrance Examination Board (CEEB) scores, and derived I.Q. scores. First of all, notice that approximately 68 percent of the distribution falls between −1 and +1 standard deviation. This is the "normal range." The farther away the scores are from the mean (50th percentile), the less frequently they will show up. In other words, many more people would be expected to achieve an I.Q. score of 100, than to score 130 or 70. If you could imagine the curve of the normal distribution as people standing on each other's shoulders according to the scores they achieved on a given test, then you have the idea of how the general population is represented by this graphic.

For convenience, most standardized test scores are reported in numbers that are based on the standard deviation, but are transformed to be more easily understood. As mentioned, if you were to obtain an I.Q. score of 130, you immediately know where you stand relative to the general population. Your score would put you at the second standard deviation (+) and that would mean that only 2.14 percent of all people who have taken the test scored higher.

Various other methods for reporting standard scores are used by test publishers. While not all are included in our graphic, the most popular ones are represented. Many test results are expressed as percentiles, but it is usually easier to deal with a specific number for reporting purposes. For example, many tests have methods for converting "raw scores" to T scores. As you can see, a T score of 50 is at the mean, and the scores either ascend or descend by 10 points with each standard deviation. Likewise, the College Entrance Examination Board reports results in hundreds, with 500 being at the mean, and the scores increasing or deceasing by 100 with each standard deviation. You probably remember your SAT examination. If, for example, you had a combined score on the two parts of the exam of 1000, then your score was precisely at the mean. On the other hand, if you scored a 1200, you were at the first standard deviation plus, and approximately at the 84th percentile.

Making Sense of Test Results

We hope these measurement fundamentals will prove helpful to you as you consider using psychological tests and interpreting their results. You will want to make sure the test you plan to use is reliable and valid for the use intended. It is also essential that the norm group for a standardized test be well defined and relevant for the interpretations that are to be made. Likewise, when interpreting an individual's score on a psychological or educational test, you will want to be cognizant of any systematic or random error contributing to this particular score and make your decisions accordingly.

Thorndike (1982) noted that the test score does not yield conclusions, but only provides raw material that must be processed through the judgment and insight of skilled professionals before it can be used in making decisions. Tests should be but one source of data in making decisions that affect an individual's life. You will need to use multiple sources of information and multiple variables from each of the data sources as you attempt to create a map of your client's functioning (Posavac & Carey, 2003). In essence, you will combine the "objective" data of the test and blend it with your refined clinical impressions. You will then have attained a more holistic picture of your client's functioning.

Psychological tests tend to be obtrusive measures of a variable because the process of observation and measurement lets the client know what is

EXPERIENTIAL LEARNING

Imagine that you have been given the task of completing a comprehensive assessment of an eight-year-old boy referred to counseling because of "anger management issues." Develop a plan for providing a detailed and holistic assessment of this boy's functioning.

1. What, specifically, would you want to know about him?

2. How will you find this information?

3. Would you use an assessment instrument? If so, how might you go about finding an appropriate test?

4. Share your plan with your peers.

happening; it potentially interferes with the natural process of behaving (Webb et al., 1971). Thus, you are encouraged to also employ non-reactive or unobtrusive measures, those procedures that minimize the possibility that the client will be reacting to the measure itself. For example, a survey of individuals regarding their level of alcohol use will give you one—probably biased—perspective on their behavior, but actual observations within a confined territory, say a university campus, may yield still other data. Tests (including surveys) can often yield valuable information that will assist you in helping your clients function better. It is important to remember, however, that even the best instruments have limited utility. Only when you combine test results with clinical observations, along with the establishment of a genuine helping relationship, can you expect to gain information that approaches the client's true pattern of behavior and the operations of his or her inner life. Tests have their place. So long as your goal is helping, there should be no reason for you to avoid their use.

Types of Tests

As indicated above, tests come in two major categories: standardized and non-standardized. If a test is standardized, this means that the norm group has been established prior to publication of the test. Most published tests with which you are familiar will be standardized and will be accompanied by a test manual that explains the populations on which the test was normed. Non-standardized tests can include structured observations, behavioral assessment, or questionnaires designed to elicit specific information from clients. One strength of a non-standardized approach is that it is flexible and can be tailored to specific clients and specific situations. You could, for example, construct a questionnaire for a specific population or for addressing the unique questions you wanted to have answered. At the time of this writing, elementary and middle school students in some parts of the country are wearing variously colored plastic "sex-bracelets." Each color is said to indicate the type of sex practice the child is interested in. You could construct a questionnaire asking about the relationship of wearing a bracelet of a certain color to the child's actual sexual experiences. If well-constructed, and anonymously responded to, your non-standardized instrument might yield useful information. (On the Internet, go to **www.google.com** and type in "sex bracelets.") Or, if the sex bracelet topic is not your area of interest, you might create a rating sheet that described the "off-task" behaviors of a third-grader in the classroom, including frequency and duration. This record could be used as a baseline measure for assessing aspects of the child's psychological and academic situation prior to working to improve the child's on-task time.

Standardized tests have the advantage of containing information on reliability and validity, the specific groups for which they are intended, and an objective scoring method for yielding results. What follows is a list of general categories of standardized tests.

Ability Tests

These include tests of *achievement*, or the measure of what people have learned; or they can be tests of *aptitude*, meaning that they purport to assess general cognitive ability, special talent, or multiple abilities. One example of a test of special ability is the Torrance Test of Creative Thinking, which assesses people's thought processes in the areas of originality, fluency, flexibility, and elaboration. All of these areas, which are distinct from the more convergent types of thinking measured by I.Q. tests, are thought to promote creative ideas.

Personality Tests

These can include the so-called objective instruments, such as the MMPI-II or the 16 PF, or they can include projective instruments such as the Rorschach or the House-Tree-Person technique. The Rorschach is the test that asks people to say what they see in ten ambiguous ink-blots that are presented to them. While there have been attempts to devise objective scoring techniques for the Rorschach, we once heard it said that it takes three to four years to get good at administering and recording a Rorschach, and a lifetime to get good at interpreting one. It is unlikely that you will want to spend that much time learning this test, but you should become familiar with the general ideas involved in its interpretation.

Interest Inventories

Over 3,000,000 interest inventories are administered each year as an adjunct to career counseling (Neukrug, 2003). The main idea of an interest inventory is that the client's responses are correlated with those of people in various areas of work who are satisfied with their career choice. Some of the most popular are the Strong Vocational Interest Inventory and the Self-Directed Search (SDS). Also in popular use is the Kuder Occupational Interest Survey. The Kuder is a forced-choice format in which respondents are asked to choose which of a group of three items is most appealing. The results place someone's preferences within ten broad interest areas: "Outdoor, Mechanical, Computational, Scientific, Persuasive, Artistic, Literary, Musical, Social Science, and Clerical" (Anastasi & Urbina, 1997, p. 398). As a counselor in training, you would probably be more likely to score higher in Social Science, Persuasive, or Artistic, than in Mechanical, Computational, or Clerical.

Intelligence Tests

These tests are, of course, meant to assess ability (as above), but they usually are predicated on the assumption that they are tapping some innate ability that is not influenced by culture or education. This assumption has been extremely controversial and the subject of legal battles and social criticism. For example, in the early part of the twentieth century, immigrants coming from Europe were administered the Stanford Binet intelligence test in order to keep "morons" from entering the country and threatening the gene pool of the United States (Schultz & Schultz, 2000). Of course, these people were culturally different and did not possess great facility with English. Even though translators were used in the testing, the testing found that most of the immigrants were "mentally defective . . . 87 percent of Russians, 83 percent of Jews, 80 percent of Hungarians, and 79 percent of Italians—were feeble-minded, with a mental age of 12" (p. 216). Obviously, there was something wrong with the testing procedure! Obtained scores on similar instruments have also victimized other cultural groups. Black and Hispanic students have sometimes been placed in special education classrooms because of low scores on intelligence tests that were actually the result of culturally bias in the test. Although many attempts have been made to create "culturally fair" intelligence tests, these efforts appear to have fallen short.

Miscellaneous Tests

Go to the library and ask to see the *Buros Mental Measurement Yearbook* or *Tests in Print,* and you will likely be amazed at how thick these books are and how many tests currently exist in publication. Just about every dimension of human behavior (musical talent, religiosity, depression, all areas of education) has been targeted for evaluation by some test publisher. You will also find information on tests in professional journals, in textbooks on assessment, and in the catalogs of test publishers. It is unlikely that you could name an area for which a test does not already exist.

Tests Most Frequently Used in Clinical Settings

In the 1970s, mental health agencies and hospitals throughout the United States were surveyed as to which categories of tests were most frequently used in their evaluations of clients and patients (Aiken, 1988). Personality tests were the most frequently used, followed by "vocations" tests, miscellaneous tests, and intelligence and scholastic aptitude tests. Later, the *American Psychologist* published a listing of specific instruments employed in clinical settings during five decades of testing (Lubin, Larsen, & Matarazzo, 1984). The Wechsler Adult Intelligence Scale, Minnesota Multiphasic Personality Inventory (MMPI), Bender Visual Motor Gestalt Test, and the Rorschach Inkblot Test were the first four listed. Of the complete list of thirty tests, ten were tests of general intelligence, nine were tests of personality, five were tests of specific abilities, three were interest inventories, two were tests of developmental level, and one was a test of language ability.

You can see from these listings that you would be wise to familiarize yourself with the specific instruments in popular use today and at least become a sophisticated consumer of test information, if not a skilled administrator and interpreter of such instruments. The reality is that you will find yourself feeling comfortable using some tests, while others will seem less relevant to your practice and your clients. Either way, general standards of effective practice would suggest that you stay aware of tests available to you, including revisions to existing tests, and that you be prepared to defend your use of, or failure to use, a specific assessment instrument.

CLINICAL JUDGMENT: THE STRUCTURED DIAGNOSTIC INTERVIEW

One of the most commonly employed assessment techniques of the community counselor is the *structured diagnostic interview,* or "Intake." The purpose of this interview is to gather information about the nature and severity of the client's presenting concerns so that appropriate interventions can be formulated. This meeting often represents a person's first contact with a counselor and thus is very important for confirming to the client that he or she has made the right decision to seek help.

As community counselors we must keep in mind that many people who have never before had contact with a mental health professional feel significant ambivalence about seeking help for their troubles. For the new client, showing up for the first session may represent the result of a long, painful, or frightening process of deciding whether or not to seek assistance. The client's anxiety may involve the fear of facing the emotional pain of current life events or old injuries. The client may also harbor unrealistic and unpleasant expectations of being criticized, misunderstood, or punished. These expectations usually derive from a history of problems in interpersonal relationships, and you must be alert to how they might show up in the first meeting. For example, a person who has often been criticized or ridiculed by others will be reluctant to give a forthright picture of himself or herself in the first meeting with you. Or the client may be court-ordered to receive counseling. In that case, the client will likely feel resentful and perhaps angry about meeting with you. Conversely, the new client may imagine that you will be perfectly nurturing, understanding, able to rectify problems immediately, and leap tall buildings in a single bound. In such situations, you must be attuned to the expectations and unconscious wishes or fantasies of the client so that the new relationship can get off to a good start.

Goals of the Structured Diagnostic Interview

Though there are multiple goals to the structured interview, the three most essential things to remember as you meet your new client are: (1) Establish Rapport, (2) Establish Rapport, and (3) Establish Rapport! Even though your goal is to gather information about the client and his or her concerns, this goal does not negate the necessity of providing a warm and empathic receptivity to the client. The last thing you want your client to feel is that he or she is being psychologically x-rayed and treated as a "patient" rather than a person. The relationship between counselor and client is the most important aspect in counseling. All the information in the world is useless if your client does not come back for a second meeting!

Presenting Concerns

Establishing rapport can best be achieved by helping the client explain the nature of his or her distress and reasons for seeking help—his or her *presenting concerns*. You must maintain an empathic and receptive demeanor, remembering to use the "LUV Triangle" as mentioned in Chapter 5, in which you *listen* to, *understand* and *Validate* the client's situation and concerns (Presbury, Echterling, & McKee, 2002). In short, the goal is to help clients to tell their "story" and to feel as if you have understood the story. As the client unfolds the tale, you must also remember to use your observational skills in this process, taking in the client's verbal and nonverbal communications, physical appearance, manner of speech and posture. Even the client's manner of speaking on the phone, behavior in the waiting room, or manner of dress can provide useful information. The client's attitude toward you as the counselor is also very important, because often the factors that contribute to the individual's distress also get in the way of the client's ability to engage in a potentially helpful therapy relationship.

Responding to Crisis

Most often, as the client's story unfolds, you will be able to get a thorough picture of the client's concerns and then formulate an appropriate response. However, among mental health professionals, community counselors are often the ones "in the trenches," the first responders, and therefore must be prepared to assess and respond to any immediate crisis. Suicidal potential and the possibility that the client intends to harm another person are obviously two problems that will take precedence over completion of the usual intake procedures. In the first case you may need to arrange for immediate hospitalization; in the second you need to alert the authorities. Likewise, information regarding any child or elder abuse will alter the normal course of the interview as the counselor follows up with the client regarding details and explains that it is the counselor's responsibility to report the abuse. Such cases of abuse must be reported to your supervisor and to the proper authorities, such as Child Protective Services agencies, within the time frame specified by your state—usually in less than seventy-two hours. An actively psychotic person will also need special treatment. If the client cannot be stabilized during the interview and cannot safely transport himself or herself to the hospital, it may be necessary for you to arrange an emergency hospitalization. Clients who are acutely decompensated, chronically unstable, or who have serious substance abuse problems may not be appropriate candidates for help in many community agencies.

Gathering Information

While the client is telling his or her story, you will artfully ask certain questions designed to gather additional and relevant information. The client's motivation to tell his or her story in response to your communication of empathy is what propels the initial session forward. At the same time, you must also have one ear attuned to parts of the story that flesh out the clinical picture. If the client does not spontaneously mention something you need to know, you can weave the question into the dialogue in a way that does not feel jarring to the client. You could, of course, just go down a list of questions and request answers from the client, but such a method does little to cement the relationship, and usually the data gathered are without nuance.

In order to place the client's problems in full context, you will want to know about the historical onset of the problems and the person's history and life circumstances. Factoring in cultural dissimilarities, including the potential presence of factors such as societal oppression, racism, or heterosexism is critical at this stage of the assessment process. Also important are the client's historical and present relationships, employment, and whether the client has experienced any recent or identifiable trauma that gave rise to the problem. Other background information such as possible substance abuse, physical health concerns, previous therapy, or involvement with the legal system is also vital.

You should keep in mind that the structured interview need not be overly rigid in how it is conducted. Discretion, clinical judgment, and sensitivity to presenting issues will all influence the course of an interview. You must keep an ear open for the *most relevant* clinical information and structure the interview around these most important issues, rather than sticking doggedly to a protocol.

The Mental Status Exam

The Mental Status Exam (MSE) is commonly used by community counselors as a component of the structured diagnosis interview. The MSE is a tool for providing fairly comprehensive information about a client's level of functioning. Often considered an integral part of the intake interview, the MSE assesses appearance, attitude, activity, mood and affect, speech and language, thought processes, cognition, and insight and judgment (Polanski & Hinkle, 2000). The MSE is fairly straightforward and offers a framework for providing descriptive information about the client. During staffing meetings in some agencies, counselors will begin their discussions of their new clients by sharing a report of the MSE.

Although direct and clearly outlined, we have found that counselors feel more comfortable working with the MSE if they have practiced administering it in both a formal and informal manner. As with other aspects of the structured diagnostic interview, the most effective counselors are able to be spontaneous and use immediacy when administering the MSE. Acknowledging a client's discomfort or hesitation, for instance, can help establish rapport and build the therapeutic alliance. On the other hand, going through the questions in a rote manner, with your eyes glued to your clipboard and without conveying your own personality and style, is likely to limit your genuine understanding of the client's concerns and capabilities. The more comfort you gain with the MSE, the easier it will be for you to administer it in a manner best designed to meet the needs and presentation of your clients.

DSM-IV: Making a Diagnosis

One important aspect of the structured interview is the necessity, in many community agencies, of making an accurate diagnosis of the client's problems. During the course of your training as a counselor, you will become familiar with the Diagnostic and Statistical Manual of Mental Disorders-IV-Text Revision or DSM-IV-TR (APA, 2000). The DSM-IV-TR contains the criteria for the wide variety of mental disorders that you will encounter. Often, you will

EXPERIENTIAL LEARNING

If you haven't already done so, take time to pair up with a classmate and practice completing an intake interview that includes a Mental Status Exam. Your campus clinic or practicum site is likely to have a common intake form, so use that form for your practice. Tape your session or ask for observers, and practice until you become adept at balancing the question-asking aspect of assessment with your ability to maintain a focused, listening stance. Keep in mind that if you're writing the entire time you're with a client, all the client will see is the top of your head. That image is not usually conducive to building a solid therapeutic relationship.

find in gathering information that the client's difficulties have characteristics that fall within an identifiable overarching DSM-IV-TR diagnostic category such as a mood disorder, psychotic disorder or personality disorder. Each of these broad categories includes specific diagnoses such as Major Depressive Disorder, Schizophrenia, or Borderline Personality Disorder. Gathering detailed information in the structured interview will help you make a specific diagnosis that has important implications for the client. The DSM-IV-TR (2000) criteria for Major Depressive Disorder are presented on pages 197–198.

The diagnostic process is very important because, as with all forms of assessment, it helps to structure the kind of interventions that will follow. For instance, the diagnosis may be helpful in appropriately assigning the case to a counselor with a specialization in treating eating disorders or depression. The diagnosis may also be useful for making an external referral to a psychiatrist, nutritionist, drug rehab center, or other professional who will play an important supportive role in treatment. Most often the diagnosis will be used as a way of conceptualizing the client's problems as a kind of "shorthand" for communicating with other mental health professionals. Sometimes the diagnosis is needed for the simple, mundane, and discouraging reason that insurance companies demand a diagnosis for all claims for reimbursement. This issue has ethical implications for diagnosis that are addressed later in this chapter.

The DSM-IV-TR organizes diagnoses into seventeen categories, each of which contains objective criteria (Maxmen & Ward, 1995). The DSM-IV-TR uses a multiaxial diagnostic system, meaning that counselors assess five areas: clinical disorders (Axis I), personality disorders and mental retardation (Axis II), general medical conditions (Axis III), psychosocial and emotional problems (Axis IV), and global assessment of functioning (GAF; Axis IV) (APA, 2000).

Criteria for Major Depressive Episode

A. Five (or more) of the following symptoms have been present during the same 2-week period and represent a change from previous functioning; at least one of the symptoms is either (1) depressed mood or (2) loss of interest or pleasure.

Note: Do not include symptoms that are clearly due to a general medical condition, or mood-incongruent delusions or hallucinations.

1. Depressed mood most of the day, nearly every day, as indicated by either subjective report (e.g., feels sad or empty) or observation made by others (e.g., appears tearful)

   Note: In children and adolescents, can be irritable mood.

2. Markedly diminished interest or pleasure in all, or almost all, activities most of the day, nearly every day (as indicated by either subjective account or observation made by others)

3. Significant weight loss when not dieting or weight gain (e.g., a change of more than 5 percent of body weight in a month), or decrease or increase in appetite nearly every day

   Note: In children, consider failure to make expected weight gains.

4. Insomnia or hypersomnia nearly every day

5. Psychomotor agitation or retardation nearly every day (observable by others, not merely subjective feelings of restlessness or being slowed down)

6. Fatigue or loss of energy nearly every day

7. Feelings of worthlessness or excessive or inappropriate guilt (which may be delusional) nearly every day (not merely self-reproach or guilt about being sick)

8. Diminished ability to think or concentrate, or indecisiveness, nearly every day (either by subjective account or as observed by others)

9. Recurrent thoughts of death (not just fear of dying), recurrent suicidal ideation without a specific plan, or a suicide attempt or a specific plan for committing suicide

B. The symptoms do not meet criteria for a Mixed Episode.
C. The symptoms cause clinically significant distress or impairment in social, occupational, or other important areas of functioning.
D. The symptoms are not due to the direct physiological effects of a substance (e.g., a drug of abuse, a medication) or a general medical condition (e.g., hypothyroidism).

(continued)

(Criteria for Major Depressive Episode, continued)

E. The symptoms are not better accounted for by Bereavement, i.e., after the loss of a loved one, the symptoms persist for longer than 2 months or are characterized by marked functional impairment, morbid preoccupation with worthlessness, suicidal ideation, psychotic symptoms, or psychomotor retardation.
(DSM-IV-TR, p. 356)

The multiaxial system allows you to take a comprehensive view of the client while providing specific information about the client's current concerns. Through this process you can then begin to formulate diagnoses and develop treatment plans. The DSM-IV-TR is always a work in progress (the DSM-V is expected to be produced by 2006), so you are advised to remember that diagnosis is not necessarily a precise act. However, the DSM-IV-TR does provide a nosology that can be invaluable for the general assessment and conceptualization process.

As you learn the various criteria for different disorders in the DSM-IV-TR, you may find yourself having a negative reaction to the idea of assigning clients a diagnosis. A diagnosis is an impersonal, clinical label that seems to reduce the client to a number of discrete symptoms that have little to do with this *particular* client's life or circumstances. Your reaction would not be unusual. The diagnosis process of the DSM-IV-TR is very much a "medical model" orientation: You reduce identifiable symptoms into a pattern to make better sense of the client's difficulties. Those of us who are counselors, in our desire to preserve the essential humanity of those with whom we work, know that when we "break a person into parts," we are no longer addressing the experiencing being that is the person.

Another difficulty with the diagnostic process is that the criteria are categorical "either-or" sorts of measures. Either the client has some symptom or behavior or she doesn't. Needless to say, most living, breathing people's self-experience is on a continuum between various complex and subtle self-states. When you are diagnosing a client, the person must be made to fit the category. Perhaps you recall the story of Procrustes who invited unwary travelers into his home to stay the night. Those visitors who were too short for the bed he offered them were stretched to match its length, while those who were too long were chopped up to fit so that their feet wouldn't hang over. Sometimes the DSM-IV-TR categories seem like a "one size fits all" sort of Procrustean bed. Those persons who fall outside of the "normal" profile, such as minority, immigrant, or non-mainstream clients of any type, may be over- or under-diagnosed. For instance, in some subcultures of Latina women, it is not unusual for psychological or emotional distress to be described as physical symptoms. These women know that they are using body metaphors to describe emotional pain. Some counselors, however, may not understand these culturally specific meanings. Because the client presents with various and diffuse bodily symptoms and complaints for which there are no medical causes, a counselor may then diagnose the client with some form of somatization disorder, a diagnosis given to people whose tendency is to translate psychological distress into subjectively real bodily symptoms.

On the other hand, because some clients' problems do fall into identifiable patterns, it is useful to recognize when this occurs. For instance, one of the authors of this book had a client who had suffered with a bipolar disorder for many years. Because her difficulties had always been interpreted as "personality problems" she had never received any medication to treat the disorder. When she was properly diagnosed, referred to a psychiatrist for medication, and treated with a combination of psychopharmacology and counseling, her life improved dramatically.

The point is that counselors must find a way to balance the necessity of preserving the *person* of the client in the therapeutic relationship with recognizing and responding to symptoms that cohere into meaningful patterns. Bipolar disorder has a strong genetic loading and has come to be understood as primarily a biologically based disorder. Without proper diagnosis and intervention, clients may suffer needlessly, even when the counselor who is disinclined to make a particular diagnosis is well meaning.

You can begin to practice the process of making DSM diagnoses by looking in the table of contents of the DSM-IV-TR and locating the pages for the "decision trees." These decision trees show how to ask and answer certain questions that will rule in or out the possibility of some disorders. By following the "yes" or "no" decision points, you will become better able to more clearly understand the procedures for arriving at a particular diagnosis. We have found this exercise helpful to our counseling students as they navigate the complex route to diagnosis and treatment planning.

ASSESSING SUICIDE RISK

Talk of suicide often stimulates both strong feelings of responsibility and intense dread in a counselor. There are few situations that you will encounter with clients that will seem more urgent, ambiguous, and sobering. There is never a way to know for sure whether a client who is talking of suicide is seriously contemplating it. Furthermore, clients who actually attempt suicide sometimes offer only vague clues or hints that should, in fact, be read as an imminent threat. As a community counselor, you would be well advised to adopt

Case Study: Rob's Habit

On the surface Rob seemed to be a success. He was a twenty-seven-year-old warehouse manager for a successful trucking company. He made a decent income and lived in an attractive apartment. But despite appearances, he had a secret life. He had been in three serious relationships since he received his Associate's Degree at the local community college, but they had all ended unhappily. He was not currently seeing anyone, despite his parents nagging him to find a nice girl. He worked long hours and brought the company laptop home with him every night. He had an Internet addiction to games and gambling that probably began about the time he finished high school. The trucking company had its own internal network and he was plugged in every day, all day, from the moment he arrived in the morning until he left in the evening. Whenever possible, he would indulge in an illicit trip to cyberspace, especially when work got stressful or hectic.

None of his managers or supervisors ever said anything about those little indiscretions at first, but as the months went by those stolen moments increased. Finally, Rob was called on the carpet when things began to get out of control. He was shown a computer printout of all of the minutes he had engaged in this questionable activity. At first Rob thought he was going to be fired, but his manager happened to be the person who hired him. She had always been very supportive of Rob. He was given a stern lecture, then a serious suggestion about seeking help from a counselor. Later Rob felt depressed and anxious about not being able to play at work and tried to rationalize that it was the best thing anyway. Besides, he reasoned, he had plenty of time when he got home.

That very evening while surfing the 'net he discovered an organization called Massive Multiplayer Online Role-Playing Gamers, or MMORPG. The more he read about MMORPG, the more excited he became. That very night he signed up, paid the fee, received his password, and became a member of the multiplayer computer role-playing group that advertised itself as enabling thousands of players to play in an evolving virtual world at the same time over the Internet.

Soon, Rob found himself rushing home every evening to begin or continue another session of online fantasy gaming that had become the center of his being. It took him several months, but in the game Rob gained a position of prestige and power that his ordinary, dull existence could never rival. Rob sometimes became so involved in his character's steamy romances and extraordinary heroics that he forgot to eat, lost track of time, and, on more than one occasion, had to call in sick. Several other times he was late for work because he was exhausted from playing the game until late at night.

Rob's new world finally came crashing down one morning when he was asked to report directly to a senior

(continued)

(Case Study: Rob's Habit, continued)

supervisor. He had made some serious mistakes that could have cost the company money and client faith. He was saved once again by his favorite supervisor, but she was simultaneously being reprimanded for not reporting his "computer gaming addiction" earlier.

Questions for Reflection

1. Do you think Rob should be given another chance at work?

2. If yes, what should be the conditions of his probation?

3. If he were to show up at your agency for help, what diagnosis would you give him?

4. What treatment would you suggest for him?

5. Should there be a DSM classification for computer, Internet, or gaming addiction?

---

the attitude of "belief." In other words, if the client speaks of suicide, do not dismiss such talk as manipulative or merely a manifestation of a personality disorder. To do so would be to disconfirm the client's experience and communicate that you will only allow certain types of content to pass between you and the client. It is better to believe the client is seriously considering suicide and be wrong, than to ignore signs of suicidal risk and be wrong.

Being able to assess the risk of suicide in your clients will depend more on your refined clinical judgment than on any objective method. While so-called "objective" protocols exist for assessing suicide risk, still you must also trust your intuition when clients mention suicide. We know that accurately predicting suicide is impossible, but performing an adequate screening is well within your grasp.

Perhaps the first step toward improved comfort in dealing with suicidal clients is to rid yourself of myths concerning suicide. Laypeople will sometimes state the suicidal gestures are simply attention-getting devices. A suicide attempt may certainly be a cry for help, but it may also be a sincere attempt to end one's life. Either way, the person needs help. Some people fear that bringing up the topic of suicide with a person who appears depressed may cause that person to commit suicide. On the contrary, the process of talking about the depth of one's despair may actually be therapeutic. In fact, according to the American Association of Suicidology (2002), feelings of hopelessness are more suggestive of suicide risk than a diagnosis of depression alone. Feeling unheard and isolated is likely to contribute to the sense of hopelessness that a suicidal person may be experiencing. If you were to communicate tacitly to your client that you do not wish to talk about feelings of suicide, you may actually be contributing to the client's experience of isolation.

The American Association of Suicidology has compiled fact sheets that detail statistics and research findings regarding suicide in the United States. For instance, the majority of people who are suicidal exhibit warning signs and give clues as to their intention. Specific diagnoses have been identified as particularly at risk for suicide, including depression, schizophrenia, drug dependency, and, among adolescents, conduct disorders. Even with all this information, working with a potentially suicidal client will leave you feeling uncertain. It is demanding and exhausting work. You must learn all you can about suicide, but keep in mind that we simply cannot fully predict another person's future behavior.

So, how can you make a judgment regarding the probability of a suicide attempt by your client? Menninger (1973) once declared, "There is a little . . . suicide dwelling in everybody's heart" (p. 142). If you are honest, you can probably recall a time in your life when things got so overwhelming that you fleetingly thought that death might be better than the situation you were going through. Of course, for most of us, such notions remain ideas and do not result in action. But for some people, their suffering is so great that they begin to view death as a way out, an end to suffering, or the only obvious solution to their problems.

Remember that the risk of suicide is not an either/or condition. Shneidman (1999) stated that the probability that someone may take his or her own life is on a continuum, ranging from low, through moderate, to high levels of risk. However, the self-preservation instinct is profoundly deep and abiding (Echterling, Presbury, & McKee, 2005). As long as the client is talking to you, he or she probably feels some ambivalence about taking this drastic, final step. If you suspect that your client may be thinking about suicide, then you need to address this issue. Ignoring your suspicions and avoiding the issue can be disastrous.

However, addressing the issue does not mean that you should engage the person in a debate in an attempt to talk them out of this option. Saying things like, "But you don't realize just how fortunate you are" or "You have so much to live for" does not change someone's mind about suicide. Such statements only serve to invalidate the person's strong sense of discouragement and may sabotage your working alliance (DeJong & Berg, 2002). Clients who are feeling suicidal are also feeling that the only control they have over their situation is to escape the agony through death. When you debate with them, they may feel that you are trying to control them.

Using the skills that you are acquiring as a caring listener, you must explore the client's world and the extent to which the idea of leaving that world through death may seem attractive to him or her. One important thing you must learn is whether the client has a detailed plan in mind. Having a plan is an indication that the person has considered how to accomplish the suicide.

Consideration of the following factors may help you determine the level of threat:

- Does the plan seem vague and unrealistic, or is it well-organized and possible? The more detailed the plan, the more seriously you should take it.

- What is the method discussed by the client? The most lethal methods are jumping, hanging, and shooting. If the client has any of these in mind, death would be the likely outcome if such methods were used.

- Has the client experienced a recent major loss? Situations such as unwanted retirement or sudden job loss, major illness, intractable pain, or the loss of a loved one can be seen as risk factors.

- Has the client previously attempted suicide? People who have tried to kill themselves before are at higher risk because they have eliminated unsuccessful strategies and have desensitized themselves to performing such an act.

- Is the person unmarried, alone, isolated, or without much social support? The lack of meaningful contact with others is a risk factor.

- Does the person's history suggest a lack of self-control or impulsivity at times? Such behavior could contribute to a snap judgment to commit suicide.

- Does the person use drugs or alcohol to excess? Being "under the influence" lowers people's inhibitions.

- Do you consider the person as meeting the DSM-IV-TR criteria for a mental disorder? As indicated above, certain mental disorders increase the likelihood of suicide.

- Is the client a middle-aged (or older) male?

- Is the person a college student? These are statistically the higher-risk groups.

Taken together, the questions listed above can comprise a heuristic for assessing suicide risk in your clients. Though each of the above-mentioned factors is thought to contribute to the risk of suicide (Sommers-Flanagan & Sommers-Flanagan, 2002), this list is not exhaustive, nor does it take into consideration the unique factors associated with any individual's situation. We offer it as a reference aid when dealing with a client who may be suicidal.

But there is good news concerning suicide risk. The annual incidence of suicide in the United States is 11.2 per 100,000 (Moscicki, 1999). In other words, 99.989 percent of Americans demonstrate their will to survive by not committing suicide in any given year (Echterling, Presbury, & McKee, 2005).

Mood disorders are one of the demographic factors most highly related to suicide risk. In fact, people with mood disorders have been found to be eight times more likely to commit suicide—an incidence rate of about 90 per 100,000 each year. However, given that suicide is such a low frequency occurrence, this significantly higher suicide rate means that, in any given year, about 99.91 percent of people with mood disorders still do not kill themselves (Jacobs, Brewer, & Klein-Benheim, 1999). If this percentage seems too high, you may want to do the math yourself. It is vital that you recognize that the vast majority of people struggling with the serious challenges of a mood disorder are nevertheless resilient enough to choose life. Keep these statistics in mind when you are dealing with a client you consider to be suicidal. Otherwise, you may suffer the countertransference of despair and helplessness that is afflicting your client. In order to be truly helpful, you need to remain optimistic in such situations. Furthermore, in the general population, the ratio of attempts to completed suicides is at least ten to one (Hendin, 1995). In other words, even when people make a serious suicide attempt, the great majority of them survive.

Suicide: Assessment as Intervention

Many forms of assessment take place as the result of a referral. A physician, school official, court official, or other third party wishes to know something about a person, so they send the person to you. You perform your assessment and communicate your results to the referring agent by phone or written report. Suicide assessment is different from other forms of assessment, in that your assessment and your intervention will take place in the same session. Once you determine that the person you are assessing is at risk for suicide, you quickly move from assessor to helper in hopes of preventing the suicidal behavior. Echterling, Presbury, and McKee (2005) offered a model for working with someone in such a crisis. They called their model the BASICS. This acronym stands for Behavioral, Affective, Somatic, Interpersonal, Cognitive, and Spiritual factors involved in the client's experience leading to suicidal thoughts. As you consider intervening on the side of life, you may find it useful to follow this acronym.

Behavioral. What is the person doing that promotes or sabotages survivability? Instead of exploring options to resolve the situation positively, the person may be openly threatening suicide or merely hinting at the possibility. Once he or she directly or indirectly introduces the issue of suicide, you must accept this invitation to address this serious matter.

If the person openly threatens suicide by telling you, for example, "I'm considering killing myself," you can respond not only to the words, but to the action of honestly sharing this intention with you. By responding this way, you intervene by validating the pain and anguish beneath those words while seeking to affirm the client. You might say, "It takes a lot of courage to come in here and talk about this" (p. 154).

Instead of an overt threat, the person may bring up the issue of suicide by merely giving a vague hint. For example, after describing his or her difficulties and concerns, someone may say, "Oh well, at least I won't have to worry about these things much longer." In this case, your response can be to ask simply, "I'm not sure I understand. What do you mean that you 'won't have to worry about these things much longer'"? (p. 154).

When someone discusses the possibility of suicide, you need to explore how the person has handled crises in the past. As previously stated, people who have made earlier suicide attempts pose a greater risk of committing suicide. You should be direct in your questioning by simply asking, "Have you ever tried to hurt or kill yourself in the past?" If the answer is "yes," then you can ask how the person prevented himself or herself from going through with it at that time. This may give you clues as to what there is about life that the person values. You should also ask about the method that the person selected. Poisons or sleeping pills are slow-acting or less effective than more immediately lethal methods. As a result, the person had more opportunities for second thoughts or rescue. When asked about his or her survival, however, the client might simply say that someone else came upon the scene before death took place, disclaiming responsibility for choosing life. In this case, you can ask what has kept the client going since that incident. In yet other circumstances, the person may report telling someone or phoning a help center hot line before the poison or pills could do their work. In this case, the person acted to prevent his or her own death. You could then ask, "What came to your mind that told you that you wanted to live, and how did you get yourself to contact others for help?"

Affective. As previously stated, the person who is feeling overwhelmed by depression, overcome by hopelessness, or burdened by a powerful sense of guilt is at high risk for suicide. If you are sensing such bleak affective themes in the person's crisis story, then you should check for thoughts about suicide. You could say, for example, "When people are feeling as bad as you have been feeling, thoughts of suicide sometimes pass through their minds. What about you?"

Scaling can be an excellent way to assess someone's sense of hope. "On a scale of 1 to 10, with one being the least hopeful you've ever felt and ten being the most hopeful, where are you now?" If, for example, the client responds with a "3," you then can follow up with, "What would be different that would let you know that you are on your way to a 4?" Furthermore, you can capitalize on any number above a 1 that the client names. You could ask, "Wow, so you have been able to keep yourself from sliding down to a 1. How did you get yourself to do that?"

Somatic. Someone who recently has been struck by a seriously debilitating condition or life-threatening illness can pose a higher suicide risk. If the crisis event involves such an illness or condition, then you can invite the person to talk about survival potential. For example, you might say, "Now that you're dealing with this illness that threatens to end your life, how are you finding the will to continue on?"

Somatic concerns also include intoxication. Intoxication is a significant risk factor for suicide, particularly among young people (American Association of Suicidology, 2002; Fowler, Rich, & Young, 1986). Individuals who are intoxicated have impaired judgment and lowered impulse control. Combining these two conditions with suicidal thoughts can have deadly results. You can check your impressions with the person by saying, in a nonjudgmental tone of voice, "I'm having some trouble understanding what you're saying because your words seem to be slurred. Have you been drinking or taking anything?"

Interpersonal. The fewer significant people—lovers, relatives, or friends—in the person's life, the higher the suicide potential (Jacobs, Brewer, & Klein-Benheim, 1999). Further, if the person's support network has been recently struck by serious conflict or tragic loss, there is a greater potential for suicide. You can assess this factor by asking, "Who are the important people in your life?" Or you may inquire, "How are the important people in your life involved in this situation?"

While suicide clusters—the dramatic increase of suicides in a community— are rare in the United States, the experience of encountering, either directly or through the media, the suicide of a friend, peer, relative, or public figure increases the suicide risk of vulnerable young people (Moscicki, 1999). People in the media call this "copycat" suicide. The loss of someone with whom the client has become extremely identified, whether personally knowing this individual or not, sometimes produces despair and a sympathetic desire to end life.

One approach you can use to intervene is hypothetical-circular questioning. Such questions can explore the interpersonal dimension to the person's view of the world and help him or her to take a broader perspective of the situation. An example of a hypothetical question is, "When you get past this crisis and have handled this situation in a way that others notice, how will you be different? What will they say that they have seen in you that makes them feel better about your commitment to living?"

Cognitive. Occasional, vague, and fleeting episodes of suicidal ideation are not unusual during times of crisis. Nevertheless, it is essential that you assess risk and the will to survive whenever someone mentions thinking—no matter how briefly—about suicide.

If the client has a carefully worked out plan of when, where, and how to commit suicide, along with a highly lethal method, his or her survival potential plummets dramatically. If a client mentions the possibility of suicide, then you can immediately follow up by asking, "You said that you have considered killing yourself. How have you thought about doing that?" Notice that you do not use presumptive language here. In other words, you do not want to suggest that you fully expect the person to have developed a suicide plan. You do not, for example, ask, "How *will* you . . ." You reserve the use of presumptive language for exceptions to concerns and visions of survival. "What is happening at those times when you think that you'd rather live?" or "How will you be feeling once you get past this crisis and no longer wish to commit suicide?"

The person who thinks that there are alternatives to suicide for resolving a crisis has greater potential for surviving. In contrast, the individual posing a higher risk of suicide seems to be wearing cognitive blinders. Such a person will see the current negative situation as unchangeable or unendurable and may view escape through suicide as the only option. Even so, you can always count on the fact that a commitment to suicide is never absolute. You can suggest something like, "I get the feeling that while part of you wants to carry this out, another part of you is trying to figure out a way to live. What is that part saying to you?"

Spiritual. It is a particularly troubling sign of high risk if someone with strong religious or spiritual convictions expresses the belief that life no longer has any meaning, that his or her situation is irredeemable, or that life is not worth living. Someone who is feeling a profound sense of spiritual alienation may see suicide as the only salvation. If this theme is emerging in the crisis story, you can follow the strategy of acknowledging, normalizing, and checking. You might say, "After all that's just happened, it sounds like you're wondering if there's any point to life right now. What would need to be happening for you to begin feeling better about going on with your life?"

Sometimes, people in a spiritual crisis are feeling sinful or guilty for some real or imagined act on their part. They may see suicide as appropriate punishment for their infraction. You will want to know about their spiritual and religious beliefs. If they see themselves as belonging to a particular faith, you might ask, "What is the way that people in your faith go about getting forgiveness for their misdeeds?"

Reducing Suicide Risk and Promoting Survival

By engaging in a counseling alliance, co-constructing a survival story, and helping clients to envision a future, you are both reducing clients' suicidal risk and promoting survival. While you are asking questions that are assessing the level of threat to the client, you are, at the same time, posing many of these questions in such a way as to open up the possibility that the client will choose life. There are still other practical strategies that you can pursue. One

EXPERIENTIAL LEARNING

Are there any circumstances in which a client should have the right to commit suicide without interference? Can you imagine encountering a situation in which a client would be suicidal and you did not intervene? If you believe there are criteria for such a situation, how would you assess a suicidal client to determine whether she met the criteria? Discuss these ideas, and your opinions, with your classmates.

is to encourage the person to remove the means of suicide. For example, you might get a commitment that guns will be given to a relative, rather than kept at home. Another is to "establish a lifeline" (Wainrib & Bloch, 1998, p. 138) by linking the person in crisis with others who are committed to keeping the person alive. A third strategy is to develop a contract with the person. See if you can get him or her to agree not to kill himself or herself until sometime after your next meeting, or to phone you if the suicidal thoughts get too intense. All these strategies attempt to give the client some form of control over his or her life without suicide being seen as the only option.

If, in spite of your interventions, you find that someone continues to threaten suicide, then you need to carry out emergency procedures for voluntary hospitalization or, as a last resort, involuntary commitment if the person presents an imminent danger to self (Clark, 1998).

ETHICAL AND LEGAL ISSUES IN PRACTICE

The ethical and legal implications associated with assessment in counseling are significant. It is unlikely that during your training to become a community counselor you will take enough courses in testing to be expert in the use of some instruments. For example, in order to be able to effectively administer and score individual intelligence tests such as the Wechsler Scales or the Stanford-Binet, you would probably need to take a course and to be supervised on as many as twenty-five administrations. Some personality assessment tests, such as the MMPI or the Rorschach, require similar, extensive training. You will, however, be expert enough to become a well-informed consumer of information on test reports from other professionals, and you will be able to use many so-called "objective" paper-and-pencil tests in your practice.

You may find it useful to get further training and supervision in the use of some test instruments. In most community counseling work, sooner or later, part of your responsibilities may include assessment of clients for various purposes. Our own experience in agencies included giving batteries of tests (including the Wechsler Scales, MMPI, Rorschach, Bender Gestalt, etc.) as part of our agency's contract with local schools, for Social Security eligibility determinations, and other purposes, such as "competency to stand trial" assessments. If you plan to have a private practice, the ability to offer such test batteries can put a floor under your financial circumstances. The going rates for the administration and scoring of such instruments is in the hundreds of dollars.

If you become licensed as a Professional Counselor (LPC), you must not offer services for which you are not qualified. The ACA Code of Ethics is clear. This mandate is especially important in the area of assessment, since accuracy in obtaining correct scores and interpretations on test instruments is crucial, and since reports of the results are often sent to users who will regard these results as literal depictions of your clients.

A Hypothetical Ethical Dilemma

Imagine that you are testing a client who has applied for Social Security disability benefits on the basis of his cognitive limitations. His name is Ralph and he is thirty years old. He is brought to you by his grandmother, who has cared for him for years. She is now quite old and worried that without income from the government, Ralph will be destitute once she passes on. Ralph has no current income, no other family support, and only went to the sixth grade in school. He has never held a job and has no marketable skills. The Social Security Administration requires that Ralph must score less than a 70 I.Q. on an individual intelligence test in order to qualify for a cognitive disability. After interviewing Ralph, you believe that he is not likely to be able to function well on his own after the death of his grandmother. You administer the Wechsler Adult Intelligence Scale to Ralph. He finds the testing situation stressful and he cries several times during the administration and asks to stop. You persevere and are able to finally complete the assessment. Later, when you score the instrument, you find that his obtained score is an I.Q. of 71.

You are bound by your ethics to accurately administer and score the instruments that you use. But you also know that the standard error of measurement on the Wechsler Scales is 5, which means that Ralph's true score would fall somewhere between 66 and 76 at least 68 percent of the time. If you wanted to be closer to being absolutely certain of his true score (99 percent), the range would be even greater. According to Anastasi and Urbina (1997), at this level of confidence, there is a "13 point range" on either side of the obtained score (p. 108). At the lower end of this range, Ralph would certainly qualify for a Social Security disability.

You don't want to bring Ralph back in for another two-hour testing situation. You will, of course, include in your report to the Social Security Administration your impressions of Ralph's functioning, his history of inability to cope on his own, and the difficulties involved in the test administration itself. However, you know from experience that the clerical person who reads the report is going to only be interested in Ralph's score—71. On this basis, Ralph does not qualify for Supplemental Security Income (SSI) benefits. What do you do? Do you shave a couple of points off his score? Do you bring him back for another ordeal of testing? Or do you submit the report as is?

We know this situation may seem difficult to resolve comfortably and in the best interests of all concerned. It is, however, realistic. In responding to any ethical dilemma, you are encouraged to proceed through a formal ethical decision-making process that includes consultation with colleagues. Thankfully, many counselors find that taking a step back from the situation, combined with the good advice and guidance of other experienced professionals, will enable them to achieve the perspective they need to make reasoned decisions.

Computers as an Ethical Problem

Increasingly, computers are being used in clinical assessment. Test publishers are offering multiple-use licenses to agencies and private practitioners for tests that are frequently used by counselors and psychologists. Some of the instruments that were once scored by hand using tables in the test manual are now automatically scored by the computer. Tests that were once mailed to the publisher for a narrative interpretation of the results now are printed out with complete scoring and interpretations. In many cases, an automated narrative describing the person who took the test is also produced.

There is good news and bad news regarding the use of computers in assessment. The good news is that computers save counselors precious time. There is little doubt that obtaining tests over the Internet will greatly increase during the twenty-first century. The ease of access and the efficiency of scoring and reporting may have a downside, however. The possibility exists that some clinicians will give over their clinical intuitions and judgments to the presumed "expertise" of the machine.

We know of a psychologist (no longer practicing) who regularly had his clients sit at the computer and take the MMPI during their first visit. Often, a third party seeking information on the person's functioning had referred these clients. Once the client, sitting at the computer, had responded to the over 500 true-false items on the MMPI, the computer would score the results and produce a graphic frequency polygon of the standard scores on the three validity scales, the ten basic scales, and several supplementary scales. Then, a report was produced, based on the algorithms of the computer program. Instead of using these data as an aid to understanding his client, and checking it against his own impressions of the client, this psychologist simply printed out the total results, including the narrative description of the client, signed his name, and mailed it to the referring third party! We offer this example as the paradigm case for the unethical use of tests. The computer is certainly a useful instrument, and as the software becomes more sophisticated, so-called artificial intelligence will become a useful aide to your counseling practice. The computer will not, however, ever become more valuable than your clinical judgment and your ethical behavior.

Multicultural Appropriateness of Tests

As has previously been stated, many standardized tests have been normed on groups of people who are culturally different than the client you may be attempting to assess. It is your job to ensure that the tests you use are appropriate for your clients. You should understand the idea of cultural bias and know, prior to using a test, whether or not it has been normed for your client population. The history of the testing movement shows that many people have suffered discrimination and injury through the use of psychological tests.

For example, shortly after World War I many states began passing compulsory sterilization laws. By 1932, over 12,000 people in thirty states had been sterilized as a result of the American eugenics movement, which supported "good breeding" and the sterilization of those with poor protoplasm (Schultz & Schultz, 2000). Bogus research studies on the genealogy of families and testing to identify "morons" were used to support the notion that people who were poor or culturally different from the mainstream were that way because of bad genes.

The Lynchburg Colony in Lynchburg, Virginia, was an institution that housed people who were thought to be feebleminded, epileptic, or to have criminal potential. These people were largely poor whites from the Appalachian Mountains, so-called "hillbillies." Occasionally, entire families were sent to Lynchburg, and children who were simply orphaned were sometimes incarcerated there. Of course, according to the Social Darwinists, the mere lack of success in life was prima facie evidence of impaired intelligence. Smart folks got wealthy; stupid folks tended to remain poor. Impoverished people who appeared as though they might be feebleminded or future troublemakers were prime candidates for the Lynchburg Colony, and they were regularly sterilized for their "health."

The famous case of a young woman named Carrie Buck went all the way to the U. S. Supreme Court (Gould, 1996). Carrie was a resident of Charlottesville, Virginia, who had borne a child out of wedlock after being raped by a relative.

During the 1920s in Virginia, such apparent sexual promiscuity was considered scandalous and grounds, according to some, for incarceration in institutions such as the Lynchburg Colony. Carrie's child was taken away from her, and she was institutionalized. However, Carrie Buck challenged the legality of her forced incarceration. When the case of *Buck* v. *Bell* was argued in Supreme Court, Justice Oliver Wendell Holmes, speaking for the majority opinion said, "[I]nstead of waiting to execute degenerate offspring for crime, or . . . let them starve for their imbecility, society can prevent those who are manifestly unfit from continuing their kind. . . . Three generations of imbeciles are enough" (p. 198). Thus, in 1927 the Supreme Court declared the states' sterilization laws to be constitutional.

The sterilization law in Virginia remained on the books until 1972, by which time over 7,500 Virginians had been sterilized. The *Washington Post* broke the story in 1980 of the Lynchburg sterilizations and reported that Carrie Buck, then in her late 70s, was again living near Charlottesville with her widowed sister Doris. Reporters who had visited Carrie and Doris stated that they were both, despite their lack of formal education, women of normal intelligence and ability. Both had been sterilized in 1928. Doris had married a plumber by the name of Matthew Figgins, and she and Matthew had tried for years to conceive a child. Doris had no idea that her Fallopian tubes had been severed. She said her caretakers had explained that the operation was for a ruptured appendix. When she finally learned the truth, she grieved openly. She said that she and her husband had tried for years to have a baby, and that she had no idea of what the people in the institution had done to her (Gould, 1996).

This chilling example highlights the dire need for counselors to understand not only the various constructs they are assessing in their clients, but the basics of measurement theory as well. The use of I.Q. tests in the early twentieth century for the purpose of maintaining a certain social order was clearly wrong. As a community counselor, you must stand against unethical use of assessment and advocate for your clients. The potential to harm clients with faulty assessment and diagnosis is real, so we encourage you to ensure that your own use of assessment with clients is reasoned and appropriate.

Although we have focused above on the ethical issues associated with assessment, you should realize that any of the issues we have mentioned could have legal implications for the counselor as well. Clients are entitled to accurate diagnosis. Counselors who fail to diagnose properly, those who fail to use appropriate assessment instruments, those who use inappropriate tests for the client or client's needs, or who inaccurately interpret test results, could find themselves charged with malpractice. Furthermore, counselors who fail to adequately screen for suicide and/or who fail to follow through on suicidal threats according to basic standards of care may be found civilly liable. As with all other aspects of the community-counseling role, counselors must ensure that they know their ethical and legal responsibilities and act accordingly.

CONCLUDING THOUGHTS

Community counselors must be able to assess their clients accurately and thoroughly in order to design appropriate interventions. Regardless of your initial response to the idea of testing and measuring clients, keep in mind that assessment need not be a "test them and tell them" endeavor. Rather, assessment is a critical and ongoing aspect of counseling that requires the best use of one's advanced listening skills, critical thought, and systemic analysis. As well as being the essential first step in the counseling process, assessment can be one of the most intriguing aspects of community counseling.

RECOMMENDED RESOURCES

We recommend that you consider keeping your assessment textbooks to ensure you remember, and can put into layman's terms, concepts such as reliability, validity, and standard error of measurement. We have found the following to be particularly helpful:

Anastasi, A. & Urbina, S. (1997). *Psychological testing* (7th ed.). Upper Saddle River, NJ: Prentice-Hall.

Also, to ensure that you remember the potential bias inherent in assessment, read through the following:

Gould, S. J. (1996). *The mismeasure of man* (revised and expanded). New York: W. W. Norton.

Tseng, W. S., & Streltzer, J. (Eds.). (1997). *Culture and psychopathology: A guide to clinical assessment.* Philadelphia, PA: Brunner/Mazel.

If you're hesitant about how to best use the DSM-IV-TR, we recommend the useful text

Maxmen, J. S., & Ward, N. G. (1995). *Essential psychopathology and its treatment* (2nd ed.). New York: Norton.

Finally, the Association for Assessment in Counseling and Education, a division of ACA, provides current and relevant information on aspects of assessment in counseling. Of particular interest are AACE's resources, which include explanations of the responsibility of users of standardized tests, standards for multicultural assessment, and test takers' rights and responsibilities.

Other Resources

Sylvia Plath's book *The Bell Jar* is an intriguing look into the mind of a woman struggling with mental illness, and *Lucky,* by Alice Sebold, reveals the author's reactions to her own rape. The disturbing film *Equus,* as well as the classics *Sybil* and *The Three*

Faces of Eve, provide the viewer with multiple opportunities to practice assessment as they piece together elements of a troubled person's life. If you watch these movies and read these books, imagine how you might work through the diagnostic decision-making process with the various main characters, what judgment you would make of the client's current situation, and what prognoses you would offer.

REFERENCES

Aiken, L. R. (1988). *Psychological testing and assessment* (6th ed.). Boston: Allyn and Bacon.

American Association of Suicidology (2002). *Suicide in the U.S.A.* Retrieved July 8, 2005, from **http://www.suicidology.org/index.cfm.**

American Psychiatric Association (2000). *Diagnostic and statistical manual of mental disorders* (4th ed., text rev.). Washington, DC: Author.

Anastasi, A., & Urbina, S. (1997). *Psychological testing* (7th ed.). Upper Saddle River, NJ: Prentice-Hall.

Baron-Cohen, S. (1996). *Mindblindness: An essay on autism and theory of mind.* Cambridge, MA: The MIT Press.

Clark, D. C. (1998). The evaluation and management of the suicidal patient. In P. M. Kleespies (Ed.), *Emergencies in mental health practice* (pp. 75–94). New York: Guilford.

DeJong, P., & Berg, I. K. (2002). *Interviewing for solutions* (2nd ed.). Pacific Grove, CA: Brooks/Cole.

Echterling, L. G., Presbury, J. H., & McKee, J. E. (2005). *Crisis intervention: Promoting resilience and resolution in troubled times.* Upper Saddle River, NJ: Merrill Prentice Hall.

Fowler, R. C., Rich, C. L., & Young, D. (1986). San Diego suicide study: Substance abuse in young cases. *Archives of General Psychiatry, 43,* 962–965.

Gould, S. J. (1996). *The mismeasure of man* (revised and expanded). New York: W. W. Norton.

Hendin, H. (1995). *Suicide in America.* New York: W. W. Norton.

Hood, A. B., & Johnson, R. W. (2002). *Assessment in counseling: A guide to the use of psychological assessment procedures* (3rd ed.). Alexandria, VA: ACA.

Jacobs, D. G., Brewer, M., & Klein-Benheim, M. (1999). Suicide assessment: An overview and recommended protocol. In D. G. Jacobs (Ed.), *The Harvard Medical School guide to suicide assessment and intervention* (pp. 3–39). San Francisco: Jossey-Bass.

Lubin, B., Larsen, R. M., & Matarazzo, J. D. (1984). Patterns of psychological test usage in the United States: 1935–1982. *American Psychologist, 39,* 451–454.

Maxmen, J. S., & Ward, N. G. (1995). *Essential psychopathology and its treatment* (2nd ed.). New York: Norton.

Menninger, K. (1973). *Sparks*. New York: Crowell.

Moscicki, E. K. (1999). Epidemiology of suicide. In D. G. Jacobs (Ed.), *The Harvard Medical School guide to suicide assessment and intervention* (pp. 40–51). San Francisco: Jossey-Bass.

Neukrug, E. (2003). *The world of the counselor: An introduction to the counseling profession* (2nd ed.). Pacific Grove, CA: Brooks/Cole.

Nunnally, J. C. (1978). *Psychometric theory* (2nd ed.). New York: McGraw-Hill.

Polanski, P. J., & Hinkle, J. S. (2000). The mental status examination: Its use by professional counselors. *Journal of Counseling and Development, 78,* 357–364.

Posavac, E. J., & Carey, R. G. (2003). *Program evaluation: Methods and case studies* (6th ed.). Upper Saddle River, NJ: Prentice-Hall.

Presbury, J. H., & Benson, A. J. (1994). Professional transitioning with expert systems: Beyond the "cognitive" process. *Report to Virginia Center for Innovative Technology, College of Integrated Science and Technology,* James Madison University, 59–72.

Presbury, J. H., Echterling, L. G., & McKee, J. E. (2002). *Ideas and tools for brief counseling*. Upper Saddle River, NJ: Merrill/Prentice Hall.

Shneidman, E. (1999). Perturbation and lethality: A psychological approach to assessment and intervention. In D. G. Jacobs (Ed.), *The Harvard Medical School guide to suicide assessment and intervention* (pp. 83–97). San Francisco: Jossey-Bass.

Schultz, D. P., & Schultz, S. E. (2000). *A modern history of psychology* (7th ed.). Fort Worth, TX: Harcourt College Publishers.

Sommers-Flanagan, J., & Sommers-Flanagan, R. (2002). *Clinical interviewing* (3rd ed.). New York: John Wiley & Sons.

Thorndike, R. L. (1982). *Applied psychometrics*. Boston: Houghton Mifflin.

Wainrib, B. R., & Bloch, E. L. (1998). *Crisis intervention and trauma response: Theory and practice*. New York: Springer.

Webb, E. J., Campbell, D. T., Schwartz, R. D., & Sechrest, L. (1971). *Unobtrusive measures: Nonreactive research in the social sciences*. Chicago: Rand-McNally.

Whiston, S. C. (2000). *Principles and applications of assessment in counseling*. Belmont, CA: Wadsworth.

Young, M. E. (2001). *Learning the art of helping: Building blocks and techniques* (2nd ed.). Upper Saddle River, NJ: Merrill/Prentice Hall.

Chapter 7

Viewing the Community Kaleidoscope: Embracing Diversity in Counseling

Difference is . . . the condition requisite to all dignity and to all liberation. To be aware of oneself is to be aware of oneself as different. To be is to be different.

Albert Memmi

When we attend to different worldviews, our horizons expand.

Jennifer Rudkin

GOALS

Reading and exploring the ideas in this chapter will help you:

- Comprehend the concept of culture and its relevance to community counseling
- Enhance your understanding of difference
- Gain self-awareness regarding diversity issues
- Explore counseling and community-oriented responses to diversity-related issues

---

OVERVIEW

This chapter presents information on multicultural trends, counselor attitudes regarding diversity, counseling strategies for working with diverse groups, relevant theories, counselors' roles in social justice and advocacy, and ethical and legal considerations. The chapter is intended to help you explore the concept of diversity as it relates to community counseling. Diversity, simply put, is variety. To be diverse means to differ from each other. This definition sounds so simple and straightforward, yet few topics create as much hesitation, apprehension, and distress as this issue. In conversations about such topics as racism, affirmative action, immigration issues, or gay/lesbian/bisexual concerns, people often find that their hearts start beating more quickly. Their mouths become dry. They become frustrated and uncomfortable. What's going on here?

The answer to this question is complex. In response, we begin by presenting the impact of diversity on the United States. Then we explore how diversity affects the counseling relationship and the ways in which counselors can pursue multicultural competence. Finally, we offer several counseling and community-related responses intended to enhance the provision of culturally relevant services.

JENNIFER'S DEFINING MOMENT: Aren't We Both Human?

Jennifer was in the second year of her counselor training program. She had a grueling schedule and wound up taking a multicultural counseling course and counseling process course on the same day. By the time she left school on those days, she felt emotionally and intellectually drained. In the multicultural course, she was learning how power and privilege influence the counseling process. Jennifer struggled for several weeks to understand that, as a heterosexual European American woman, her experience of life in the United States was different than that of an African American woman's, a lesbian's, or someone with a disability. Once she began to explore the concept she felt overwhelmed and guilty. She felt paralyzed by what she read about unearned privilege and was confused about how to make sense of her status as a member of the power majority in the United States.

The biggest challenge came at the end of one of her multicultural classes. Jennifer said in class that she had always believed that people were all from the same race—the human race—and that people's similarities transcended their differences. Trenae, a fellow student, approached Jennifer after class to say that her comments belittled Trenae's experience as an African American woman. In fact, Trenae said, Jennifer's words revealed an insensitivity that suggested that Jennifer couldn't genuinely empathize with an ethnic minority.

Jennifer left the encounter feeling both angry and ashamed. By the time she arrived at her counseling process class, she also felt hopeless. She looked at William, a Korean-American peer, and said, "You and I have such different realities. I just don't know if I could ever know what it's like to be you."

William looked at her with confusion. "Aren't we both human?" he said. "Can't we relate on that dimension?"

Jennifer was floored. "I just can't win in this conversation," she said. "I have no idea how to make sense of this multicultural stuff."

Questions for Reflection

1. How do you feel about talking openly with others about diversity issues?

2. What are some of the reasons that discussions about topics such as ethnicity, class, and sexual orientation are often difficult?

3. What is your obligation, as a community counselor, in appreciating and accepting individual differences?

4. Can a bigot be a good counselor?

IMPLICATIONS OF DIVERSITY IN THE UNITED STATES

Perhaps one of the confounding factors in our efforts to fully understand and accept diversity is that in the United States the true benefits of diversity are not yet ingrained in our consciousness. Many of us, in fact probably most of us, suspect that great goals can be obtained by sincerely embracing each other and our differences. However, the act of genuinely exploring what diversity means for each of us is challenging and stressful. We might discover some things about ourselves or others that would be painful to face. Further, as Weinrach and Thomas (1996) affirm, we relate most easily to people who are like us. The more similar we are, the more comfortable we feel.

When speaking of diversity in the United States, we are usually referring to any difference from the mainstream or majority culture. By mainstream we typically mean light-skinned people who are of Western European descent, middle-class, heterosexual, able-bodied, and Christian. Thus, diversity for our purposes includes those who are ethnic minorities, poor, gay, lesbian, bisexual, transgendered, disabled, and religious minorities. Although there are many other types of difference, such as being introverted rather than extroverted, or Southern versus Northern, these differences have not traditionally resulted in discrimination toward those who differ. Children and elderly people are also sometimes considered to be culturally different from the mainstream in that their needs are not always accounted for by traditional agency services or policies.

Dimensions of Difference: Race, Ethnicity, and Culture

We should begin here by clarifying the use of terms relevant to discussions of diversity in the United States: race, ethnicity, and culture. Race and ethnicity are often treated as synonymous concepts. However, many sociologists and anthropologists agree that *race* is a form of ethnicity rather than a legitimate physiological concept in its own right (Smelser, Wilson, & Mitchell, 2001). Race is a social construction based on appearance. Ethnicity is a social definition that includes people who share a common national or tribal heritage. Ethnicity is a more universally accepted, inclusive, and therefore useful concept, but race is the more commonly used descriptor for ethnic difference in the United States (Mayo, 2000). In this chapter we intend the term *ethnic minorities* to include the concept of race. In doing so, we recognize that even the term *ethnicity* is flawed and fails to acknowledge the complex ways in which people prefer to be identified.

Culture, then, is an even broader concept. Fundamentally, culture, as Diller pointed out, gives our lives its "content" (2004, p. 59). Our culture shows us how to act and what to expect. Counselors and clients bring their cultural heritage into their sessions every time they meet. In fact, culture is such a part of us that we tend to take it for granted. We're only aware of it when some jolt, often some *difference,* brings it into focus for us.

In the most general sense, cultural groups include any group whose members share organizing beliefs or similarities (Axelson, 1993). Gordon (1964), in a classic work on assimilation, described culture as including the beliefs, behaviors, and traditions that groups use to organize life and interpret their experience. Culture and cultural expectations, in particular, are transmitted from one generation to another, or in some cases from one group member to another. Thus, there is a culture of ethnicity, gender, sexual orientation, age, and, of course, community. Further, a given culture changes over time, in reaction to the various cultures that surround it.

A Deeper Exploration of Culture

Conceptualizing culture in the broadest sense provides an *etic* or universal view of people. An *etic* standpoint allows us to look for commonalities among individuals, such as emphasizing the basic needs and emotions of all people, highlighting the importance of community and family, and focusing on whatever "universals" can be found. In some ways the *etic* view mirrors the "Can't we all just get along?" approach to difference. In the Defining Moment at the beginning of this chapter, Jennifer applied an etic view in her statement that all people are simply part of the human race. Interestingly, according to Steinberg (2000), as the United States has become more diverse, our agencies have begun to adopt universal principles in responding to clients' needs. However, in following universal principles, we run the risk of ignoring contextual and unique cultural factors, such as discrimination and oppression.

The opposite, an *emic* or indigenous view, emphasizes the unique, individual characteristics that differentiate people (Castillo, 1997). In this view, mental health is conceptualized as mental health for a specific population, so healthy family or communal life is defined as healthy specifically for a certain group of people. This *emic* view allows counselors to avoid making sweeping generalizations that limit their practice. However, an exclusively *emic* approach can lose a sense of societal context and relevance, and cloud the counselor's ability to adequately assess client functioning. For instance, in the "Defining Moment" when Jennifer was talking with William, she seemed unable to look beyond the emic approach to difference. In her effort to understand others, she was frustratingly buffeted between the two extremes.

One way to strike a balance is to consider the following reminders:

- Culture is manifest in *unique* ways by every individual, based on characteristics such as age, socioeconomic status, race, ethnicity, gender, and personality. For example, two Latina immigrants from Colombia who are the same age who live in the same U.S. city may lead drastically different lives, with different aspirations, lifestyles, and worldviews. Culture, in reality, must accommodate heterogeneity.

- *Everyone* is influenced by his or her culture. By definition, our culture affects us daily. We are not always conscious, however, of that influence.

- Our clients (as well as our friends and colleagues) will determine for *themselves* which group identities are most salient for them. We must then work to understand and respect that self-determination. For instance, a Chinese-American lesbian may feel that her identity as a Chinese-American is more influential in her daily life than her identity as a lesbian. This woman's unique culture is enacted by her, regardless of how we may conceptualize her (Weinrach & Thomas, 2004).

- Each culture is *not* equally valued by mainstream society. Generally speaking, the culture of Protestantism is more easily accepted by most people in the United States than the culture of Islam. The culture of heterosexual identity is more highly valued in U.S. society than the culture of bisexual identity.

This last point is critical. In the overview of this chapter, we mentioned that the topic of diversity often becomes emotionally charged. One of the reasons for this charge is the fact that people of different cultures are treated differently in the United States, often as a result of their cultural membership.

One of the difficulties we face in understanding culture is comprehending accurately the reality of our *own* culture and how it continuously influences us. Our culture covers us like a veil—we see everything through it (Sue, 2004). It has a profound impact on our interactions and beliefs. Yet we're so accustomed to it that we often forget it's there. Thus, when many counselors talk about "cultural differences" with clients, they're talking only about their clients, not themselves. They are forgetting that their own culture is also an important variable in the counseling room. If we fail to examine our own culture, we can't begin to understand how it truly influences us as we interact with our clients.

EXPERIENTIAL LEARNING

Explore your culture by responding to the following items:

1. How do you define the word *culture?*

2. Describe your culture.

3. How does it influence you on a regular basis?

4. What has your culture taught you about difference, specifically difference in ethnicity, gender, sexual orientation, age, ability, or religion?

5. What group identities are encompassed in your description of your own culture?

6. What role, if any, does ethnicity play in your own culture?

Look back over your answers. As you continue to read, keep in mind that you are perceiving your life through the veil of your culture. Your culture creates for you a unique reality, just as your clients' different cultures create for them a unique reality.

REALITIES FACING MINORITY CLIENTS

Regardless of how difficult it may be for us to discuss diversity, this topic is critical for community counselors. Heterosexism and sexism affect our clients daily. Our neighborhoods are still segregated along color lines. Ethnic minorities still experience higher rates of poverty and unemployment than do European American people (Steinberg, 2000). Ethnic disparities exist in access to and provision of healthcare (Appiah & Guttman, 1996). The educational and thus achievement gap between European Americans and ethnic minorities is still present. Furthermore, many U.S. social problems, including inadequate schooling, gang violence, drug abuse, crime, and poverty, are often more pronounced and detrimental in communities consisting primarily of ethnic minorities (Boger & Wegner, 1996; Reed, 1999).

Mental Health Concerns for Ethnic Minorities

The U.S. Department of Health and Human Services (USDHHS, 2001) has produced a compelling report detailing mental health problems for ethnic minorities. The report acknowledges several facts relevant to the work of community counselors, such as the pervasive influence of European American, Judeo-Christian values on institutions such as mental health facilities. As the report acknowledges, although European values have influenced the United States for most of its history, the U.S. population is changing. As a result, clients who differ from this traditional majority have systematically been treated differently than its members, often facing limited access to appropriate care or receiving substandard care (USDHHS, 2001).

The report provides information regarding the need for mental health-care; availability, accessibility, and utilization of mental health services; and appropriateness and outcomes of mental health services for African Americans, American Indians and Alaska Natives, Asian Americans and Pacific Islanders, and "Hispanic Americans." (Note that the term *Hispanic Americans* was created by the U.S. government to identify people whose ancestry is from Spanish-speaking countries or regions. The term *Latino* is now a more popular term and is usually the descriptor preferred by Latinos themselves.) Significant concerns for many minorities include unwillingness or delay in seeking mental health services, mistrust of the mental health system, and belief in the idea that mental illness is a stigma. Further, many minority individuals who do seek mental healthcare will first go to a primary provider, usually a physician, who may or may not have adequate training to treat mental illness or provide appropriate referrals. Then, those who do seek counseling services sometimes encounter counselor bias and misunderstanding or ignorance of the client's culture—all of which can negatively influence the client's treatment.

As a result of these and other factors, half as many African Americans as European Americans receive mental health treatment. Considering that many African Americans are in high-need populations, the implications of the disparity between the two groups are even more pronounced. When African Americans do receive mental health treatment, they are more likely to be incorrectly diagnosed than European Americans. Asian Americans and Pacific Islanders—an extremely heterogeneous group—utilize mental health services less than any other ethnic population. Those who do seek services tend to be experiencing more extreme disturbances. Among Latino populations, Latino youths are more likely to experience depression and anxiety, drop out of school, and contemplate suicide than European American youths.

Another issue that complicates the provision of quality mental health services to minority clients includes the amazing diversity that exists within ethnic groups. The umbrella term *Asian American,* for instance, is completely insufficient for describing the range of cultures and individuals in the United States and who come here from Asia. Also, the manifestations of mental illness and, indeed, mental health needs themselves, vary widely among ethnic groups, and even within different groups in the same cultural or ethnic category. This report suggests that many of our communities are facing critical shortcomings in their ability to provide mental health services.

Demographic Trends

The President's *Race Initiative* in 1997 indicated that the biggest domestic challenge currently facing the United States is "color" (Smelser, Wilson, & Mitchell, 2001). Future trends reveal that this report may be accurate. Demographic projections suggest that by the year 2050 the United States will have no single majority group. Indeed, in 1999 California became the first state with no one racial group claiming a numerical majority ("California," 2004). Latinos are expected to gain majority status in California by 2040, and by 2050 European Americans are expected to make up about 23 percent of the state's population, with Asian Americans comprising 12 percent and African Americans 6 percent.

We can expect the rest of the country to follow California's lead, at least to some degree. From 2000 to 2050, the Latino and Asian populations are projected to increase dramatically in the United States, with the African American population increasingly slightly (Sandefur, Martin, Eggerling-Boeck, Mannon, & Meier, 2001). By 2010, Latinos will replace African Americans as the largest minority group in the United States. European Americans are expected to be 53 percent of the U.S. population by 2050.

Demographics are also affected by fertility and family patterns (Blank, 2001). The difference between fertility rates for European Americans and African Americans has stabilized—African Americans now consistently have higher fertility rates than European Americans. The fertility rate for Latinos has been the highest of any group. In 1996, the total fertility rate of American Indians was 13 percent higher than that of European Americans. The fertility rates for Asian Americans have been calculated as 6 percent higher than for European Americans.

Another significant aspect of demographic trends is the rate of teen pregnancy. In 1997, 21 percent of European American girls became pregnant by age eighteen, and 40 percent of minority girls became pregnant by this age (Blank, 2001). Single-parent families are becoming more common, with the highest rates among African Americans, followed by Native Americans, Latinos, European Americans, and Asian Americans. Of the above mentioned groups, African Americans and Native Americans have the lowest life expectancies and the highest infant mortality rates and death rates (Blank, 2001).

These data are sobering, suggesting that our community health systems need to make significant adjustments in order to serve effectively our changing communities. Societal trends also provide compelling information (Bean & Bell-Rose, 1999; Blank, 2001). The gap between African American men's and European American men's pay has shown little progress for African American men. Latino men have experienced decreases in pay. European

EXPERIENTIAL LEARNING

Investigate the U.S. Census data for the community in which you currently live, or the city in which you plan to work after graduation. You can easily gain access to detailed information about population characteristics online by going to **www.census.gov.**

1. What diversity exists there?
2. How have the demographics of this community changed since the previous census?
3. What are the implications for you as a future community counselor in this area?

American women now earn more than Latino and African American men. African American women's pay, however, has stayed about the same since the 1980s, and Latinas' pay has decreased slightly. African Americans are poor at three times the rate of European Americans, and Latino poverty has increased since the 1980s (Frey, Abresch, & Yeasting, 2001).

Societal conditions, including oppression and lack of access to resources, tend to make some groups more vulnerable to poverty and crime. African Americans are more likely than members of any other group to be homicide victims and are more likely to be involved with the criminal justice system than European Americans (Blank, 2001). Minorities are also still more likely to live in substandard housing than European Americans. Clearly, those who are ethnic minorities in the United States face numerous societal stressors that can compound or create mental health issues.

RESPONDING TO DIVERSITY FROM A COMMUNITY COUNSELING PERSPECTIVE

Multicultural counseling has been labeled the Fourth Force in counseling, suggesting that it has a place along with psychodynamic, behaviorist, and humanist approaches in the field. Difference, as it relates to vital characteristics such as ethnicity, gender, sexual orientation, age, and ability, is clearly a vitally important concept for community counselors. If we deny difference, then we deny reality. And if we dwell only on difference, then we block any possibility for connection. Our challenge as community counselors is to find a creative tension and productive balance as we explore this concept.

The definition of *multicultural* by the Council for the Accreditation of Counseling and Related Programs (CACREP) is so broad that it suggests that *multicultural counseling* technically occurs whenever the counselor and client are different from each other. This approach seems simplistic and ignores the power differential that exists in our communities. Fortunately, several researchers have proposed specific multicultural counseling competencies and standards (Sue, Arredondo, & McDavis, 1992), which have been through several review and revision processes. In 1996 Arredondo et al. published an attempt to operationalize the multicultural standards. Then, in March 2003 the American Counseling Association voted to endorse the multicultural competencies.

The endorsed document identifies thirty-one counselor competencies, with the goal that these competencies will become the standard for practice and training in the field. The competencies describe counselor attitudes and beliefs, knowledge, and skills in the three categories of (1) Counselor Awareness of Own Cultural Values and Biases, (2) Counselor Awareness of Client's Worldview, and (3) Culturally Appropriate Intervention Strategies (Arredondo et al., 1996).

The competencies document presents a three-stage process for counselors attempting to enhance their multicultural competence. First, counselors need to understand themselves fully. Then they need to work to understand their clients' experiences and beliefs. Finally, they are expected to develop conceptualization and intervention strategies that are relevant and responsive to their clients' needs. These tasks are obviously easier said than done. We can, however, explore our counseling relationship in a systematic manner to help ensure our practice is culturally competent. We suggest that community counselors begin by:

- Analyzing the culture of the counseling relationship
- Staying informed regarding recent research
- Working to create comprehensive conceptualizations
- Attending to the nuances of the counseling process and relationship

Counselors can then put these skills into practice to craft relevant individual and community interventions. We explore each of these topics further, beginning with a look at the culture of counseling.

Analyzing the Culture of the Counseling Relationship

What is the culture of counseling? What practices do we assume will occur in a counseling session? What beliefs do we assume counselors share? Although answers to these questions may differ depending on the counselor's theoretical orientation, many would agree that the culture of counseling requires a basic level of *trust* and relies on client *self-disclosure*. These expectations warrant further examination.

As counselors work to build trusting relationships with their clients, they simultaneously recognize that their clients' experiences in the world may not engender trusting relationships. If a person has been discriminated against in the past because of her social class, for instance, she may expect the counselor to discriminate against her as well. Building trust with this client may take more time and effort than building trust with a client who is accustomed to being treated with respect and dignity (Baruth & Manning, 2003).

Some counselors find such situations especially challenging. "Of course I'll respect my client, regardless of how much money she has or what her ethnicity might be!" they think. The most difficult aspect of this scenario is not necessarily how the counselor will feel about the client, although that's undoubtedly important. The major concern is determining how to build a relationship with someone who has no real reason to trust—and may even have substantial reason to distrust—you as a helping professional. Thus, community counselors must have the capability to recognize how societal influences have affected their clients and then assess how that impact will influence the counseling relationship. Assuming that clients will automatically trust us is naïve.

Another relevant aspect of counseling culture is the belief that clients must fully self-disclose. As mentioned earlier, the ability and willingness to self-disclose is dependent, at least in part, on the trust that has been established in the relationship. Many people of various cultures have been taught that disclosing one's feelings, family concerns, or worries is inappropriate (Sue & Sue, 2003) and avoid seeking formal counseling. However many of these people, such as immigrants or refugees, may find that they are required to meet with mental health professionals in order to receive certain social services. Community counselors cannot realistically expect such a client to be enthusiastic about sharing intimate thoughts and feelings. The counselor's job is to patiently help the person to experience counseling as a safe haven— a refuge for exploration, discovery, and change.

Fostering client trust and encouraging self-disclosure have long been considered fundamental aspects of counseling. When these aspects become more specific based on the counselor's particular theoretical orientation, the potential obstacles multiply. For instance, a psychodynamic orientation stresses that insight is eventually necessary for lasting change to occur. How will counselors with this orientation work effectively with those who are unwilling to share their insights or who believe that their own reflections are irrelevant to their concerns?

Another mainstream counseling tenet is the belief that facilitating individuation is an overarching goal when working with adolescents. How then does a counselor work with a young Muslim woman who is expected by her family to immerse herself in the roles of daughter, wife, and eventually, mother? How will the counselor reconcile her own belief in the benefits of individuation with the client's desire to put others' needs before her own? In worst-case scenarios, clients in situations such as these have been misunderstood and misdiagnosed. These problems are due in part to the mismatch that may occur between the culture of counseling and the culture of the client (Castillo, 1997).

Community counselors also need to be aware of societal influences that can negatively affect the counseling relationship. These influences, all of which are potential obstacles to the relationship, include prejudice, discrimination, oppression, and society's conveyance of unearned power and privilege to European Americans.

Acknowledging Prejudice, Discrimination, and Oppression

According to Allport's (1954) classic work, *prejudice* is an inaccurate and negative way of thinking about others. All people have prejudices, and people develop and maintain prejudice with ease. Why? According to Allport, human brains are essentially categorizing machines. We quite naturally tend to group people, things, and ideas into categories. We then look for evidence to support our categorizations. Our ability to categorize also encourages us to prefer to be around people who look and sound like us. In fact, we are more likely to remember information that is presented to us by people who resemble us than information presented to us by people who are dissimilar from us.

One of the benefits of this ability is that it enables us to deal with enormous complexities. Without it there would be no science, technology, or written language. However, the drawbacks of our tendency to categorize are that it can encourage us to avoid difference and enable us to make significant errors in attribution as we assess the behavior of people who are different from us.

Community counselors also need to fully understand the concept of discrimination, as it is very likely to influence many agency clients. *Discrimination* is "the differential allocation of goods, resources, and services, and the limitation of access to full participation in society based on individual membership in a particular social group" (Adams, Bell, & Griffin, 1997, p. 88). Thus, discrimination refers to behavior as opposed to only attitudes. Discrimination, which can take many forms, is prejudice put into action (Bucher, 2004).

Prejudice and discrimination reinforce *oppression,* in which the group with power uses that power at the expense of other groups (Diller, 2004). Oppression is descriptive of the actions taken in intolerant environments that generally limit people in their ability to self-express or live life freely with equal access to resources. Prejudice and discrimination can result in oppressive systems that allow and perpetuate injustice (Adams, Bell, & Griffin, 1997).

If, as mentioned above, all people have prejudices, then we must assume that counselors have prejudices, too. Prejudice and discrimination can therefore occur in the counseling relationship, creating an oppressive environment for clients. Claiming that one is not prejudiced, or that one is "colorblind," is one way to avoid addressing prejudice in counseling. However, this claim is ineffective and usually untrue. Researchers and multicultural theorists agree (Lee, 1997; Sue & Sue, 2003) that acknowledging and addressing one's prejudices is a fundamental skill of culturally competent counselors. Therefore, examining and responding to our own prejudices should be a prerequisite for counseling practice.

Our clients' experiences with discrimination and oppression undoubtedly affect their worldviews and realities and are relevant considerations for us as community counselors. When working with our clients, we must therefore ask: How has the world treated our clients? How does that treatment affect their current concern? How do we, as counselors, mirror societal expectations? Sue and Sue (2003) suggest that, regardless of our ethnicity or minority/majority status, the fact that we're trained professionals marks us as members of "the establishment." How will that identity influence how our clients see us?

Dealing with Power and Privilege

A deeper look at the concepts of prejudice, discrimination, and oppression reveal that (1) people are treated differently in the United States based on factors such as ethnicity, class, gender, ability, age, and sexual orientation; and (2) in the United States, European Americans have more institutional power than other groups. According to Diller (2004), in the United States "the cultural form that has been adopted by and dominates all social institutions is White, Northern European culture" (pp. 43–44). European Americans in the United States have determined how our society functions. Thus, our definitions of what is good and bad, right and wrong, appropriate and inappropriate, and healthy and unhealthy are affected by European American culture. As a result, European Americans in U.S. society have unearned privilege that results, at least in part, from the color of their skin. Peggy McIntosh said it this way: "I have come to see white privilege as an invisible package of unearned assets which I can count on cashing in each day, but about which I . . . remain oblivious" (p. 10, 1989).

If you're not sure how this might manifest in your own life, take some time now to imagine how it might feel to be someone other than yourself. Imagine what it might be like to wake up every morning and think about your skin color, or sexual orientation, or specific physical disability, and wonder how that characteristic will influence your day today. Will people treat you differently because of it? Will you have to explain your motives because of it? Most European Americans do not think about their skin color every day. Some

think of it rarely, if at all, because they do not *have* to think abou.. ..
one of the privileges that comes with having white skin, or with being a member of mainstream U.S. society. For instance, many white people are unaware of the fact that their skin color will usually work for, rather than against, them in business and social settings (McIntosh, 1989). In McIntosh's view of white privilege, skin color alone is akin to currency; society allocates more worth and power to those with white skin.

Recognizing power and privilege is vitally important for community counselors as they assess their multicultural counseling relationships. Different groups are afforded different levels of power in our society, and these differences are likely to affect us all in very tangible and pervasive ways. Furthermore, the allocation of societal power and privilege can mirror the power differential that exists in many counseling relationships. Thus, clients' concerns about their own efficacy and self-worth—concerns that were developed as a result of their lack of societal power—can be exacerbated in counseling relationships in which the counselor relies on a hierarchical rather than collaborative or egalitarian relationship. Read "Randy's Story" for one student's observations regarding his own privilege.

Keeping Abreast of Relevant Theories

In addition to understanding the culture of the counseling relationship, community counselors can also enhance their multicultural competency by keeping abreast of emerging theories and other developments related to the specific populations they will be serving. For example, theories are now being refined that specifically address work with clients who are gay, lesbian, bisexual, or transgendered (Barret & Logan, 2002). Fisher and Moradi (2001) provide an overview of recent developments in research regarding racial and ethnic identity for African Americans, European Americans, Native Americans, Asian Americans, Latinos, and Jewish clients. Walsh (2000) and Atkinson, Kim, and Caldwell (1998) specifically describe theories relevant for Asian populations, and Sue, Ivey, and Pedersen (1996) have developed a comprehensive theory of multicultural counseling in general. These theories and models will be tested and evaluated, and new approaches will emerge. Connecting now with the Association for Multicultural Counseling and Development, a division of the American Counseling Association, will help you stay informed about these important professional developments. Then your job will be to see how these emerging theories and models actually relate to your work with clients.

Models of Identity Development

As evidenced by Allison's story (see the box on page 232), one struggle community counselors may have is translating training into practice. Identity

Randy's Story: What's the First Thing You Think About Yourself?

I had been keeping a journal as part of a requirement for my multicultural counseling class and was having some interesting internal dialogues regarding "diversity issues." As a European American man, I could accept the idea that women, including European American women, had fewer advantages than I did, but I had a hard time getting my head around the idea of European American privilege.

I'm a recovering alcoholic, and I feel like I've scraped and scrapped for every thing I've attained in my life. I always figured the only reason I'm still here is because I'm too determined and stubborn to die. If I can make it to graduate school, anyone can.

Then one day I was genuinely moved by a conversation I had with a fellow student, Joyce. Joyce and a couple of other students hosted a roundtable discussion regarding diversity issues. I was interested, so I attended. I was the only European American person there, so although I felt awkward at first, I appreciated the chance to talk with other students and hear about their experiences. We were talking about oppression and discrimination, and I said that as an alcoholic I felt like a minority who had special experiences that most people didn't have. "I'm different from the mainstream too," I said.

"Yes," replied Joyce, "but the difference with you, Randy, is that I can't tell you're an alcoholic by looking at you. My black skin is the first thing I think about when I look at myself in the mirror each morning. It's always there,

always present, and it automatically influences how people see me. Even white people who aren't necessarily overtly prejudiced factor in the color of my skin when they see me. I think the average person on the street sees you as just another guy, and I would bet that your white skin is not the first thing you notice about yourself when you look in the mirror in the morning."

She nailed it. I don't have to think about being white. The world I live in has been created with me in mind. That's what white privilege means.

Ever since I wrote those words in my journal, I've felt edgy and almost excited. I'm not sure what my next steps are going to be, but I know I'm beginning to see the world differently now. I have to keep saying to myself, "Okay, I know how the world has been for me. But how has it been for my clients? What's the first thing they think about when they look in the mirror in the morning?"

Understanding our different realities, and helping people articulate their unique struggles, is what I think counseling is all about.

Questions for Reflection

The significance of Randy's story lies, in part, in his realization of the uniqueness not only of Joyce's reality, but of his own as well. We're all marked by our own distinct set of experiences and characteristics.

1. Take time now to reflect on times in your own life when you've been a

(continued)

(Randy's Story: What's the First Thing You Think About Yourself? continued)

minority. How did those times affect you?

2. What about times when you've been an obvious member of the majority group? How was that different?

3. If the tables were turned for you, and you suddenly became other than you are, how would your life change? If you're a European

American woman, for instance, imagine your life as an African American man. What unique supports and challenges would exist for you then?

As you answer these questions, begin to think about the experiences of your clients. What will be the most salient issues for them?

---

development models can provide helpful categorizations for community counselors attempting to conceptualize their clients in a societal context. These models describe the sequence of assumptions and behaviors that occur as people's attitudes regarding themselves and others develop. Identity models have been developed to explain white racial identity (Helms, 1993; Rowe, Behrens, & Leach, 1995); black racial identity (Cross, 1971); minority racial identity (Atkinson, Morten, & Sue, 1989); and gay/lesbian identity (Cass, 1984; Coleman, 1985). More models exist, including those that describe feminist identity development (Downing & Rousch, 1985) and the identity development of groups as specific as biracial Japanese-Americans (Collins, 2000). With some exceptions, these models tend to share several common characteristics:

- They typically define a first stage of identity development as one that is heavily influenced by the dominant society.

- The second stage usually includes a crisis that shakes up one's worldview and results in the individual questioning prior assumptions about self and others.

- Later stages often involve the individual's quest for more information regarding one's own group, accompanied by a drawing away from other groups, and a resolution in which the person becomes more universally tolerant.

We present two models here, both developed by Janet Helms (1993; 1995), to illustrate the general process of ethnic and cultural identity development. According to her model of White Identity Development, whites move through a developmental process in which they begin to abandon racism and learn to develop a positive white identity. (Note: Although we use the term *European Americans* in this chapter to refer to mainstream individuals, we use the term *white* here in keeping with Helm's language.) Helms' model was originally

Allison's Story

Allison, a licensed professional counselor, wrote the following regarding her dissatisfaction with training in diversity-related issues:

"Soon after I started my internship, I was confronted by the challenge for which I was least prepared, and for which perhaps we're ALL least prepared. This is the experience of working with 'multiply stressed' families.

"These families are outside the social and cultural mainstream, dealing on a daily basis with situations that would sink me if I faced them. They often have values that are confusing to the 'helping community,' including educators and health practitioners, and generally they have little trust for these helpers. Nonetheless, they need to interface with mainstream society, if only because their children are required to attend school. I've been working in school-based mental health, so I straddle several of these worlds. And worlds apart they are. My highest percentage of parental turndowns for service comes from the highest-need population. The reason is simple—they don't trust us. They see a short straight line between agreeing to counseling for their child to having the child removed from their home. And I don't blame them! They haven't been treated well by very many systems.

"My professional development training never gets into these issues. It's like the elephant in the living room. I go to a fine presentation on working with adolescents and their parents. Then I'm supposed to translate from the vignette with the well-educated middle-class parents in the presentation to the elderly female relative who is caring for her two grandchildren while their mother is in jail. This is the same woman who reportedly lost her own children to the system long ago for being an 'unfit mother.' Both girls have been sexually abused in the past by male relatives. They live in a small cluster of homes in a 'subcommunity' of people who wrestle with wrenching daily anxiety about basic needs. People in this group don't necessarily trust one another much more than they trust me."

Questions for Reflection

1. Think for a few minutes about Allison's experience. How can you prepare yourself now to work with families such as those Allison describes?

2. How will you build rapport, and eventually build trust, with people who are markedly different from you?

3. How can you help your agency be responsive to the particular needs of clients who have reason to mistrust established mental health systems?

presented as a stage-based developmental model, but she later called the various levels "statuses" to reflect the dynamic nature of progression in the model.

The *contact* status represents a basic level of awareness of the implications of race. Whites who exhibit contact beliefs tend to be oblivious or deny race as a salient issue.

The next status, *disintegration,* is marked by disorientation and confusion. At this point, the white individual has been confronted with contradictions and/or evidence that indicate that racism and prejudice exist. The person therefore feels torn between maintaining a sense of loyalty to whites—and thereby denying or justifying racism—versus confronting his or her own prejudice. At this point, the white person may begin to believe that whites are actually superior to other groups.

In the *reintegration* status, she or he will engage in selective perception and may avoid contact with those who are different. The person will likely look down on other racial groups and maintain the belief that whites are superior.

The *pseudoindependence* status marks movement toward developing a more positive white identity. At this point, the person begins to accept intellectually that being white means something, and that racism and oppression do exist. The person may seek to accept other groups but is not emotionally invested in exploring her or his own role in perpetuating racism.

In the *immersion/emersion* status, people begin to become more aware, emotionally and cognitively, of the effects of racism and start to examine the personal effects of race or ethnicity on themselves. The person at this status actively seeks information about race-related issues and may engage in race-related activism.

The final status, *autonomy,* reflects a person who has made a commitment to denounce racism and give up unearned white privilege. The person at the autonomy status avoids perpetuation of oppression and racism whenever possible.

Helms expanded on Cross's original work to develop a model of Black Racial Identity that then evolved into a model describing racial identity development for People of Color (1995) in general. In this model, people of color can move through five statuses, beginning with *conformity*. People in *conformity* tend to devalue their own group while valuing whites.

At some point, many people of color have an experience that challenges their conformity. Perhaps they witness racism or experience prejudicial treatment first-hand. They may then experience *dissonance,* a status marked by confusion and ambivalence.

The *immersion/emersion* status occurs as people of color begin to idealize their own group and denigrate what is seen as white. People of color at the immersion/ emersion status may experience group pride and seek to actively avoid whites and white culture.

The *internalization* status involves a positive commitment to one's own group, coupled with the ability to be objective about the strengths and weaknesses of whites.

The final status, *integrative awareness,* suggests that the person can value her or his own identity while respecting and empathizing with other groups. The person experiencing integrative awareness is able to look beyond her or his own group to see the importance and relevance of all groups.

Models of identity development are useful for a number of reasons. First, they remind us that not all members of a group are alike. Second, these models provide us with a framework from which we can conceptualize our clients' reactions to their surrounding environments. Third, they alert us to the contextual nature of our identities and the ways in which societal influences affect us (Helms, 1995). Furthermore, models of identity development help counselors keep in mind that people's attitudes regarding their identity change over time. However, these models are not personality theories. They focus instead primarily on how one's group membership, such as sexual orientation or ethnicity, influences one's perceptions about self and others. These models are one example of the type of research being generated that can inform community counseling work.

Comprehensive Conceptualization

In their efforts to achieve multicultural competence, community counselors are expected to make accurate diagnoses, identify appropriate goals and treatment plans, and provide effective intervention and prevention strategies. These actions are predicated on the existence of an accurate and thorough conceptualization of the client in context. However, counselors must also respond to the demands of agency policies, managed health regulations, and insurance requirements which often require provisional diagnoses after the first visit.

The best way to avoid the potential pitfalls of meeting such demands is for counselors to learn and practice effective conceptualization skills. The following model for conceptualization is an example that can be adapted to the counselor's needs depending on agency setting and client characteristics.

D'Andrea and Daniels (2001) created the RESPECTFUL counseling model in an attempt to provide a comprehensive view of client dynamics. The RESPECTFUL approach suggests that counselors consider every client's:

R—Religious and spiritual identity

E—Economic class background

S—Sexual identity

P—Psychological maturity

E—Ethnic/racial identity

C—Chronological/developmental challenges

T—Trauma and threats to well-being

F—Family background

U—Unique physical characteristics

L—Location of residence and language differences

Ideally, as they glean additional information from the mental status exam and intake interview, community counselors will ensure that the above characteristics are assessed.

Counselors should then consider several additional factors. First, what is the role of the community agency and the counselor in the client's life? Has the client struggled with social service systems in the past, or is he or she a newcomer to counseling? Does the client see the agency as a place of assistance, or a bureaucratic bundle of regulations and obstacles? How does the client view the counselor? Is the counselor seen as an agent of hope, or as one more member of the establishment? Does the client want the counselor to serve as an adviser, a resource person, a confidant, or an advocate? The answers to these questions will profoundly influence the counseling relationship.

Second, is this client currently in crisis or particularly vulnerable? Although this question will be a part of every intake interview you complete, the answer has particular relevance for clients who are culturally different from the counselor. In these situations the counselor may be more likely to miss hints or suggestions that reveal intense stress. Perhaps the client has insufficient trust at this point to reveal his distress. Adherence to cultural or family characteristics may also inhibit disclosures that feel too private or personal (Sue & Sue, 2003). Furthermore, mainstream counselors must work vigilantly to ensure they adequately understand the environmental stressors that affect some culturally different clients. Personal safety, for instance, is a daily concern for many in the United States.

Third, what existing sources of support can help this client? Some African American clients, for instance, may find assistance from spiritual practices and religious figures. Hip hop and rap music are also sources of comfort to some younger African American clients. Seeking help from herb doctors, a shaman, or elders can be common forms of self-help in cultures ranging from the rural poor to Hmong clients to Quakers.

Finally, how will the counselor create and maintain a therapeutic relationship best designed to meet this client's needs? This emphasis on the relationship between the counselor and client suggests another important step toward achieving multicultural competence—attending to the culture of the counseling relationship itself.

Attending to the Counseling Process and Relationship

Pedersen (2002) identified several measures that can be helpful in ensuring that the multicultural counseling process is relevant and responsive to clients' needs. First, identifying and focusing on the poignancy of a client's story, in order to illuminate and then talk about the client's struggle, may help the counselor attend to the client's worldview in a manner consistent with the Multicultural Counseling Competencies. Further, being especially watchful for resistance, reluctance, or misunderstanding from the client may provide vitally helpful information to the community counselor in building a therapeutic alliance with a culturally different client.

Pedersen also suggests that avoiding defensive and biased responses to client diversity requires the counselor to have explored and sought understanding of her own biases, unresolved issues, and worldview. Should a culture-related problem or misunderstanding occur, the counselor is expected to use recovery skills to promptly and respectfully address the issue. Failure to do so is likely to result in clients who terminate early or who discount the potential usefulness of counseling.

Finally, counselors are encouraged to ensure that their conceptualizations are flexible, thorough, and adaptive to new information. These goals seem relevant to effective work with all clients and can help community counselors avoid fundamental mistakes in understanding clients' concerns and contexts. The above concepts form the basis for preparing to work effectively with diverse clients. We also recommend that community counselors consider the following as they work with diverse clients:

- Ask your clients to explain specifically what they want from the counseling process. Why have they come to see a counselor? What do they hope to achieve?

- Determine what your clients want from *you* as counselor. What roles do your clients want you to take? How do they want you to help them? For instance, are they expecting you to serve as a therapist, facilitator, or guide?

- Negotiate with your client an appropriate counseling culture (Castillo, 1997). Consider the ways in which what you offer as a counselor does and does not meet your clients' wants and needs. Then work with the client to figure out how you can build an effective relationship.

- Be honest with your clients. If you need clarification, ask. If you're confused about an aspect of the relationship, be immediate. Talk about the process when appropriate.

- Be flexible. Realize that your theoretical orientation may be irrelevant or poorly suited to your clients' needs. Understand that many cultures are much more communal than the European American norm of the United States. Including family in treatment and decision making is often a requisite part of effective practice.

• Work to articulate the client's struggle. Remembering that you don't have to solve a client's problem can help you achieve the perspective you need to listen, understand, and validate the client's concern.

• Know when you need help. If you don't understand how best to work with a client, seek supervision and/or consultation. Similarly, know when you need to refer.

• Be familiar with indigenous models of helping that may be appropriate for your clients. Ideally, you will have contacts with people in other cultures who can help you understand and access culturally appropriate helping processes.

• Take responsibility for learning about the cultures in your area. Expecting your clients to teach you everything about their beliefs is passive and wastes clinical time.

• Work to develop cultural empathy (Chung & Bemak, 2002), which will enable you to be sensitive to the unique experiences of your clients. Cultural empathy requires a broad level of sensitivity and respect that could perhaps be described as a type of respectful awe for the client's experience and needs—a lofty goal, perhaps, but one well worth pursuing.

CONSIDERATIONS FOR WORKING WITH SPECIFIC GROUPS

In order to become multiculturally competent in their work, community counselors are expected to draw from the aforementioned knowledge and skill areas to develop responsive and effective counseling interventions. How can we best counsel African Americans? What is the best way to work with European American men? Which techniques work best for gay/lesbian/bisexual or transgendered clients? These questions themselves are flawed, for they suggest a uniformity among people, indeed even among counselors and counseling sessions, that doesn't exist. Attempting to characterize a specific culture is a difficult and risky task. Furthermore, treating individuals as members of a group rather than as distinct individuals is ineffective and potentially unethical (Ridley, Liddle, Hill, & Li, 2001). Doing so would ignore the unique characteristics of the individual client.

However, the fact that people share a culture suggests that the people within that culture share common beliefs and practices. Further, societal treatment of individuals within cultural groups is often consistent and comprises a shared, common experience for the group. African Americans often face

...crimination, for instance, as do people with disabilities. Immigrants often face acculturative stress as they attempt to create a life for themselves in the United States. From this framework, then, we can provide an overview of different populations, highlighting potential shared areas of concerns and suggesting relevant counseling implications.

Ethnic Minorities

The largest groups of ethnic minorities in the United States are Latinos, African Americans, and Asians. These groups are extremely heterogeneous, and they share little except for their status as minorities. This status, however, suggests that members of these groups may experience more discrimination and oppression than European Americans. These factors are significant considerations for community counselors.

Furthermore, these clients may be less likely to voluntarily seek counseling services and more likely to expect direct assistance from counselors than to desire reflective, introspective counseling services (Sue & Sue, 2003). Several researchers and practitioners have developed intervention strategies that hold promise for working with specific members of these population groups. Adams and LaFromboise (2001), for instance, developed the "Mother-Daughter Relational Group Therapy" program to strengthen relationship and coping skills among one segment of the African American population. This group intervention relied on self-in-relation theory and the application of interpersonal and cognitive behavioral approaches. The women worked through a series of groups in which they explored the problems and potential in their relationships, and then worked toward developing greater empathy. Participants in the group reported that the strengthened relationships between mother and daughter seemed to moderate the effects of stress in their daily lives. This group relied on Afrocentric theory and practices that complemented cultural traditions to create an apparently effective intervention.

Several resources exist for counselors working to expand their competence with Latino clients. For instance, Santiago-Rivera, Arredondo, and Gallardo-Cooper (2002) have published a guidebook for working with Latino families. This book draws on the multicultural counseling competencies and provides specific strategies for working with Latino clients, including the appropriate use of interpreters, understanding etiquette expectations, and developing culture-centered genograms.

Similarly, Sue (1997) offers several suggestions for working with Asian Americans. Countering the notion that Asians are the "model minority," Sue states that the Chinese in America, in particular, present a bimodal distribution of success. One group is very successful, and one group is very poor.

Thus, counselors must ensure that they have accurately conceptualized their Asian clients prior to offering interventions. For example, Sue provides specific suggestions for providing appropriate assertiveness training for Chinese Americans, which include discussing culture and racism, exploring situational assertiveness, and using practice and cognitive coping strategies. Such a training experience would certainly not be appropriate for every Chinese American client.

However, of note here is Sue's emphasis on creating an intervention that relies on clear understanding of the client's own culture and the juxtaposition of that culture with the dominant U.S. culture. Further, Atkinson, Kim, and Caldwell (1998) present a compelling argument that counselors working with Asian American clients should reconsider their role as therapists. Instead, these researchers suggest that counselors expand their counseling roles to include serving as *consultants* and *facilitators* of indigenous support systems.

One important subset of ethnic minority groups includes refugees and immigrants. Refugees by definition are those who are essentially forced to leave their countries of origin. Their flight from their native countries is typically hurried and involuntary (Chung, Bemak, & Okazaki, 1997), and most experience trauma and its aftereffects. Immigrants who are not refugees, on the other hand, often come to the United States in the hope of finding a better life for themselves (Lee, 1997). Although they may not be fleeing war or genocide, many immigrants do experience hardship and sometimes trauma as they attempt to settle in the United States. Both refugees and immigrants also experience acculturative stress (Miranda & Matheny, 2000).

Some communities have agencies dedicated to assisting these clients, such as Refugee Resettlement Centers and Migrant Education and Services Centers. Community counselors should realize, however, that historical and environmental stressors on these community members are often intense (Hondageneu-Sotelo, 1999; Miranda & Matheny, 2000). Language barriers, unfamiliar cultural practices, and mistrust are potential obstacles to effective counseling services. Bemak, Chung, and Bornemann (1996) developed the Multi-Level Model to provide mental health education, therapy, cultural empowerment, and indigenous healing options to refugees. This model presents a promising, comprehensive approach to helping refugees cope with their lives in the United States.

These interventions are just a glimpse of the resources available to community counselors. They are potentially effective because they share (1) an emphasis on accurate understanding of minority culture, (2) a focus on existing client strengths, and (3) the use of culturally consistent and acceptable intervention strategies. These strategies can thus serve as a guide for counselors attempting to develop appropriate interventions in their own communities (Pope & Coleman, 2001).

Gay, Lesbian, Bisexual, and Transgendered Populations

Demographers struggle to identify the exact proportions of the U.S. society who are straight, gay, lesbian, bisexual, or transgendered. Estimates suggest that up to 15 percent of the U.S. population is gay, lesbian, bisexual, or transgendered (GLBT) (Barret & Logan, 2002). Although the ACA Code of Ethics (2005) mandates that counselors avoid discrimination against sexual minorities, counselors should realize that heterosexism, a form of discrimination in which heterosexuality is seen as normal and other sexual orientations as deviant, is common in the United States. Even more disturbing is homophobia, in which an individual expresses extreme hate or fear of gays and lesbians. These concerns are very relevant for GLBT clients and are sometimes experienced as ubiquitous environmental stressors.

Many GLBT clients also experience stress as they determine whether or not, or when, to come out to family, friends, and society. These clients face restrictions on their ability to marry or publicly commit to partners and their ability to comfortably express affection to partners in public. They are not universally protected in workplace antidiscrimination and equal employment statements.

Barret and Logan (2002) provided several guidelines for counselors hoping to effectively serve the GLBT community. Among them are the expectations that counselors understand their own beliefs regarding sexual orientation; comprehend the role of politics in the GLBT community, such as the significance of gay marriage bans, sodomy laws, and workplace discrimination; learn theories regarding homosexuality; and understand the challenges facing GLBT clients who are also ethnic minorities. Although intended specifically for work with GLBT clients, these guidelines are relevant for all multicultural counseling work. The organization *Parents, Families and Friends of Lesbians and Gays* (PFLAG, **www.pflag.org**) is a helpful starting place for counselors searching for more information and resources.

People with Disabilities

According to the U.S. Census Bureau (**www.census.gov**), people with disabilities represent 19 percent of the U.S. population over the age of five. European Americans have the lowest rate of disabilities, and the rate of disabilities tends to increase as people become older. The 1990 Americans with Disabilities Act (ADA), designed to end discrimination against people with disabilities, defines disabilities as impairments that substantially limit a major life activity, that are of importance to most people's lives, and that are permanent or long-term. Disabilities include emotional, cognitive, behavioral, and physical impairments that can be congenital or can occur as the result of illness or accident. Review this act at the ADA website, **www.ada.gov.**

EXPERIENTIAL LEARNING

The Reverend Fred Phelps, of Topeka Kansas, creator of the Westboro Baptist Church, has gained notoriety for his outspoken condemnation of gays, lesbians, bisexuals, and transgendered individuals. He has picketed the funerals of people like Matthew Shepard, a young gay man who was brutally murdered simply because he was gay. Phelps keeps an active agenda for picketing funerals and protesting programs that support GLBT issues. Imagine that Phelps plans to picket your community.

1. As a community counselor, what would your response be to Phelps' presence?

2. What effect do you think antigay activists like Phelps would have on your clients who are gay, lesbian, bisexual, or transgendered?

3. If you are straight, or heterosexual, what assumptions do you think your clients who are sexual minorities might have about you and your views on gays, lesbians, bisexuals, and transgendered people? If you are a sexual minority, what assumptions might your clients have about you that may be relevant to address in the counseling relationship?

People with disabilities face numerous stressors in addition to the stress of the disability itself. The prevalence of stereotypes regarding people with disabilities as pitiable, damaged, helpless, and heroic (Lee, 1999) undoubtedly negatively affects counselors and clients, and undermines the dignity of the individual. Furthermore, daily living skills such as mobility, self-care, and the ability to support oneself financially and physically can be very difficult for people with disabilities. Clients who have disabilities and who are also ethnic or racial minorities face distinct challenges. Bryan's (1999) coverage of the multicultural aspects of disabilities is a particularly useful tool for counselors working with this population.

In order to work most effectively with community members with disabilities, counselors are encouraged to understand federal regulations regarding disability, including the Workforce Investment Act and the Work Incentives Improvement Act, which have direct bearing on many community agencies. Further, counselors should ensure that their agency is accessible to people with disabilities; explore their own biases and prejudices regarding people with disabilities; understand the role of rehabilitation counselors, occupational therapists, and physical therapists in their clients' lives; and treat their clients with respect and dignity. The American Rehabilitation Counseling Association, a division of ACA, is a particularly helpful resource for community counselors attempting to enhance their understanding of the culture of people with disabilities.

Religious Minorities

The majority of the U.S. population, 83 percent, is Christian. Thirteen percent of the people in the United States report having no religious preference, Jews represent about 2 percent of the population, Muslims, and Buddhists each comprise about 0.5 percent, and Hindus about 0.4 percent (Kosmin & Mayer, 2001). Often, clients who are members of religious minorities are members of ethnic or racial minorities as well.

Clients who are members of religious minorities deserve special consideration in light of recent world events. The terrorist attacks of September 11, 2001, have resulted in increased visibility of the religion of Islam in the United States. Unfortunately, however, for some in the United States the Islamic religion is unilaterally, and therefore inaccurately, linked with terrorism. Islamic terrorists constitute a subset of zealots who, most feel, in no way represent the teachings of the Koran. Even so, the incidence of hate crimes against Middle Eastern people and Arabs in the United States, including those who were simply perceived to be Middle Eastern or Arabic, increased significantly after 2001 (Djupe & Olson, 2003). Clients who are religious minorities may find themselves the victims of stereotyping, discrimination, and hate crimes. Counselors are thus encouraged to assess their community's climate regarding religious tolerance. Reaching out to religious minorities and building relationships with religious leaders and administrators are critical first steps to creating inclusive, safe communities. Ideally, counselors will also educate themselves regarding religious and spiritual practices, including knowing the dates of relevant religious holidays, appreciating religious practices that influence dress and dietary habits, and respecting the manifestation of diverse religious beliefs.

The Elderly

According to the U.S. Administration on Aging (2003), 12.3 percent of the U.S. population is sixty-five years of age or older. In 2002, people who were sixty-five years of age could expect to live another nineteen years if they were female, or another sixteen years if they were male. The older population is expected to grow significantly in the future. In part because of advancements in medical care, we can expect the population of older people to swell to 20 percent of the population by 2030. The population of elderly in the United States is incredibly diverse, but many people in this category share common characteristics.

In 2002, among women aged seventy-five and over, half lived alone (Administration on Aging, 2003). Older men are more likely to be married, and older women are more likely to be widowed. A little over 8 percent of elderly European Americans were poor in 2002, compared to 23 percent of elderly African Americans and 21 percent of elderly Latinos. The poverty rate is higher for older women than for older men.

Most elderly people, regardless of ethnicity and gender, face multiple declines in mental and/or physical functioning. As they adapt to these changes, they also often have to deal with adjustment issues related to retirement, loss of loved ones, and anticipation of death (Myers & Harper, 2004). Approximately one-third of the elderly population is believed to have mental health problems such as anxiety and depression (Smyer & Qualls, 1999). Loneliness and depression are key considerations for elderly clients, as are pragmatic issues such as transportation and access to counseling services.

Counselors can best serve the elderly population in their communities by first assessing how the mental health needs of this group are currently being met. Some communities have strong networks of home health providers, aging services coalitions, and elderly protective service agencies. Other communities, however, especially in rural areas, provide services in piecemeal fashion and are apt to miss large segments of the population. Perhaps the most efficient and effective way to build connections with the elderly population is to connect with local hospitals, agencies, and physicians who work with elderly patients. These sources can provide valuable referrals.

When working with elderly clients, counselors should be prepared to assess their own feelings regarding aging, including their beliefs about and reactions to death and dying issues. According to Myers and Harper (2004), building rapport with elderly clients may be challenging, as these clients may feel hesitant to seek counseling. Elderly clients may also treat counselors as physicians, thereby expecting a directive and authoritarian relationship with the helper. Kennedy and Tanenbaum (2000) found that adapting therapy to accommodate age-related concerns is warranted and that interventions adapted for elderly clients may be as effective as those for younger clients. Thus, responding to clients' physical limitations and needs, their connections with family, and their cognitive capabilities is key. Read about Gena's experience in "'Grandma' Fowler's" story, told in the following box. Although this population has not been adequately researched, existing studies indicate that the potential exists for counseling services to be helpful for elderly clients. This potential is especially evident when the community counselor is willing to show flexibility, genuine interest, and regard when meeting with elderly clients. The American Association of Retired Persons (AARP) website, **www.aarp.org,** has numerous helpful resources.

"Grandma" Fowler

When Gena was a community counseling intern, she was assigned an outreach caseload that included several elderly clients. At the time Gena was thirty-five years old and married with children. A European American woman beginning her second career, Gena had a reasonable amount of self-confidence, both personally and professionally, and enjoyed the opportunities she had to visit with her elderly clients in their homes.

A month into her internship, Gena found that she had started to become preoccupied with one of her clients. Mrs. Fowler, also known in her neighborhood as "Grandma" Fowler, was an eighty-two-year-old African American woman who struggled with diabetes and depression. When Gena first met with Mrs. Fowler, she labeled her as "grumpy and sullen," but after a few weeks Gena realized that Mrs. Fowler's grumpy presentation was simply a façade. She was, in fact, a dynamic and alert woman who was initially slightly suspicious of the white counselor who came to visit her.

Gena talked with Mrs. Fowler about their ethnic differences, and the two developed sufficient rapport to enable Gena to more fully hear and understand Mrs. Fowler's concerns. Gena found that she began to feel protective of Mrs. Fowler, angry toward the "ungrateful" children who took her money and never visited, and impatient with the "nosy" neighbors who offered too much advice and too little assistance. In response, Gena began to expand her professional boundaries: She volunteered to call the local home health agency for Mrs. Fowler when she had a billing question. She gave Mrs. Fowler a poinsettia at Christmas. She gave Mrs. Fowler a ride to her neighbor's house, and at one point she took Mrs. Fowler on a drive so that she could see the new shopping mall being built near her home.

Gena would occasionally feel uneasy about these "extras" she provided for Mrs. Fowler, but she convinced herself that she was acting appropriately in order to meet the specific, cultural needs of her client. As an elderly African American woman, Gena reasoned, Mrs. Fowler had distinct expectations of the counseling relationship. *It would be silly for me not to comply on such minor issues,* Gena told herself.

One day as she concluded her supervision session, Gena mentioned to her supervisor in passing that Mrs. Fowler had given her an excellent recipe for pumpkin pie. Gena's supervisor looked confused. "That's interesting," he said. "How did you find yourself exchanging recipes during a counseling session?" Initially Gena felt self-righteous and slightly superior. "In multicultural situations such as this," she explained, "it's appropriate to respond to the client's cues. By allowing Mrs. Fowler to give me this recipe I was respecting her cultural need to establish a personal relationship with me."

"Really," said her supervisor. "I was just thinking that the way you describe Mrs. Fowler is the way you've described your own grandmother. Are you

(continued)

("Grandma" Fowler, continued)

responding to cultural cues or giving in to countertransference?"

Gena was dismayed to find that she couldn't answer her supervisor. She truly had no idea how to assess the professionalism of her relationship with "Grandma" Fowler.

Questions for Reflection

1. How will you identify the distinction between responding to clients' cultural needs and expectations and losing your therapeutic boundaries?

2. In the case of Gena and Mrs. Fowler, age rather than ethnicity was a salient concern affecting the relational dynamic between counselor and client. What are your stereotypes and expectations of elderly clients? How might your own experiences, or lack of experience, with the elderly influence your counseling work?

CONSIDERATIONS FOR WORKING AT THE COMMUNITY LEVEL

Clearly, community counselors who seek multicultural competence must use appropriate prevention and intervention strategies with their individual clients. We are expected to be agents of change. A critical expectation of community counselors is that we also work to enhance the communities in which we live. Although some counselors still struggle with their roles as advocates, the skill of advocacy is a foundation of community counseling work (Lewis & Bradley, 2000).

Advocacy

The 2005 ACA Code of Ethics mentions advocacy as a specific expectation for counselors. As we mentioned in Chapter 2, when working as advocates counselors speak up for the clients. They assess and attempt to anticipate their clients' needs, and then use their personal and systemic power to intervene. A key consideration in advocacy work is to ensure that the counselor never takes power from the client (Toporek & Liu, 2001). Speaking on behalf of people who can already use their own voices may actually inhibit and marginalize clients. Rather, counselors begin their advocacy work with a clear conceptualization of their clients' capabilities, and then step in to build on existing strengths. This type of advocacy can include communicating often with representatives of various social service and community agencies, such as Community Service Boards, Child Protective Services, Health Departments, Police Departments, and schools, regarding specific client populations. Sharing understanding of different client populations' characteristics and concerns can facilitate genuine preventive work (Mayo, 2000).

In some cases, this type of advocacy may take the form of secondary rather than primary prevention. For instance, a community that relied heavily on Asian immigrant farm labor endured a tragedy when a Cambodian refugee was killed by the town's SWAT team. The man, who suffered from PTSD, was drinking one evening and remembering the brutal days before his flight from Cambodia. He grabbed a gun and started firing shots into the air, shouting that he was trying to drive away evil spirits. Frightened neighbors tried to calm him and eventually called the police. The police arrived quickly, but no one in the force was able to speak the man's language. The police responded in what they felt was the only way to ensure their own and residents' safety: they killed the man in his apartment.

The response from the surrounding community was mixed and volatile. Many felt the police were too hasty, some felt that the incident "proved" that refugees were dangerous, and others felt the police had no choice but to respond with violence. Anticipating an increase in anti-immigrant and anti-refugee sentiment, and recognizing a genuine need in the community, several counselors called a community meeting to discuss the issue. At this meeting the counselors worked to dispel myths about refugees, educate citizens and agency representatives regarding the needs of the population, mourn the loss of a community member, and soothe recent immigrant and refugee citizens' fears regarding the police.

The role of the community counselor need not always be so dramatic, and most situations are not necessarily lethal. The role of advocate, however, is likely to be one of the most challenging—and potentially effective— endeavors of the community counselor.

Policy Action

Counselors can also work at the community level by initiating or influencing policy development and changes. Community counselors are in the somewhat unique position to know first-hand what environmental stressors face their clients, and to be able to clearly articulate their clients' needs. Community counselors hear from their clients, for instance, when schools and other community institutions are unresponsive to clients' concerns. They witness the effects of discrimination and see the results of inadequate housing. They know when the community is letting their clients down. Therefore, counselors are perhaps the best people to advocate for the initiation of human service and mental health programs and to speak out against restrictive or ineffective policies (Toporek & Liu, 2001).

When working at the community level, counselors can effect significant systemic change. By relying on their own expertise regarding their clients, using the participation of citizens themselves, and tapping into community

It's Not *Really* Sex

A group of counselors who specialized in providing counseling to adolescents met regularly for consultation. In discussing their cases, they discovered that they had all recently encountered an increasing number of young Latino adolescent clients who had developed oral and genital herpes. After discussing the issue among themselves and with their clients, the counselors discovered that many of the young people in their community viewed oral sex as a safe type of pseudo sex. The adolescents were unaware of the potential risks of oral sex and were living in a culture in which fear of unwanted pregnancy was of paramount concern.

In response, the counselors pushed local school and community officials to develop community-wide counseling and educational services regarding the potential hazards of unprotected oral sex. They found, however, that the school and community leaders were hesitant to specifically address the topic of oral sex. They feared that they would look like they were advocating premarital sex rather than abstinence for adolescents. The counselors felt limited in their ability to respond effectively until finally a Mexican American counselor found several Latino families who were willing to help spread the word that oral sex is not necessarily safe sex.

Questions for Reflection

1. If you were to encounter a similar situation in your community, how would you attempt to educate the client population regarding safe sex?

2. In this case, Latino families who came into contact with the community counseling agency were reluctant to talk about sex with their counselors and refused to talk about it with their children. How might you address this reluctance while maintaining a respectful relationship with your clients?

networks, they can provide an essential framework for building effective community interventions (Duffy & Wong, 2003). See "It's Not *Really* Sex" in the accompanying box for what happened when one group of counselors worked with the local community.

SUGGESTIONS FOR ONGOING PERSONAL AND PROFESSIONAL GROWTH

In essence, developing multicultural competence requires counselors to step out of their comfort zone and risk feeling awkward, uncertain, and unsettled about themselves and their relationships with others. Although it is a challenging task, the graduate training experience is the ideal setting in which to embark on this journey. Students are in the right place to live with ambiguity, accept feedback, question assumptions, and manage intense emotions.

As you work to develop and refine your skills, consider the following steps you can take toward developing multicultural counseling competence. Personally:

- Know yourself. Know your own values, as well as your own biases.
- Continue to expand your cultural awareness.
- Make every effort to confront your prejudices and stereotypes.
- Set lofty goals for your own pursuit of multicultural competency in counseling.
- Spend time with those who are different from you.
- Explore your community, and take advantage of the range of diverse experiences the community can provide for you.

Professionally:

- Become an advocate. If your clients' and other citizens' needs are not being met in your community, use your power and speak up.
- Assess the culture of the agencies and organizations in which you work. Are these places open to and welcoming of clients who live outside mainstream U.S. culture? Do they take a preventive stance in which they work toward client empowerment?
- Develop a list of community resources—people and agencies—to whom you and your clients can turn for assistance.

As you work on developing your multicultural competence, keep this dilemma in mind: The less comfortable we feel with those who are different, the more likely we are to avoid them. The more likely we are to avoid difference, the more likely we are to feel uncomfortable with difference. And so it goes. How will you break this cycle?

ETHICAL AND LEGAL ISSUES IN PRACTICE

One of the most challenging ethical issues for counselors is responding appropriately to the ambiguity inherent in many ethical dilemmas. Although ethical codes are helpful, they do not always prescribe action or help the counselor thoroughly think through the situation (Ridley, Liddle, Hill, & Li, 2001). Further, Pedersen (1997) has stated that the 1995 ACA Code of Ethics promoted the perspective of the dominant culture and failed to acknowledge the potential impact of culture. Fortunately, the revised ACA Code of Ethics (2005) addresses some of these shortcomings. For instance, multicultural and diversity considerations are specifically mentioned in the new Code in sections regarding informed consent, bartering, respecting clients' rights, nondiscrimination, diagnosis, assessment, counselor education and training, and research.

However, complicated ethical questions can become even more complicated when multicultural issues are involved. In response, Ridley, Liddle, Hill, and Li (2001) suggest the following model of ethical decision making. First, counselors must determine whether or not an ethical problem exists. Specifically, does the immediate concern reflect a conflict with ethical codes and accepted standards of practice? Second, the counselor is encouraged to make his or her own ethical perspectives explicit. Is the counselor operating from a universal approach, for instance, in which one standard exists for all, or a relativist stance? Next, counselors are encouraged to seek consultation from trusted others. Checking in with colleagues and supervisors is often helpful. Counselors are then encouraged to openly explore assumptions about culture, examining their own beliefs as well as ways in which culture impacts the overall situation. The next step involves brainstorming with the clients and others about how the issue arose and how the issue may have been avoided. This step is important in ensuring that counselors and agencies learn from and adapt to diverse cultures and the new challenges they may generate. Finally, counselors are encouraged to brainstorm solutions and analyze the feasibility and acceptability—including the cultural acceptability—of various responses. Although this model is not strikingly different from many commonly accepted approaches to ethical decision making, it includes reminders to assess the impact of culture and to conceptualize not only the client, but the entire ethical situation, from the standpoint of possible cultural difference.

The potential for legal ramifications regarding multicultural counseling is present any time services are offered in a potentially discriminatory or prejudicial manner. Using assessment instruments that are culturally biased, for instance, may result in counselors being accused of endorsing discrimination (Swenson, 1993; Cottone & Tarvydas, 1998). Further, ignorance of relevant cultural expectations may place counselors at risk for accusations of malpractice if they diagnose without considering the client's context. For instance, clients who have been systematically exposed to oppression may understandably present as hostile. If this hostility is perceived as strictly antisocial in nature, then the counselor's assessment is flawed.

Counselors are also in error if they suggest interventions that could potentially disrupt a client's lifestyle. In one instance, for example, a counselor suggested that a female Muslim client become more assertive with her husband, demanding more freedom and access to family resources. When the client did as the counselor suggested, the woman's husband beat her and threatened the counselor. Although the counselor wasn't sued, certainly her behavior did not demonstrate an adequate standard of care.

EXPERIENTIAL LEARNING

Perhaps one of the most useful actions you can take right now is to formalize your process of self-assessment and reflection regarding diversity and your own multicultural counseling competence. We invite you to complete the following self-assessment and develop your own professional development plan.

Use the following scale to evaluate your own multicultural counseling knowledge and skills:

1	2	3	4	5
Not Very	A Little	About the Same as Most People	Very	Thoroughly

_____ How knowledgeable are you about your own cultural/ethnic group?

_____ How knowledgeable are you about cultural/ethnic groups other than your own? (If you write four or above, list the groups about which you are most knowledgeable.)

_____ How comfortable do you feel discussing race relations?

_____ How comfortable are you with the idea of counseling clients who are ethnically different from you?

_____ How comfortable are you with the idea of counseling clients whose religious or spiritual beliefs are different than yours?

_____ How comfortable are you with the idea of counseling clients who are from a different socioeconomic class than yours?

_____ How comfortable are you with the idea of counseling clients who have a different sexual orientation than yours?

_____ How comfortable are you with the idea of counseling clients who have a visible physical disability?

_____ How skilled do you think you will be in counseling "culturally different" clients in general?

_____ How open are you to learning more about multicultural issues that affect you?

Take some time to think about your responses. Record any additional thoughts and reactions you may have as you select your answers. Then, based on your responses, develop a plan to enhance your personal and professional development.

Finally, when counselors and clients are dramatically different from each other, whether through culture, lifestyle, or language, the potential for misunderstandings, faulty diagnoses, or inaccurate conceptualizations can increase. Thus, as we've mentioned before, counselors are advised to know themselves and their biases, know their clients as well as they can, and find supportive and effective consultation and supervision to ensure that the most effective and appropriate care is offered.

CONCLUDING THOUGHTS

This chapter has provided a brief overview of a very complex and vital topic for community counselors. As our society continues to become more diverse, counselors are called upon to refine their skills in order to provide ethical and effective service. We encourage you to spend time now, while you're in the protected environment of your training program, to venture beyond your comfort zone, examine your own attitudes, increase your knowledge of and develop your skills for working with diverse clients.

RECOMMENDED RESOURCES

Ponterotto, Casas, Suzuki, and Alexander have edited two very helpful resources: the first and second editions of The *Handbook of Multicultural Counseling* (Ponterotto, Casas, Suzuki, & Alexander, 1995 & 2001). These books, which differ widely in their coverage, offer chapters that include empirical, conceptual, and strategy-based topics. One organization that is particularly relevant for community counselors is the *Association for Multicultural Counseling and Development,* which is a division of the American Counseling Association. Chartered in 1972, AMCD strives to improve cultural, ethnic and racial empathy and understanding to advance and sustain personal growth. The address of its webpage is **www.amcd-aca.org.** The AMCD produces *The Journal of Multicultural Counseling and Development,* which is a vital resource for community counselors.

Several divisions of ACA will also be helpful to those interested in learning more about certain populations. You may want to look into the Association for Adult Development and Aging, the Association for Gay, Lesbian, and Bisexual Issues in Counseling, the American Rehabilitation and Counseling Association, and Counselors for Social Justice. More information regarding these divisions is available on the ACA webpage **www.counseling.org.**

You may also be interested in joining a listserv that is dedicated to discussing diversity issues in counseling. To join, send an e-mail to **Listserv@listserv.american. edu.** Leave the subject line blank, and in the body of the message place the following: "Subscribe Diversegrad-L," your e-mail address, and your full name.

Other Resources

Numerous movies and books will be helpful to you as you continue to explore the concept of difference as it relates to counseling. *The Color Purple* by Alice Walker is the fascinating story of the transformation of the heroine Celie from a submissive African American adolescent into an assertive woman. *The Joy Luck Club* by Amy Tan poetically explores both the experience of immigration and the sometimes painful and always complicated dynamics of mother-daughter relationships. Ralph Ellison's *The Invisible Man* is one of the few masterpieces of American literature in the twentieth century. It is one of those rare books that grabs you from the start and can forever change your way of thinking.

We strongly recommend you view and discuss the classic films *Blue-Eyed* and *The Color of Fear*. In recent years, there have been many movies that have addressed the issues of racism, sexism, oppression, and diversity. These include *Remember the Titans, Mi Familia, Torch Song Trilogy, Malcolm X, Avalon, I Am Sam, Priest, Far from Heaven, The Hurricane,* and *Boys Don't Cry. Crash* is an exceptionally powerful film that presents a challenging and comprehensive view of our struggles to live in a diverse society.

Once Were Warriors and *Whale Rider* are powerful portrayals of the Maori people of New Zealand as they struggle to cope with oppression and to reclaim their cultural heritage. *Whale Rider* has the bonus of being one of the rare movies that has a strong, determined, and resourceful girl as the main character.

REFERENCES

Adams, M., Bell, L. A., & Griffin, P. (Eds.). (1997). *Teaching for diversity and social justice: A sourcebook.* New York: Routledge.

Adams, V. L., & LaFromboise, T. D. (2001). Self-in-relation theory and African American female development. In D. Pope-Davis & H. Coleman (Eds.), *The intersection of race, class, and gender in multicultural counseling* (pp. 25–48). Thousand Oaks, CA: Sage.

Administration on Aging. (2003). *A Profile of Older Americans.* Retrieved July 2, 2004, from the U.S. Department of Health and Human Services Administration on Aging website: **http://www.aoa.gov/prof/Statistics/profile/ 2003/2003profile.pdf.**

Allport, G. W. (1954). *The nature of prejudice.* New York: Doubleday.

American Counseling Association. (2005). *ACA Code of Ethics.* Retrieved August 22, 2005, from **www.counseling.org/Content/NavigationMenu/ RESOURCES/ETHICS/ACA_Code_of_Ethics.htm.**

Appiah, K. A., & Gutmann, A. (1996). *Color conscious.* Princeton, NJ: Princeton University Press.

Arredondo, P., Toporek, R., Brown, S. P., Jones, J., Locke, D. C., Sanchez, J., & Stadler, H. (1996). Operationalization of the multicultural counseling competencies. *Journal of Multicultural Counseling and Development, 3*, 42–78.

Atkinson, D. R., Kim, B. S. K., & Caldwell, R. (1998). Ratings of helper roles by multicultural psychologists and Asian American students: Initial support for the three-dimensional model of multicultural counseling. *Journal of Counseling Psychology, 45*, 414–423.

Atkinson, D. R., Morten, G., & Sue, D. W. (1989). A minority identity development model. In D. R. Atkinson, G. Morten, & D. W. Sue (Eds.), *Counseling American Minorities* (pp. 35–52). Dubuque, IA: W. C. Brown.

Axelson, J. A. (1993). *Counseling and development in a multicultural society.* Pacific Grove, CA: Brooks/Cole.

Barret, B., & Logan, C. (2002). *Counseling gay men and lesbians: A practice primer.* Pacific Grove, CA: Brooks/Cole.

Baruth, L. G., & Manning, M. L. (2003). *Multicultural counseling and psychotherapy: A lifespan perspective* (3rd ed.). Upper Saddle River, NJ: Prentice Hall.

Bean, F. D., & Bell-Rose, S. (Eds.). (1999). *Immigration and opportunity: Race, ethnicity, and employment in the United States.* New York: Russell Sage Foundation.

Bemak, F., Chung, R., & Bornemann, T. (1996). Counseling and therapy with refugees. In P. Pedersen, J. Dragun, W. Lonner, & J. Trimble (Eds.), *Counseling across cultures* (4th ed., pp. 243–265). Thousand Oaks, CA: Sage.

Blank, R. M. (2001). An overview of trends in social and economic well-being, by race. In N. Smelser, W. Wilson, & F. Mitchell (Eds.), *America becoming: Racial trends and their consequences: Vol. 1* (pp. 21–39). Washington, DC: National Academy Press.

Boger, J. C., & Wegner, J. W. (Eds.). (1996). *Race, poverty and American cities.* Chapel Hill: University of North Carolina Press.

Bryan, W. V. (1999). *Multicultural aspects of disabilities.* Springfield, IL: Charles C. Thomas.

Bucher, R. D. (2004). *Diversity consciousness: Opening our minds to people, cultures, and opportunities* (2nd ed.). Upper Saddle River, NJ: Prentice Hall.

California by the numbers. (2004, May 23). *The Washington Post,* p. A2.

Cass, V. C. (1984). Homosexual identity formation: Testing a theoretical model. *Journal of Sex Research, 20*(2), 143–167.

Castillo, R. J. (1997). *Culture and mental illness: A client-centered approach.* Pacific Grove, CA: Brooks/Cole.

Chung, R. C., & Bemak, F. (2002). The relationship of culture and empathy in cross-cultural counseling. *Journal of Counseling and Development, 80,* 154–159.

Chung, R. C., Bemak, F., & Okazaki, S. (1997). Counseling Americans of Southeast Asian descent: The impact of the refugee experience. In C. Lee (Ed.), *Multicultural issues in counseling: New approaches to diversity* (2nd ed., pp. 207–232). Alexandria, VA: American Counseling Association.

Coleman, E. (1985). Developmental stages of the coming out process. In J. C. Gonsiorek (Ed.), *A guide to psychotherapy with gay and lesbian clients* (pp. 31–43). New York: Harrington Park.

Collins, J. F. (2000). Biracial Japanese American identity: An evolving process. *Cultural Diversity and Ethnic Minority Psychology, 7*(2), 115–120.

Cottone, R. R., & Tarvydas, V. M. (1998). *Ethical and professional issues in counseling.* Upper Saddle River, NJ: Merrill.

Cross, W. E. (1971). The Negro-to-Black conversion experience: Toward a psychology of Black liberation. *Black World, 20*(9), 13–27.

D'Andrea, M., & Daniels, J. (2001). RESPECTFUL counseling: An integrative model for counselors. In D. Pope-Davis & H. Coleman (Eds.), *The interface of class, culture, and gender in counseling* (pp. 417–466). Thousand Oaks, CA: Sage.

Diller, J. V. (2004). *Cultural diversity: A primer for the human services.* Belmont, CA: Brooks/Cole.

Djupe, P. A., & Olson, L. R. (2003). *Encyclopedia of American Religion and Politics.* New York: Facts on File.

Downing, N. E., & Roush, K. L. (1985). From passive acceptance to active commitment: A model of feminist identity development for women. *Counseling Psychologist, 13*(4), 695–709.

Duffy, K. G., & Wong, F. Y. (2003). *Community psychology* (3rd ed.). Boston: Allyn & Bacon.

Fisher, A. R., & Moradi, B. (2001). Racial and ethnic identity: Recent developments and needed directions. In J. Ponterotto, J. Casas, L. Suzuki, & C. Alexander (Eds.), *Handbook of multicultural counseling* (2nd ed., pp. 341–370). Thousand Oaks, CA: Sage.

Frey, W. H., Abresch, B., & Yeasting, J. (2001). *America by the numbers: A field guide to the U.S. Population.* New York: New Press.

Gordon, M. (1964). *Assimilation in American life.* New York: Oxford University Press.

Helms, J. E. (1993). *Black and European American racial identity: Theory, research, and practice.* Westport, CT: Praeger.

Helms, J. E. (1995). An update of Helms's European American and People of Color racial identity models. In J. Ponterotto, J. M. Casa, L. A. Suzuki, & C. M. Alexander (Eds.), *Handbook of multicultural counseling* (pp. 181–198). Thousand Oaks, CA: Sage.

Hondageneu-Sotelo, P. (1999). Women and children first: New directions in anti-immigrant politics. In S. Coontz, M. Parson, & Raley, G. (Eds.), *American families: A multicultural reader* (pp. 288–304). New York: Routledge.

Kennedy, G. J., & Tanenbaum, S. (2000). Psychotherapy with older adults. *American Journal of Psychotherapy, 54,* 386–407.

Kosmin, B. A., Mayer, E., & Keysar, A. (2001). *American religious identification survey*. Retrieved July 2, 2004, from The Graduate Center, The City University of New York website: **http://www.gc.cuny.edu/studies/ aris_part_two.htm.**

Lee, C. C. (Ed.). (1997). *Multicultural issues in counseling: New approaches to diversity*. Alexandria, VA: American Counseling Association.

Lee, W. M. L. (1999). *An introduction to multicultural counseling*. Ann Arbor, MI: Taylor & Francis.

Lewis, J., & Bradley, L. (Eds.). (2000). *Advocacy in counseling: Counselors, clients, and community.* Greensboro, NC: ERIC Counseling and Student Services Clearinghouse.

Mayo, M. (2000). *Cultures, communities, identities: Cultural strategies for participation and empowerment*. New York: Palgrave.

McIntosh, P. (1989, July/August). European American privilege: Unpacking the invisible knapsack. *Peace & Freedom,* 10–12.

Miranda, A. O., & Matheny, K. B. (2000). Socio-psychological predictors of acculturative stress among Latino adults. *Journal of Mental Health Counseling, 22*(4), 306–317.

Myers, J. E., & Harper, M. C. (2004). Evidence-based effective practices with older adults. *Journal of Counseling and Development, 82,* 207–218.

Pedersen, P. B. (1997). The cultural context of American Counseling Association Code of Ethics. *Journal of Counseling and Development, 76,* 23–28.

Pedersen, P. B. (2002). Ethics, competence, and other professional issues in culture-centered counseling. In P. B. Pedersen, J. G. Draguns, W. J. Lonner, & J. E. Trimble (Eds.), *Counseling across cultures* (5th ed., pp. 3–27). Thousand Oaks, CA: Sage.

Ponterotto, J. G., Casas, J. M., Suzuki, L. A., & Alexander, C. M. (Eds.). (1995). *Handbook of multicultural counseling.* Thousand Oaks, CA: Sage.

Ponterotto, J. G., Casas, J. M., Suzuki, L. A., & Alexander, C. M. (Eds.). (2001). *Handbook of multicultural counseling* (2nd ed.). Thousand Oaks, CA: Sage.

Pope, D. B., & Coleman, H. L. K. (2001). *The intersection of race, class, and gender in multicultural counseling.* Thousand Oaks, CA: Sage.

Reed, A., Jr. (Ed.). (1999). *Without justice for all.* Boulder, CO: Westview Press.

Ridley, C., Liddle, M., Hill, C., & Li, L. (2001). Ethical decision making in multicultural counseling. In J. Ponterotto, J. Casas, L. Suzuki, & C. Alexander (Eds.), *Handbook of multicultural counseling* (2nd ed., pp. 165–188). Thousand Oaks, CA: Sage.

Rowe, W., Behrens, J. T., & Leach, M. M. (1995). Racial/ethnic identity and racial consciousness: Looking back and looking forward. In J. G. Ponterotto, J. M. Casas, L. A. Suzuki, & C. M. Alexander (Eds.), *Handbook of multicultural counseling* (pp. 218–235). Thousand Oaks, CA: Sage.

Sandefur, G., Martin, M., Eggerling-Boeck, J., Mannon, S., & Meier, A. (2001). An overview of racial and ethnic demographic trends. In N. Smelser, W. Wilson, & F. Mitchell (Eds.), *America becoming: Racial trends and their consequences: Vol. 1* (pp. 40–102). Washington, DC: National Academy Press.

Santiago-Rivera, A., Arredondo, P., & Gallardo-Cooper, M. (2002). *Counseling Latinos and la familia: A practical guide.* Thousand Oaks, CA: Sage.

Smelser, N. J., Wilson, W. J., & Mitchell, F. (Eds.). (2001). *America becoming: Racial trends and their consequences, Volume 1* (pp. 1–530). Washington, DC: National Academy Press.

Smyer, M. A., & Qualls, S. H. (1999). *Aging and mental health.* Malden, MA: Blackwell.

Steinberg, S. (Ed.). (2000). *Race and ethnicity in the United States.* Malden, MA: Blackwell.

Sue, D. (1997). Counseling strategies for Chinese Americans. In C. Lee (Ed.), *Multicultural issues in counseling* (pp. 173–188). Alexandria, VA: American Counseling Association.

Sue, D. (2004). European Americanness and ethnocentric monoculturalism: Making the "invisible" visible. *American Psychologist, 59,* 761–769.

Sue, D. W., Arredondo, A., & McDavis, R. J. (1992). Multicultural counseling competencies and standards: A call to the profession. *Journal of Counseling and Development, 70,* 477–486.

Sue, D. W., Ivey, A. E., & Pedersen, P. B. (1996). *A theory of multicultural counseling and therapy.* Pacific Grove, CA: Brooks Cole.

Sue, D. W., & Sue, D. (2003). *Counseling the culturally different: Theory and practice* (4th ed.). New York: Wiley.

Swenson, L. C. (1993). *Psychology and law for the helping professions.* Pacific Grove, CA: Brooks/Cole.

Toporek, R. L., & Liu, W. M. (2001). Advocacy in counseling: Addressing race, class, and gender oppression. In D. Pope-Davis & H. Coleman (Eds.), *The intersection of race, class, and gender in multicultural counseling* (pp. 385–416). Thousand Oaks, CA: Sage.

U.S. Department of Health and Human Services. (2001). *Mental health: Culture, race and ethnicity: A supplement to Mental Health: A report of the Surgeon General.* Rockville, MD: U.S. Department of Health and Human Services.

Walsh, R. (2000). Asian psychotherapies. In R. J. Corsini & D. Wedding (Eds.), *Current psychotherapies* (6th ed., pp. 407–444). Itasca, IL: F. E. Peacock.

Weinrach, S. G., & Thomas, K. R. (1996). The counseling profession's commitment to diversity-sensitive counseling: A critical reassessment. *Journal of Counseling and Development, 73,* 472–477.

Weinrach, S. G., & Thomas, K. R. (2004). The AMCD multicultural counseling competencies: A critically flawed initiative. *Journal of Mental Health Counseling, 26,* 81–93.

Chapter 8

Responding to Change: Lifespan Development

All growth depends upon activity. There is no development physically or intellectually without effort, and effort means work.

Calvin Coolidge

If every day is an awakening, you will never grow old. You will just keep growing.

Gail Sheehy

GOALS

Reading and exploring the ideas in this chapter will help you

- Understand the theories of individual and family development across the life-span
- Gain greater knowledge of the various levels of personality as well as cognitive, moral-ethical, interpersonal, faith, and family development
- Begin to clarify your own perspective as you attempt a better understanding of other people and the way they see the world
- Realize that all concerns that people experience are in some way associated with their level of human development

---

OVERVIEW

This chapter presents information on individual and family development and transitions across the lifespan, including theories relevant for work with individuals and families. Human beings, by their very nature, are neither static nor stagnant. They are wired to be constantly changing, emerging, and dynamic beings. Having a developmental perspective is essential to your professional identity. It is the conceptual foundation, guiding principle, and very heart of your counseling work, so it is not surprising that an entire chapter of this introductory text is devoted to human development. Most summaries of human development concentrate only on the individual, but because community counselors also work at the systemic level, we include a section on the development of the most important system of all—the family. By focusing on both individual development and family transitions, you work to facilitate personal growth, enrich family life, promote wellness, and prevent potential problems before they start.

Understanding the course of human growth is also vital because you will be interacting with people at different stages of life. How you deal with a five-year-old child coping with the death of a parent is very different than how you work with a fifty-year-old adult struggling with this same event. Children are not merely miniature adults. They differ dramatically from adults in how they interpret the world, approach problems, deal with emotions, interact with others, and even in how they experience life. We have also discovered that human development is a process that is much richer and more complex than simply growing older. The only way you can effectively understand and successfully work with your clients is to recognize the many facets of human development. The intention of this chapter is not to provide you with an exhaustively detailed discussion of how infants are transformed into grown-ups. After all, later in your training, you will have an entire course devoted to this subject. Our immediate purpose here is to familiarize you with basic developmental concepts that are fundamental and essential to your daily work as a community counselor.

We wish to end this introductory overview on one last point. Whatever your background, whatever your current situation, and whatever your future plans, we can guarantee two things—you are at a particular developmental point along life's journey, and your family system is also at a certain stage. Therefore, you bring to this chapter a wealth of personal and family experiences. As you read this material, apply the concepts to your own life and family situation. What insights do these theoretical perspectives offer about yourself and your relationships? Relating these ideas to yourself and your family is more than just a technique for learning developmental theories. These models can help you to chart your own continuing course of growth and serve as beacons for future progress. They may also challenge you to examine your self and take a closer look at your family's dynamics. All counselors face their own developmental crises. Failing to deal with them can impair your effectiveness with clients. However, successfully making your way through these stages can help you in becoming a more mature, sensitive, and empathic counselor.

MARTHA'S DEFINING MOMENT: Three Calls

Martha was in the second month of her first job as a community counselor. Although she enjoyed her work, she was still struggling to manage her heavy case load. She occasionally felt pushed to the level of her competence, and at times she was overwhelmed by the range of issues that her clients presented. One Monday morning she was taking advantage of a few moments of "free time" to get caught up on paperwork. She cursed under her breath as the first call of the day came in; she knew that the call could start a chain of events that would undoubtedly complicate her day.

She picked up the phone and listened, uttering occasional encouragements and soothing words to the caller. The mother of a family with whom Martha was working was going into minute detail to explain how her fifteen-year-old daughter had painted satanic symbols on her arms with red fingernail polish, kicked a hole in her bedroom door, and then skipped school for the day. Earlier in the week Martha had spent several hours with this family in their home, talking about the ways in which they deal with crisis. After setting a time for them to meet again, Martha hung up the phone.

Call number two came fifteen minutes later as Martha was preparing to meet with her first client of the day. The call was from Jay, a client who was twenty-eight years old and had been in recovery for two years. He had recently gotten married and was excited about the positive changes in his life. Jay began reporting in a belligerent tone that he and his wife were getting separated, he was blowing off his appointment for the day, and he was getting ready to go score some crank. "Just wanted you to know what a waste I am," he said before hanging up the phone.

Martha immediately started searching for Jay's cell phone number as she received call number three. *I can't handle this,* she thought. *These clients are making me crazy.* She thought about letting the phone ring while she gathered her thoughts, but she immediately felt guilty and grabbed the receiver. Her heart sank as she heard the querulous voice of one of her elderly clients, nicknamed Philly. Philly was seeing Martha because of her depression, but she had recently begun to develop panic symptoms as well. Philly's husband was beginning to show signs of dementia, and Philly's physical health was deteriorating. Philly apologized for calling, but said she needed Martha to know that her husband had disappeared some time during the night. Philly wanted to know if she should call the police, and if Martha could please help her. Martha immediately envisioned her own grandmother experiencing this type of stress and promised to come to Philly's apartment as soon as she could.

Martha took a deep breath and found herself beginning to respond almost reflexively. She reassured Philly that she would make the phone calls. She encouraged Philly to ask her nearby neighbor to come and stay with her until a representative from either Elderly Protective Services or the police arrived. Martha herself would then check in with Philly as soon as she had talked with Elderly Protective Services. As she was dialing the phone, Martha flipped through Jay's file and was relieved to see that she had his cell phone number. She would call him as soon as she had reported the disappearance of Philly's husband and checked on Philly. *I'm not giving up on you yet, Jay,* she thought.

As Martha waited for her phone call to be answered, she was slightly surprised to find that her annoyance and frustration were gone. She felt a surge of energy, even of empowerment, as she realized that perhaps she could handle these different clients' needs after all.

Questions for Reflection

1. How might their various developmental levels affect not only Martha's clients, but Martha's reaction to her clients?

2. As you think about Martha's clients, which age group and family situation would be most compelling for you?

3. Which age group or family situation would be most difficult for you?

4. How do you imagine your own growth and development will influence your work as a counselor? What advantages and disadvantages do you think you will experience as you age?

BASICS OF HUMAN DEVELOPMENT

Researchers have proposed numerous and sometimes conflicting ways of understanding and, to some degree, predicting human development. However, there are certain assumptions that most developmental theorists hold in common. Human development is usually seen as unfolding in an orderly, continual process. The processes of development are sequential and identifiable, and they ultimately involve change. Even though the word development *implies* change, the core nature of the individual nevertheless remains the same. Thus we are able to talk with our clients about the past, present, and future and understand that although change is inevitable, we all do have a fundamental sense of self that anchors our understanding of the world.

One of the issues we constantly encounter as community counselors is the fact that once people become accustomed to a certain way of living and viewing the world, they often resist change. Change throws us into ambiguity and confusion; we often experience change as loss (Ivey, Ivey, Myers, & Sweeney, 2005). As we grow into adults and make our way into the world, we learn, as author Thomas Wolfe (1934) said, "You can't go home again." Becoming an autonomous adult suggests positive growth, but at the same time it implies losing the safe haven of childhood. Every transition we make in the course of our lifetime thus contains the good news and the bad news. The good news is that we are able to understand, perform, and accommodate to life with more skill and assuredness. The bad news is that we must give up some of the safety that the previous stage of life may have afforded.

At every transition point in life, if people are able to successfully deal with the developmental task required, they become better able to cope. One important variable for successful coping will be whether they are supported in this process. Most of us have adapted to the increasing demands of life with the help of family or friends. But sometimes people seek counseling in order to understand and accommodate to the changes they are experiencing.

The code of ethics of the American Counseling Association states that counselors are dedicated to assisting people in this process and to the enhancement of human development over the client's lifespan (2005). As a community counselor, with the aid of the theories discussed in this chapter, you will be able to assess your client's level of development in the various domains and help him or her toward achievement of the next level. When you see clients who are in distress, you will find it useful to think of their problems as difficulties in development. With human development as your basic clinical assumption, your orientation to counseling will then remain preventive, optimistic, and wellness-oriented—all fundamental approaches to the work of community counseling.

Influences of Nurture and Nature

It is possible that, back when you were taking your first psychology class, you came across the "nature-nurture" debate. The "nature" argument is that what and who a person becomes is mostly the result of the genes that the individual was given at conception. This is the "biology is destiny" stance. The "nurture" argument, on the other hand, states that people are largely "blank slates" when they are born and that who they become is the result of their learning (Pinker, 2003). If their environment is rich and nurturing, they will develop more optimally than someone who is born into an intellectually impoverished or neglectful environment.

Developmental theories often seem to view people as "time release capsules" in whom certain possibilities will emerge based on their chronological age. Their physical abilities, personality characteristics, and cognitive skills will "unfold" within an expected window of time. Furthermore, these emergent abilities occur in sequence. You don't, for example, usually learn to read or drive a car before you learn to walk or talk. However, as these developmental "windows" open at various stages in the person's growth, there also needs to be a "fit" between the individual's developmental need and what the environment can provide. Developmental problems can be traced not only to physiology, but to the failure of an opportunity to learn necessary survival and relationship skills.

Clearly, the answer to the question, "Is it nature or is it nurture?" is that it is both. As a counselor, you can do little about your client's genetic inheritance, but you can provide a nurturing condition in which he or she can learn or relearn ways to become a more fully functioning person. In this way, you will be helping clients change what appears to be their nature. You will be helped in this effort by a greater understanding of normal development and of what can go wrong at the various stages of a person's growth.

In the next section, following a brief consideration of genetics and some of the ways in which it can be a factor in counseling, we will discuss some of the prominent theories of development and their relevance to counseling.

Genetics as an Element in Counseling

To begin with the beginning—you began life as a single cell, a fertilized egg which contained forty-six chromosomes (Sroufe, Cooper, DeHart, & Marshall, 1996). Copies of these original chromosomes are still to be found in every cell of your body today. From a physiological standpoint, the genetic instructions contained in your chromosomes have made you who you are. Furthermore, these genes maintain you over your lifetime, despite the fact that the cells of your body are constantly dying and being replaced. But are you now who you were when you were, say, two years old, or twelve years old? Of course not. You have changed physically and psychologically over the years, even though your basic chromosomal structure has not. How is it possible that people change, yet stay the same, during the course of their lives? This remains one of life's mysteries.

From the moment of conception until birth, environmental toxic substances, known as teratogens, can alter our physiology. The nervous system of the embryo is at its most vulnerable period during the first six weeks of pregnancy, so alcohol, tobacco, or other drug ingestion could be injurious to the baby's brain even before the mother knows she's pregnant. In addition, maternal stress during pregnancy, poor nutrition of the mother, genetic or chromosomal mistakes, physical insult, or other as yet unknown anomalies may militate against normal physical and psychological development.

Why would these details be important to community counselors? If you are indeed committed to assuming a preventive and wellness-oriented approach in your work with clients, you need to understand the importance of early development. Although you are primarily concerned with the psychological aspects of the human being, you have to know how physiology can dramatically affect people's thoughts, feelings, and actions.

For example, your clients may be expecting parents who will bring to the session concerns about the pregnancy. The birth of an infant is a common developmental milestone, but many regard it with anxiety and apprehension. Perhaps the pregnancy will be unwanted and your client will be contemplating abortion. Or maybe your client will be a mother struggling with a drug problem that will have an impact on the infant's development. Another dilemma arises when an amniocentesis or other procedure has revealed a malformation of the fetus, and the parents are deciding whether to terminate the pregnancy. You can also expect to see parents who have long attempted to become pregnant and failed, or who have experienced multiple miscarriages. Still other clients will know the horror and tragedy of stillbirth. Even when a birth takes place, parents may be seeing you because the infant is experiencing a life-threatening condition or is unexpectedly malformed. Perhaps the mother has lapsed into a postpartum depression. Whatever the presenting circumstances, you need to learn as much as you can about development of both the fetus and the parents during this crucial life stage of pregnancy. Furthermore, you must clarify your own values because you may find many of your clients' issues to be challenging to your beliefs.

Now that the human genome has been mapped, many biotech companies are attempting to reprogram genes in the laboratory. Prospective parents in the future will face complex issues such as choosing the physical characteristics, increasing intelligence, and altering the personalities of their children. Already, people like James Watson (1999), the co-discoverer of the double helix structure of DNA, are stating that even a psychological attribute such as low-to-average intelligence can be considered a birth defect, and that we should begin to contemplate the prospect of designer-children based on gene selection. He stated that while the "dream" of producing "humans with talents and characteristics far superior to those of twentieth-century denizens" may yet be far off, "we must not lack the courage to use science to challenge the all too often grossly unfair courses of human evolution" (pp. 296–298). As your counseling career stretches into the future, you will need to keep abreast of biotechnology and its effects on your clients. You will also need to continually reappraise your stance on future biomedical

EXPERIENTIAL LEARNING

We suggest that you develop a chart or mnemonic system to help you learn about the different theories and how they are similar to each other. Be creative, invent a procedure, or develop a group project. Then compare your results with others in the class. Whenever possible, indicate on your chart or system the cultural limitations of the theories.

ethical issues, and decide how to deal with clients whose value systems differ from your own.

Developmental Theories

The next section on human development theories contains a significant amount of valuable information. Although with time and practice you will naturally become better able to remember the various approaches to understanding development, these concepts need to be immediately available to you in your work with clients. At the same time, realize that there are limitations to these theories. They typically reflect a predominantly Western European way of conceptualizing development. Working with clients from other cultures will require community counselors to broaden their understanding of what constitutes "normal" developmental. See the Experiential Learning box for some suggestions.

Personality Development: Erikson

Perhaps the defining aspect of a human being is his or her personality, "the sum total of enduring characteristics that differentiate one individual from another" (Feldman, 2000, p. 201). One of the most influential theorists to detail the stages through which a child travels toward his or her mature personality was Erik Erikson. Erikson (1963) is best known for introducing the concept of the "identity crisis." Ironically, it was Erikson's own series of crises of identity that may have led him to this notion. He acknowledged this in the following statement: "My best friends will insist that I needed to name this crisis and see it in everybody else in order to really come to terms with it in myself" (Erikson, 1975, pp. 25–26).

Erikson was named Erik Homburger for his stepfather, whom he thought was his biological parent until later in life. As the stepson of a Jewish man in twentieth-century German culture, Erik was not accepted by many of his classmates, while at the same time, his Jewish classmates shunned him because of his blond, Aryan appearance. After leaving Gymnasium (German high school), he "spent several years wandering about Europe in search of his true self" (Schultz & Schultz, 2000, p. 450). Though he had no formal education beyond high school, he eventually came to the United States, changed his last name to Erikson, and taught for years at Harvard University. Having been psychoanalyzed by Anna Freud, Erikson took the foundation of his developmental theory from Anna's father Sigmund. Erikson elaborated upon Freud's original idea of oral, anal, phallic, and genital psychosexual stages and created eight stages of development from birth to old age.

Erikson conceptualized the entire span of life as a series of stages, each of which involved a particular developmental crisis. His framework has had a profound impact on the counseling profession because it alerted practitioners to the different opportunities and challenges that their clients face at each phase of life. A basic premise of his model is that by successfully resolving each crisis, a person continues to mature, grow, and develop. However, if someone experiences a trauma, lacks the essential support of others, or fails to resolve the crisis, then the developmental process is derailed, the person stagnates, and the potential for fulfillment is compromised.

At the first stage, the infant deals with the issue of *Basic Trust Versus Mistrust,* and if the baby is successful at this level of development, then he or she has gained a fundamental faith in others and a deep belief in the goodness of life. Moving on to the second stage, *Autonomy Versus Shame and Doubt,* the toddler has the opportunity to develop a sense of confidence and personal will. Preschoolers, roughly between three and five years old, then undergo the stage of *Initiative Versus Guilt,* which can lead to a sense of enterprise and resourcefulness. School-age children typically experience *Industry Versus Inferiority,* which, if successfully completed, will leave a child with the feeling of competence, diligence, and activity. Adolescents then face the stage of *Identity Versus Role Confusion,* in which they begin to define their unique, integrated, and continuous personalities before they become adults.

Ideally, adolescence in Western culture affords a period of moratorium. The adolescent is not yet called upon to make commitments of an adult nature and may be able to leisurely explore the "who am I?" question and the consolidation of the ego. "Identity, then, is a dynamic fitting together of parts of the personality with the realities of the social world so that a person has a sense both of internal coherence and meaningful relatedness to the real world" (Josselson, 1987, pp. 12–13). This identity structure is continually updated as new experiences and information are encountered. One of Erickson's (1950) definitions of identity was that it is "the accrued confidence [in] the inner sameness and continuity of one's meaning for others" (p. 235).

As one's identity develops, three elements emerge as necessary for consolidation (Patterson, Sochting, & Marcia, 1992). First, the person begins to experience an inner sameness, an integrity of action and decision making, so that his or her behaviors do not appear to be random. Second, this inner sameness is experienced as continuous and extending over time: actions in the past and expectations of the future seem to be tied to the self as it is experienced today. Third, this identity is perceived to exist within a social context: relationships and roles serve to sustain and enhance the integrated and continuous identity.

James Marcia (1966, 1980) followed up on Erikson's descriptions of the "identity crisis" with additional research that revealed other facets, or "identity statuses." The identity struggle can turn out in one of several ways. Obviously, the best outcome would be the achieved identity. But other outcomes are possible.

Identity diffusion is the least advanced status that the identity struggle can produce. In this status, the commitment to a set of values and goals is virtually absent, and personal exploration is either quite shallow or missing altogether. "People in identity diffusion tend to follow the path of least resistance, and may present as having a carefree, cosmopolitan lifestyle or as being empty and dissatisfied" (p. 11). Although one may imagine that a client at the identity diffusion status will likely be young and inexperienced, counselors often find that their clients who have personality disorders, who are using or abusing substances, or who have other mental disorders may present at the identity diffusion status.

Identity foreclosure status is a high level of commitment, but without the personal exploration for its consolidation. Many people will foreclose early in their lives, but will later explore and achieve a more realistic identity. For example, children who in elementary school are committed to being a rock star or famous athlete, and adolescents who are committed to be what their parents envision for them, may later find personal value in other pursuits and beliefs. If this re-exploration does not take place, then foreclosure tends to produce a less developed state than either *moratorium* or *identity achievement*.

The *moratorium* status is a sort of protracted adolescence. The person in this stage is intensely exploring, but has not resolved the identity struggle. The *identity achievement* status is the autonomous resolution of identity: the making of commitments to personal values and goals. "It is the exploration of the moratorium period that distinguishes the flexible strength of the identity achievement from the rigid strength of identity foreclosure" (p. 12).

Then, in early adulthood, an individual faces the developmental crisis of *Intimacy Versus Isolation*. At this stage, one must be able to establish a close personal relationship with another person without losing the hard-won sense of identity. Failing this task, the person may end up with an inability to form and maintain a close relationship and will likely experience the sense of loneliness that follows this failure.

In midlife, the stage a person must deal with is called *Generativity Versus Self-absorption*. In this stage, one must turn from former preoccupations with self and begin to engage in helping others who have not yet reached this level of development. Reaching out to the next generation is significant in this stage, for Erikson felt that creating a legacy was of utmost importance for middle-aged adults. Parenting, for instance, is a common task of generativity. Finally, in late adulthood, it is time to take inventory of one's life and make sure that it has been lived in accordance with one's values. This stage, called *Ego Integrity Versus Despair,* is when the person must assess whether he or she has made a contribution to humanity. Some refer to this stage as "leaving the world a better place than how you found it."

Every stage of Erikson's developmental theory involves social relationships (Brown & Srebalus, 2003). Parents and family are most important in the first three stages, the peer group is the focus in adolescence, and partners and lasting connections with others mark the final stages. The fact that all stages, if not successfully negotiated, can involve relationship problems makes Erikson's theory quite useful to counselors attempting to conceptualize their clients' concerns in the context of the client's developmental history and current environment.

However, there are limitations that exist in any application of theory to practice. Gilligan (1982), for instance, arguing from a feminist perspective, believed that Erikson placed too much emphasis on autonomy and suggested that women may proceed in a slightly different pattern of development than men. This suggestion certainly makes intuitive sense, especially considering the different expectations that society has for men and women. Furthermore, the presentation of and response to various developmental tasks will be heavily influenced by multiple factors in clients' lives, including issues such as poverty, level of cognitive functioning, and environmental supports such as access to education and resources. Nevertheless, you may find that this theory provides at least a decent anchor for making sense of the concerns of clients at different ages.

Cognitive Development: Piaget

Swiss psychologist Jean Piaget is credited with establishing the first useful model of stages involved in cognitive development. Although his initial formulations were published in Europe during the 1920's, they were not well known in the United States due to the hegemony of Behaviorism during that time (Schultz & Schultz, 2000). In the 1960s, when cognitive psychology became well established in the United States, theorists, researchers and practitioners began to recognize the brilliance of Piaget's ideas. However, even after Piaget's theory was becoming popular, some critics complained that it was

EXPERIENTIAL LEARNING

Interview someone who is facing either the middle or late adulthood stage of life with regard to the following questions:
- In what ways has this person's perspective changed in recent years?

- Who were the significant people who have helped this individual to become the person she or he is?
- What is this person's life mission?
- What advice does this person have for you?

based on anecdotal observations of his own children and was, therefore, not scientifically based. Nevertheless, Piaget has made a great impact on our understanding of the stages involved in cognitive development. His theory is a constructivist one, meaning that the focus is on how people take in, and make sense of, their experience of the world. In the constructivist sense, everyone's reality is a personal reality, not reality per se.

As people learn about their world, two complementary processes are taking place in the mind. These processes are known as "assimilation" and "accommodation." Benjafield (1992) described the assimilation process as a subjective process. We assimilate information when we adjust our perceptions to fit our existing schema. If a child pretends a broomstick is a horse and jumps on, then the broomstick is changed by the child into something that suits the child's needs at that moment. In this situation, the child has assimilated the broomstick into his or her existing mental "scheme." An adult who expects people to be friendly toward her may assimilate when she meets strangers by treating them as friendly, even though she has no existing evidence that they are likely to be friendly in return. On the other hand, when the child changes himself or herself to fit into an existing situation, this is the process of accommodation. Such accommodation can be seen in a child's tendency to imitate. If a child copies a parent by using the broom to sweep the floor, the child is essentially changing the self to be more like something else—the parent. Similarly, if the friendly adult mentioned above encounters multiple unfriendly people, she may accommodate by modifying her existing scheme and becoming surly in return.

According to Piaget, successful adaptation requires that the processes of assimilation and accommodation be kept in balance. Continually tailoring perceptions to suit ourselves (assimilation) would result in an "unrealistic" picture of the world. On the other hand, chronically changing ourselves to fit the perceived reality (accommodation) could result in our not knowing who we are or what we want. The balance that must exist between these two processes is termed "equilibration." Maintaining this balance is the essence of how we learn about the world and come to an understanding of ourselves in that world. Regardless of the stage of one's development, assimilation and accommodation always present a person with the dialectical struggle for equilibration.

Between birth and age two, Piaget (1963) considered the child to be in the *sensory motor period* of development. This beginning stage is seen in the child's attempt to adapt to the world through physical action. The world is schematized as a place of sensations and immediate actions. By the end of this stage, the child has learned to move around the environment and to solve problems in a variety of ways. As the physical body develops greater abilities, such as crawling, walking, or grasping small objects between the thumb and forefinger, and the toddler's language develops, his or her behavioral repertoire increases along with a more fine-grained view of the world.

Between the ages of approximately two and seven, the child is in the *preoperational period* of development. Children can now think about their sensory motor coordination, but all conclusions are based on their primitive perceptions and their narcissistic desires. Nothing like a standard logic yet exists in their minds. Bjorklund (1989) stated that the concepts at this age are formed in what he called an idiosyncratic style, also known as "fiat equivalence." An example of this style of association is when the child says, "Cat and chair go together because a cat meows and you sit in a chair" or "Shovel and dog go together because I like shovels and I like dogs" (p. 114). This period is critically important for community counselors who work with children and their parents. Often, one of the most basic educational aspects of a counselor's work is helping parents understand the cognitive capabilities of their children. When children "misbehave," for instance, they may simply be exhibiting their inability to understand the parent's reasoning.

According to Piaget, when children reach the *concrete operations period* between the ages of seven and eleven years, they better understand how classes of things and events are related, but this understanding is still tied to concrete objects in the world. Early on in this stage, children are forming concepts based on common descriptive characteristics of perceived objects. For example, they might say, "Cat and squirrel go together because they both have long tails" or "Train and ship go together because they're both big," but later, they will form concepts according to what Bjorklund called a *complementary* style. In this style, the child draws on *associative* relationships in order to form categories: "Cat and milk go together because a cat drinks milk" or "Cowboy, horse, and pants go together because a cowboy needs pants to ride a horse" (p. 114). Still later in this stage, concepts are formed on a *functional* basis. "An apple and an orange are alike because you can eat them both." Concrete operations is an "iconic" stage for the child, meaning that he or she may be able to make a mental map of how to get to a friend's house, but would be less likely to follow a series of verbal instructions as to how to get there.

In Piaget's *formal operations period,* which emerges and becomes increasingly refined in children between the ages of twelve and fifteen, their thinking begins to allow them to contemplate objects that do not exist in their perception. Abstract concepts such as democracy, capitalism, or totalitarianism, for example, can begin to take on real meaning for the formal operational child. In addition, conceptual objects now are sorted according to more sophisticated categories. In this model of thought, things are associated because they are considered to "possess" common attributes: knife, fork, and spoon go together because they are all eating utensils. Beyond the sorting of concrete objects, children may now be able to grasp the fact that abstract ideas such as "monarchy" and "oligarchy" can be placed in the same category because they are systems of governing.

Once the child is able to perform such mental operations, he or she becomes a full-fledged member of the intellectual community. Adult people everywhere seem to group objects and ideas into categories and then arrange these categories into hierarchies (Gardner, 1991). The more organized the categories are, the better the thinking one can do with them. If I know, for example, that this furry, purring object that I am observing belongs to the category "cat," and that all the objects in the cat category belong to the category "feline," and these in turn belong within the category "animal," then my hierarchy allows me to make good inferences about such creatures. The essence of good thinking is having everything in its proper category and having the categories properly stacked, like Russian dolls, with the more abstract categories containing those that are more concrete. This is a system of clearly bounded superordinate and subordinate categories. In addition, the child who has reached this level of cognitive development can understand metaphors and symbolic language, test hypotheses, and can think about the world and specific problems in multiple ways. On completion of the formal operations stage of development, the individual is capable of critical and logical thought.

Piaget's beliefs are still widely cited and used as general benchmarks for understanding cognitive development. However, more recent theories have contradicted and expanded on his ideas (Bee & Boyd, 2003). Neo-Piagetians, for instance, combine information processing principles with Piaget's stages to provide a more complex and refined understanding of cognitive development.

Further, it should be noted that the stated ages at which people arrive at the above cognitive stages are ideal and are not set.

Regardless of how you choose to conceptualize cognitive development, you need to understand the developmental levels of your clients so that your way of communicating does not go "over their heads" or make them feel "talked down to" as well as to ensure that your interventions are on target. You would not, for example, employ many abstract concepts in your conversation with someone who is still in the concrete operations stage of development.

You will likely also find that models such as Piaget's will be helpful in your role as consultant to parents and families. Helping parents understand, for instance, the potential limitations of a toddler's ability to grasp issues such as responsibility and fairness can be vital in ensuring that parents have reasonable expectations for their children. Several counseling students used Piaget's and several other theorists' models to create straightforward charts detailing typical child development. They then displayed these charts at a local free clinic and a daycare center. Parents of children at the daycare center were interested enough in the information that the director of the center invited the counseling students to conduct a brief workshop for the parents on "Understanding Your Child's Needs and Abilities." Interventions such as this one, although fairly concrete and direct, can be powerful preventive measures.

In the example above, the counseling students worked to ensure that the information they presented was in language and format appropriate to the needs of their audience. The majority of the parents and caregivers at this particular day care were relatively young, and most had completed several years of high school. Ensuring that the intervention or program is responsive to the clients' needs is a critical concern. Ivey, Ivey, Myers, and Sweeney (2005) have established a counseling theory that details how you might approach clients based on their level of cognitive development. Focusing on wellness over the lifespan as well as culturally competent practice, the authors emphasize appropriate developmental assessment and the use of developmentally appropriate interventions and strategies to work toward positive change. You may find their writing on this subject helpful as you think about counseling people at these different levels.

Moral Development: Kohlberg and Gilligan

Lawrence Kohlberg (1984) studied the ways in which people of differing ages make moral decisions. He presented his subjects with stories of dilemmas in which a protagonist must decide on an action with moral implications. He then asked his subjects what they would do in such circumstances. Kohlberg was not so much interested in their decision, but rather, their reasons for the

EXPERIENTIAL LEARNING

Design a flyer, brochure, or chart for parents that explains in concrete, specific language the various stages of cognitive development. Include in your flyer or brochure an explanation and example of children's behaviors that might be associated with the various stages.

moral choice. From this work, he developed a model of developmental morality. He found that people's moral reasoning tended to change predictably through stages as they grew older and experienced more of life.

Kohlberg's theory showed people developing through three major levels: preconventional, conventional, and postconventional. Within each level, he identified two stages, which means that there were, in all, six stages of moral development through which people's reasoning progressed.

Stage One: Punishment and Obedience Orientation—Right actions are defined by physical consequences and the perception of physical power, and the child's desire to avoid punishment. Even as adults, people sometimes regress to this level if they make a moral choice based on whether they think they will get caught.

Stage Two: Instrumental and Relativity Orientation—Right actions are defined by their instrumental value to attain pleasure; the needs of others are considered a means to realizing the child's needs. This could be called the "horse trader mentality." Children and adults functioning at this stage do not take into account the needs or feelings of others. Social exchanges are pragmatic, meaning that they operate on the reciprocity principle of "You scratch my back, and I might scratch yours—so long as I have a chance of maximizing my gain."

Stage Three: Interpersonal Concordance Orientation—Right actions are defined by the expectations of one's role relative to the group. At this stage, moral choices are made with the hope of gaining the approval of significant others, or avoiding their disapproval. A child at this level of development (usually before age thirteen) will often choose to engage in a behavior that he or she believes is wrong if others are doing it. Parents with children at this stage usually ask, "Well, if everyone chose to jump off a cliff, would you do it?" (Of course, this is a useless strategy on the part of the parent.)

Stage Four: Law and Order Orientation—Right actions are defined by one's relationship to greater authority; the exception is where there is conflict with other fixed group duties. At this stage, some kids will decide that it's not okay to smoke in the bathrooms at school because smoking is simply against the rules. Although this stage does not necessarily exhibit a complex way of reasoning, many community counselors have found to their relief that a law and order orientation has prevented some of their child clients from engaging in illegal behavior.

Stage Five: Social Contract Orientation—Right action involves fair ways of resolving disagreements; all values are relative and should be tolerated. The welfare and social good of individuals drives moral decision making. Someone at this stage will be concerned whether the needs of each person in a group are met, and if not, then the group needs may require modification. All members must have a voice or an advocate. People at this stage are willing to question precedents and laws that are not good for society.

Stage Six: Universal Ethical Principles Orientation—Right action is action in accord with consistent, comprehensive, universal moral principles; these are used to evaluate all other principles, including democratic consensus. Someone at this stage may commit civil disobedience, for instance, if she believes that her action will address an unjust situation or preserve someone else's rights.

Kohlberg found that some adults had not mastered moral thinking at the *conventional* level (stages three and four), much less reaching third level of *postconventional* moral reasoning. Furthermore, there was an implication in his results that women usually only rose to stage five, while men sometimes attained stage six. This seemed to suggest that, on average, women were either intellectually or morally inferior to men.

Reacting to the research of Kohlberg, Carol Gilligan (1982) conducted her own investigation of moral attitudes. Noting that most of Kohlberg's subjects had been males, Gilligan set out to study both sexes equally. Her findings revealed that, rather than the differences between male and female moral reasoning being hierarchical, there are two distinct and equal orientations to ethical behavior. In other words, at some point in the moral reasoning progression, boys and girls begin to branch in the way they arrive at ethical decisions. Gilligan called these orientations "voices." One voice has come to be known as the "justice perspective" and the other the "care perspective" (p. ii).

In general, boys tend to adopt the justice perspective as their default style, while girls favor the care perspective. Males at high levels of moral development seem to favor autonomy and individuality, and moral choices are made so as to not violate the boundaries of others. High-level females, on the other hand, tended to stress the value of connectedness and relationship

when making moral choices. The difference in these perspectives was illustrated by an event in which school children were asked to write essays on
how to improve their city. For the boys, improving the city meant "more
parks, new buildings, renovations, better streets, more lighting" (p. i). The
girls, however, took improving the city to mean that relationships should
be strengthened between the people by identifying those in need and taking
action to help them.

Many studies have been conducted on the differences in these two "focus
phenomena" of moral reasoning. The results have suggested that while both
males and females are generally capable of reasoning in both modes, boys
focus more often on the justice perspective, while girls focus on the care
perspective. Gilligan (1982) took issue with Kohlberg's assertion that boys
attained a higher level of moral development, and suggested that what may
be happening is that girls are resisting the detached and dispassionate attitudes that accompany abstract and formal reasoning. In addition, Gilligan
pointed out that any story can be told from different angles, and events can be
seen in different lights. Someone who focuses on justice will see human relationships in terms of equality and the balancing of scales. The moral ideals of
reciprocity, equal respect, and the avoidance of oppression are paramount in
this view. The care perspective, on the other hand, stresses responsiveness,
engagement, emotional attachment to others, and a web of interpersonal
connection that remains resilient. From a care perspective, the detached
objective stance adopted by those who wish to reason dispassionately is seen
as indifference and abandonment.

Perhaps the most important issue for community counselors regarding
these issues is the constant demand that the counselor respond appropriately
and effectively to the client's needs. A counselor who misreads a client's
strong personal connections to others as excessive dependence, for instance,
runs the risk of providing faulty diagnosis and ineffective treatment. As with
all issues of difference, counselors must engage in critical self-reflection and
consider the importance of societal influences, including sexism and gender-
role socialization, in their conceptualizations. See "Dealing with Don" on
pages 275–276.

Perspective-Taking and Empathy: Flavell

The term *empathy* has traditionally been associated with the feeling of an
emotional response on the part of someone who is sensing the state of
another person (Eisenberg, Murphy, & Shepard, 1997). As we mentioned in
Chapter 4, the more contemporary cognitive term for understanding others
is "perspective-taking." Researchers have distinguished between cognitive
perspective-taking (the ability to *understand* another's thoughts or mental

Dealing with Don

Kate had been on the staff of a community counseling agency for two years when she met Don. Don was twenty-four years old. He was handsome, intelligent, and had a well-paying job. He also had a significant problem—he chose to "date" only very young women. Accused of statutory rape by the parents of a fifteen-year-old girl, Don was convicted, put on probation, and ordered by the court to receive counseling. Kate was his designated counselor.

Kate found Don intriguing but, over time, incredibly annoying. When discussing his attraction for underage women, Don simply replied that they were "compliant, eager to please, and easy to control," and "they make me look good." Women such as Kate, he said, were too demanding and, "no offense intended," just not his type.

Kate was dismayed to find that she did indeed take offense at Don's comment. She found herself wanting to confront Don in inappropriate ways, such as exclaiming that in her opinion dating young teenagers made him look foolish and immature, not "good," and that adult men shouldn't need to choose their mates based on features such as "compliance."

Kate also found that she had trouble gleaning anything of significance from Don's background. He started to feel like an enigma to her, and a very unwelcome one at that. In their most recent session, Don acknowledged that he understood that if he kept dating young girls he'd just keep getting in trouble, so he was determined to take a new approach to dating. "I'm just going to start looking for women my own age who are either needy or not too bright," he said. "Sorry," he grinned at Kate, "I guess that still leaves you out. You must be fairly smart, since you've been to graduate school."

Kate boiled silently, feeling like a failure. How could she possibly get through to Don while dealing with her own very negative reactions to him? After consulting with a colleague, Kate realized that she was fundamentally confused by Don's personality and his level of moral development. He was unaware of the effects of his behavior in general and his comments to her in particular. Although Kate felt insulted by his views, she was deeply disappointed in herself for reacting so negatively to Don's dismissive attitude toward intelligent and mature women. In spite of her efforts, Kate failed in her attempts to dredge up any empathy for her client. Unable to build a therapeutic alliance, their sessions together never explored Don's likely sense of insecurity, lack of trust in others, feelings of vulnerability, identity diffusion, and fear of genuine intimacy. Instead, for much of their time together in session, Kate would seethe in a quiet but raw rage.

Questions for Reflection

1. What areas of development (personality, cognitive, moral) would you want to explore more completely with Don?

(continued)

(Dealing with Don, continued)

2. What would you want to know about his childhood and family?

3. How do you think you would personally feel about working with

Don? If you had a negative reaction as strong as Kate's, what would you do to ensure you continued to practice effectively?

---

states) and affective empathy, or emotional contagion (the ability to *sense* another's emotional state).

Flavell (1992) identified four levels of the acquisition of perspective-taking in children. The first is the recognition that mental states exist. The second is the realization that certain situations call for the need to acquire information about the mental states of others. The third is the ability to make inferences about others' mental states. Finally, some gain the ability to apply this skill appropriately in some given situation. Piaget's (1926) early experiments on the failure of young children to perspective-take are well known. His notion of "egocentrism" suggested that before a certain age, children cannot escape their own experience and focus on what others might see from their perspective.

As children begin to understand what might be going on with other people, they develop an important set of social abilities. By the age of two they know that a boy who has lost his pet will likely be sad, and one who has received a gift might be happy. A question that is often debated is whether children use these contextual cues by imagining how they would feel in the situation and then projecting those feelings onto another, or whether they are actually evaluating the other's experience. When children write stories, they provide a much richer description of the protagonist's internal state—with whom they identify—than of the other characters in the story. Only in later stages of development do they write more elaborate descriptions of the mental states of others (Presbury, Benson, Fitch, & Torrance, 1991). The fact that children's understanding of their own feelings and thoughts precedes an understanding of others has been cited as reason for believing that children use themselves as templates for evaluating others.

It is possible, however, that empathic understanding is present long before the ability to verbalize it. According to Buck and Ginsburg (1997), empathic ability is a biologically inherited predisposition to communicate with others. Their position is that these are "wired-in" social abilities that have evolved over the eons and are suited to the condition of our being social animals. They regard the above abilities "as emergent properties of a primordial biological capacity for communication that inheres in the genes" (p. 19).

Even Charles Darwin (1872/1955) speculated that this empathic predisposition provided the biological basis for ethics and religion in humans. According to Darwin, the function of the emotional communication process is to maintain the social order.

Although the development of empathy does not follow the same stages as perspective-taking, Hoffman (1984) and others have described the growth of empathy over time. At approximately the age of one year, the child begins to enter a stage that Hoffman called "egocentric empathy"; the child understands that the distress of another person is not his or her own. However, the child offers a comfort based on his or her own experience—not on the distressed person's experience. For example, the child might offer a toy that has served to soothe him or her, but which might be refused because the toy does not serve the same function for the other child.

Beginning at about two to three years of age, the child becomes capable of adding the beginnings of a perspective-taking ability to his or her empathic response, but it will not be until much later that the full realization of the other person as possessing a separate identity occurs. Aron, Aron, Tudor, and Nelson (1991) stated that when we feel close to other people, "much of our cognition about the other in a close relationship is cognition in which the other is treated as self or confused with self" (p. 242). We realize a closer connectedness with the other so as to be temporarily merged with them. The now clichéd expression of this merging experience, "I feel your pain," conveys that the observer experiences the agony of the other person as if it is his or her own.

Davis (1994) argued that when the observer adopts the perspective of the other person (through interpersonal accuracy and attributional judgments), this will likely produce empathic concern. Davis goes on to assert that both affective empathy and perspective-taking must be present in the observer for the full empathic response. In this view, both cognition and emotion must be present to combine perspective-taking with genuine empathy. The result is an empathy accuracy that can enhance our clients,' and our own, relationships.

Attachment: Ainsworth and Bowlby

Researchers in the area of social intelligence have suggested that infants who have experienced adequate caregiving are more likely to become securely attached to their primary caregiver. Securely attached children are then more likely to develop into well-adjusted adults (Ainsworth, Bell, & Stayton, 1971). Davis (1994) found the evidence to be quite strong that close and secure family relationships are positively correlated with heightened affective responsivity to the experiences of others. Of course, the converse is also true: Insecurely attached individuals seem to be less empathic and—in some cases—less able to predict the behavior of others.

The work of John Bowlby (1969/1982, 1973, 1980), perhaps more than the writing of anyone else, has influenced current thinking on the phenomenon of "attachment." The notion that a human infant requires certain responses from a primary caregiver in order to fully develop psychologically is now generally accepted and "solidly embedded in developmental psychology" (West & Sheldon-Keller, 1997, p. 1). Attachment theory claims that human infants at birth exhibit care-seeking behaviors, and if these are met with adequate caregiving, then the infant will progress successfully to later stages of development. In subsequent stages as well, the child will be in need of certain types of responses from the caregiver in order to actualize the full potential of his or her psychological repertoire. If there is failure in this interaction between caregiver and child, then disorders of adult personality are the likely result. As Bowlby (1977) put it: "Whilst especially evident during early childhood, attachment behavior is held to characterize human beings from the cradle to the grave" (p. 129).

Weiss (1991) identified the three central criteria that define attachment behavior in infancy. They are as follows:

1. Proximity seeking: an attempt to remain within protective range of the attachment figure
2. Secure base: when the attachment figure is present, the child appears to be comfortable and secure
3. Separation protest: displays of sadness, anxiety, or rage when the attachment figure cannot be located

These are also reliable criteria on which to measure attachment in adults. One of the most compelling implications of attachment is the fact that our clients' attitudes toward significant others, including their own children, will be influenced by their own early attachment experiences. Understanding the influence of attachment can help counselors accurately assess and treat clients' interpersonal and family concerns.

Theory of Mind: Baron-Cohen

Theories of mind are explanations for how children understand other minds. Like other developmental theorists, those who study this ability suggest that it progresses in relatively predictable stages. Taylor (1996) stated that "theory of mind" has recently evolved from being a topic of small and specialized interest, to being a major research enterprise in the area of social cognitive development. Central to this area of study is the developing child's understanding of the intentional states of others, particularly as regards their beliefs and desires.

As children grow, they become better able to predict the behaviors of others through an accumulating set of heuristics, and eventually a full-fledged theory of what goes on in the minds of others. Taylor acknowledged Piaget's

(1926) interest in children's theory of mind, but claimed that it was Premack and Woodruff (1978) who got the ball rolling in this area of study. Premack and Woodruff had studied this sort of understanding in chimpanzees and offered the following: "In saying that an individual has a theory of mind, we mean that the individual imputes mental states to himself and to others" (p. 515). This theory is then used to predict what others may do in certain situations. While a child's ability to make such predictions may be greatly refined through experience, this theory of mind mechanism (Leslie, 1994) exists from an early age.

Baron-Cohen (1996) considered four components of our "mind-reading" system to be essential:

1. ID: the Intentionality Detector

2. EDD: the Eye-Direction Detector

3. SAM: the Shared-Attention Mechanism

4. ToMM: the Theory of Mind Mechanism

In naming his intentionality detector "ID," Baron-Cohen apologized to Freud in case he still held the "copyright" on this term. Baron-Cohen's ID is a perceptual device that interprets motion stimuli in terms of the volitional states of goal and desire. In other words, using what Dennett (1991) called the "intentional stance," movement attracts attention and ID attempts to determine whether this movement comes from a self-propelled agent. If it is determined to be an agent, then the assumption is made that it moved because of some goal or desire. If the movement turns out to be the waving of a tree branch in the wind or the ripple of a waterfall, then ID withdraws intentional agent status from it.

The survival value of such a device is obvious: When our ancestors went to the water-hole for a drink, it would have been crucial for them to distinguish inanimate non-agents from, say, saber-toothed tigers. With such a device as the ID, we will often experience "false positives," we may mistakenly take something to be an agent when it is not. This default is, however, superior to its alternative—for example, mistaking a real saber-toothed tiger for a tree branch. "In evolutionary terms, it is better to spot a potential agent, and start checking its goals and desires, than to ignore it. In the game of survival, it is best not to miss a single trick" (Baron-Cohen, 1996, p. 35).

The second component identified by Baron-Cohen is the Eye-Direction Detector (EDD). Newborn humans almost immediately look at faces and search for eyes. Likewise, your dog looks at your eyes, instead of your kneecap, which is closer to its eye level. The three basic functions of EDD are as follows: "[I]t detects the presence of eyes . . . it computes whether eyes are directed toward it or toward something else, and it infers . . . that the organism sees that thing" (pp. 38–39).

EXPERIENTIAL LEARNING

One way to assess and hone your own ToMM is to use a variation of Interpersonal Process Recall (Kagan, 1980) in your counseling techniques or process class.

- Make a videotape or DVD of a counseling session in which students counsel each other regarding real issues.
- After the session, the counselor and the client should spend some time alone thinking or writing about their intentions during the session as well as general reactions to how the session progressed.
- The next step requires the counselor and client to watch the taped session together. Counselor and client take turns stopping the tape, asking what the other person was thinking at that moment in the counseling session, and sharing their own reactions. The process can be a powerful tool for learning more about others' thoughts while offering a useful peer supervision session. As you engage in this process, pay particular attention to those times in which you were right on target regarding the other person's thoughts and the times when you were off base. What may have been going on during those particular moments in the session?

SAM (shared-attention mechanism) detects triadic relationships among an agent, the self, and a (third) object. This is the "do you see what I see?" mechanism. Around nine months of age, children will detect the gaze of a parent and then look to see what the object of that gaze might be. Shortly afterward, toddlers will employ a "protodeclarative pointing gesture" to call the parent's attention to what they see and find interesting.

From these three basic mechanisms, the child begins to develop ToMM, a theory of mind mechanism. The child can then imagine the intentional dynamics taking place within another individual and thereby predict what they are likely to do next. Some people are very good at this, while others are abysmally deficient in this ability. The ability to "read other minds" is largely based on the level of sophistication of one's ToMM; it is the ability to predict behavior based on what one assumes to be the other person's beliefs and desires. We know that people with autism are poor mind readers, and it has been suggested that some crucial circuit in the brain is responsible. However, most community counselors we have known are very good mind readers. Given that one possesses a merely adequate brain, this ability seems to be one that can be perfected in a training environment.

Adult Development: Kegan and Perry

As previously discussed, Piaget considered the attainment of abstract and logical ability to be the quintessence of cognitive development. Once a person had achieved this *formal operations* level, then critical and scientific thought could take place. This stage of development, usually completed by the end of adolescence, would stay much the same for the rest of someone's life. But Labouvie-Vief (1980) argued for a stage beyond formal operations, which she called *postformal*. Her assertion was that life events do not present themselves in logical, black-and-white terms and that mere logic cannot sustain a person in most real-world situations.

Feldman (2000) offered an example of how people need to think beyond formal operations in order to understand life events. He asked us to imagine that John, who is married to Mary, is a heavy drinker and has, on several occasions, come home drunk after being out with his buddies. Mary is fed up and gives him an ultimatum: If he comes home in this condition again, she will leave him, take the children, and sue for divorce. Tonight, John arrives home late after an office party, and Mary is waiting up for him. She immediately sees that he is drunk.

Does she leave him, as she had threatened? Sheer logic will not help us to know in advance what Mary will do. We are aware that there are many variables that will influence her decision. There is no "right" thing to do. As Aristotle pointed out over two millennia ago, reasons are not the same as causes. Life is complicated. As Feldman put it, as adults begin to deal with the contingencies of life beyond formal operations, they must confront paradoxes and think in metaphors. For this reason, when dealing with adults in counseling situations, it is important that you understand how they are making sense of their relationships and how they view events in their world. Two theories of development that focus primarily on how adults make sense of the world are Kegan's (1982) *constructive development theory* and Perry's (1970) theory of *epistemological reflection*. These theories are presented in brief below.

Kegan asserted that we construct reality in different ways as we grow older and have more experience. At each transition between developmental stages, some challenge exists which necessitates our giving up our former worldview. He posited that we pass through six stages over the lifespan, with stages zero to four being experienced in childhood. The child is born into stage zero, which is similar to Piaget's sensory-motor period. At this level, the child has no sense of self as separate from the outside world. In the spirit of Freud's oral stage, Kegan calls this the *incorporative stage*.

Stage one, the *impulsive stage,* is when the two-year-old reaches the "terrible twos" and begins to "disembed" the self from the environment. As we mentioned in Chapter 4, this is the age at which the child first recognizes herself in the mirror as shown by the so-called "rouge test," in which a dab of rouge is placed on the child's forehead and the child is set before a mirror. Prior to this birth of self-recognition, the child sees a baby in the mirror, not realizing who the baby is.

Stage two is the *imperial stage* in which the desires and needs of the child become paramount. The child then "wants what she wants when she wants it." Acquisition becomes the main enterprise of the child.

Stage three, according to Kegan, marks the transition into adulthood. This is the *interpersonal stage* which can be seen in adolescence, but is maintained by many adults. In this stage, one's needs and wishes are met through a relationship with another person. One sees oneself only through the eyes of the other. Think of how many songs you have heard with the theme of "without you I am nothing," and you will instantly recognize the main theme of this level of development.

In stage four, the *institutional stage,* the person begins to move toward greater autonomy. While relationships remain important, they no longer are crucial to the establishment and maintenance of the person's identity. They feel what they feel, know what they know, and may not hesitate to share their thoughts.

Finally arriving at Kegan's (1982) stage five, the *interindividual* level, the person is able to freely share with and learn from others. This level appears to resemble Erikson's "intimacy." Having established a personal identity, the individual is now capable of entering into meaningful relationships with others without threat to his or her sense of self. In fact, the person may seek out information about him- or herself from others. While a person at this level will modify his or her behavior in reference to this feedback, he or she enjoys a sense of personal integrity and boundary that has been achieved in the developmental struggle. The person might exclaim, "I finally know who I am!"

Perry (1970), like many of the other developmental theorists discussed in this chapter, conducted his research at Harvard University. Because his subject-group was made up of primarily white, male college students, his research has sometimes been criticized, but it has remained robust in its influence on people who track the cognitive development of college students from admission to graduation. Perry found that most entering students employed Piaget's formal operations in their thinking. This was Perry's first stage, which he called the *dualistic,* right or wrong, attitude in which the students approached their learning in a somewhat perfectionistic manner. In general, people at this stage reasoned that things were right or wrong, or good or bad. These people had little tolerance for ambiguity and wanted to know the "truth" of things. They tended to believe what their professors told them and to treat as gospel what was written in books.

As they began to be exposed to ideas other than their own and hear other points of view, their dualism gradually declined. This next level of thought, known as the *multiplistic* stage, was marked by the realization that issues can have more than one plausible interpretation and by a decrease in their reliance on authority for answers. They slowly began to trust their own opinions and to be able to argue their position in justification of their thinking. They became more interested in understanding other people's way of viewing things.

Finally, the students entered a phase of cognitive development Perry (1970) called *relativistic*. At this stage, they began to tailor their responses to the circumstances at hand, realizing that there are "different strokes for different folks." They became more eclectic or transtheoretical in their intellectual attitudes, and instead of viewing other people as ignorant or misguided, they began to understand the circumstances that had brought them to their current beliefs. This did not mean that the relativistic thinker's own beliefs were so malleable as to be subject to "any old wind that blows." They could maintain their worldview in the face of differing opinions, but their beliefs and values were no longer rigid as they had been in the dualistic phase. They realized that different cultures, for instance, could have different standards that are all equally valid (Feldman, 2000).

Perry and Kegan's contributions can, at the very least, be tools for you in conceptualizing your clients' development and concerns. As such, your understanding of your clients will then suggest your interventions. As you learn more about these theories in your course work, and as you gain practice with clients, you will likely find that the more information you have that can suggest possible explanations for human behavior, the better equipped you will be to understand and respond to your clients.

Faith Development: Fowler

It could be said that most issues brought by clients to a counselor are problems of spirituality and faith. Spirituality, in its broadest sense, is involved in the effort to create personal meaning. As people grow and develop, they become increasingly concerned with what life means, how they can live it well, and unless they have a firm set of beliefs (a faith) to live by, people can be adrift in life. You may think that faith issues are better left to the clergy or the philosophers. But, since all humans are basically spiritual creatures, it is important that you understand how faith develops over the lifespan and how crises of faith affect people's lives.

"Faith" in this discussion refers to the way in which people make sense of their human condition and arrive at a set of personal values. The content of one's beliefs, the "what" of people's faith is not our focus. And when we say that people are spiritual, we are regarding spirituality as Ceasar and Miranti (2001) defined it. They stated that "spirituality includes one's capacity for creativity, growth, and the development of a value system" (p. 210).

James Fowler (1981/1995) developed a theory of faith development based on the work of Erikson, Piaget, and Kohlberg. In Fowler's view, faith is of concern to everyone, regardless of whether they are religious in the orthodox sense. Fowler, a Methodist minister, began teaching at Harvard in 1972 and was a student of Lawrence Kohlberg, along with Carol Gilligan and Robert Kegan. It is obvious that his theory has been influenced by the milieu in which he found himself at that time. His scheme of development is hierarchical, and he saw impetus for progression from one stage to another in the same way that Erikson conceived of it. In each stage, as "disequilibrium" arises, one can either move to a higher stage or become arrested in personal growth. (Someone has called this the "no pain, no gain" theoretical approach to human development.)

Fowler's stage zero, called *primary faith,* is the way the infant comes to view self, others, and the world. If children have successfully mastered this stage, which is based on Erikson's basic "trust versus mistrust" stage, they will lay the foundation for trust in later relationships. If the child in the infant-toddler stage has experienced adequate nurturing from the primary caregiver, then the beginnings of a solid sense of self, a secure attachment to others, and an optimistic view of life will ensue. On the other hand, neglected or abused children with an "attachment disorder" will not trust themselves, other people, or the world. They will have lost faith at the outset of life.

Fowler's next stage of faith development, stage one, *intuitive-projective faith*, begins sometime after age four. While in this stage, children live in a world of feelings, images, and stories. It is a stage based on Piaget's preoperational level, and is also akin to what Bruner, Goodnow, and Austin (1956) identified as the "iconic" stage of development. According to Gardner (1982), children in this stage often produce unaware metaphors such as describing a bald man as having a "barefoot head," a cloud as "a scar in the sky," or the ocean waves making ridges on the sand as "like a little girl's hair being combed." Their world is a storied environment (for good or ill) and the developing child is vulnerable to the influences of others. It is not uncommon to hear parents warning children against undesired behaviors by saying that a policeman, a bogeyman, or God will get them if they don't behave. They may be repeatedly told that they are bad or sinful, or that they should be sure to say the "If I should die before I wake" prayer, because one never knows how things will turn out. These are not situations that are designed to strengthen one's level of trust in self, others, or the way the world goes. Conversely, if the child at this stage is exposed to optimistic stories containing benign animals and humans as characters, and the stories end happily, the child's faith is more likely to be strengthened.

According to Fowler, stage two, the *mythic-literal* period of faith, commences between the ages of six-and-a-half and eight. Children at this age are at the beginnings of Piaget's concrete operational phase of development. They still rely on adult authority to convey information, but they are beginning to figure out for themselves concepts such as causation and the way things work in their experience. Cognitively, they are "either-or" thinkers. At this stage, the children are struggling to reconcile what they have been told to believe about the world and their own personal experience of events.

In Fowler's stage three (around ages twelve or thirteen), the *synthetic-conventional* stage, children are developing an ideology for the first time, although they are not completely aware of their newly constructed beliefs. This event corresponds to the initial phases of Piaget's formal operations. According to Piper (2002), it is stage three that represents a watershed in the child's development of a personal worldview and value system. Fox, Fitzgerald, Erricker, Logan, Logan, and Ota (1995) stated that for many adults, stage three becomes "a permanent resting place." These authors see many dangers existing at this stage of one's development that may militate against progression to more complex levels of faith.

As is obvious in the developing adolescent, he or she is strongly influenced by the beliefs and attitudes of peers. This influence is manifested by the need to belong and to show this by having the right clothing, hairstyle, music, jargon, and by being seen in the right places with the right people. Even though the adolescent's values are strongly felt, they are still in a stage of "hero worship" and can model the beliefs and values of sports figures, rock stars, and other celebrities. People at this age are beginning to struggle with the "Who am I?" question, so their values are vulnerable to the influence of others. Outside their peer group, they may be troubled by questions and doubts that they cannot fully articulate. This is a time of great upheaval in life: raging hormones, greater freedom and responsibility, and the true transition period between childhood and adulthood. To believe and decide on one's own is to risk losing the support of the group. Some choose group membership over personal freedom. Fowler's research data suggested that one-fourth of people twenty-one and older remain at this level of faith development (Piper, 2002).

Sometimes, the person or group with which the stage three person is identified may let the individual down in some way. Because people's faith at this level is largely centered outside themselves and based on their identification with the esteemed person or group, when their illusion is betrayed they may enter into a period of despondency and despair. During the Nixon administration in the 1970s, the Watergate Scandal caused many Americans to become disaffected and cynical regarding politics and to develop a mistrust of government. More recently, a series of scandals have surfaced in the Roman Catholic Church, in which a number of parishioners have come forward to reveal that their priests had sexually abused them as children. For people whose faith development was arrested at the stage three level, this revelation that their priests had violated their trust was experienced as a crisis of faith. These "true believers" were left with a sense of "spiritual homelessness" (Steere, 1997). They were experiencing what Janoff-Bulman (1992) called "shattered assumptions." In many cases, however, such disillusionment may propel a person toward a more complex level of faith development. With the proper environmental support, together with benign development, instead of becoming victims of this crisis of loss, resilient people can move on to become survivors and reach a new level of awareness (Echterling, Presbury, & McKee, 2005).

It is around the age of eighteen or nineteen that the person may enter Fowler's stage four, the *individuative-reflexive* level of faith development. It's here that the person can then throw off the yoke of the "tyranny of the they" (Fox et al., 1995). While other people's opinions and judgments remain important, the person at this level can independently come to conclusions that may differ from those of others. This does not necessarily mean that the content of one's beliefs must change from stage three to stage four, but that the person now begins to "own" the set of values and meanings. It is possible, however, that the person may reject what was formerly believed and be seen by others as rebellious. They may, because of their new-found sense of freedom and its accompanying feeling of exhilaration, seek to convert others to their way of thinking.

It is unusual for anyone before midlife to reach Fowler's stage five, *paradoxical-conjunctive faith*. In this stage, the person attains what Perry (1970) referred to as "commitment in relativism." The person understands that she doesn't know or understand everything, that others' views are valid, and that she is able to rely on a core sense of belief or knowledge that informs her life (Fox et al., 1995). Instead of leading to an immobilizing sense of nihilism, successful mastery of this stage of faith can lead to an increased level of comfort with ambiguity, a greater tolerance of others, and a realization that the opposite of a truth may also be a truth.

Few people ever reach stage six, *universalizing faith*. At this level the person would attain the level of development akin to Maslow's (1970) "self-actualizing person." In such an ideal state, a person would achieve what Fowler (1981/1995) called a "decentration" from self—the ability to understand the views and experiences of others at a truly empathic level and to fully take in their perspective. Martin Luther King and Mother Teresa are among those seen to have achieved this stage (Fox et al., 1995).

It should be noted that Fowler's theory has met with a good deal of criticism, mostly from the "religious right" (Piper, 2002). And in much the same way that Gilligan took issue with the idea of hierarchical stages in Kohlberg's model, Piper has found fault with certain aspects of Fowler's theory. He, like Gilligan, suggested that "higher" is not always necessarily better. Because most developmental theories have been predicated on studies of European-American males by male researchers with decidedly Western views, they therefore lack a universal validity. They are narrow from both a cultural and gender standpoint.

However, if we, as counselors, view these theories of individual development as "reasonable fictions," and not as falsifiable theories, we can use them as guideposts to help us better understand what is happening in our clients' mental lives as they pass through "stages of development." You should regard these theories as tools, rather than as canon. Further, we encourage you to keep abreast of recent research regarding faith and other aspects of human development by regularly reading scholarly journals. Our field is evolving; significant findings are reported frequently that can substantially influence our practice. For instance, all community counselors need to be vigilant in seeking more knowledge regarding diverse cultures in order to ensure that they are not imposing European American standards on clients who have distinctly different expectations regarding lifespan development.

FAMILY DEVELOPMENT

Most community counselors realize quickly that their work with individual clients requires them to conceptualize their clients in the context of their families. As individuals develop, they are influenced by and in return influence their families (Carter & McGoldrick, 1999), creating a dynamic that is inextricably related to the individual's current level of functioning. Thus, counselors are encouraged to combine models of individual development with those of family development in order to develop a more comprehensive understanding of their clients' needs.

Several family theorists have offered models of the developmental process through which "normal" families are thought to proceed (Becvar & Becvar, 1999; Carter & McGoldrick, 1980; Hill, 1970). No such family truly exists, of course, although the idea of a typical family life cycle has been accepted as fact in the counseling field for years (Rice, 1994). The Becvars (2006) caution that as most general family life cycle models depict the progress of a couple through the traditional pattern of marriage, child-bearing, and child rearing, they present a stereotype, and such models can only approximate the development of the diverse configurations of what may constitute a "family." For instance, single-parent families, stepfamilies, gay families, and unmarried families will all face unique challenges and crises, but in general, they will also have

to deal with some of the difficulties listed below. Similarly, members of different ethnic groups and cultures have different notions of families and are likely
to exhibit different developmental stages. Nevertheless, the general process
depicted below has some utility for counselors attempting to understand the
stressors their clients may face as members of families.

Early Stages of the Family Life Cycle

A general overview of the family life cycle, which combines the work of
Carter and McGoldrick (1999) and Becvar and Becvar (2006), suggests that
the family development story begins with Erikson's individual (1963), who
may be still dealing with the identity crisis, or who may be in the next phase
of "intimacy versus isolation." At this point the individual is struggling with
how to preserve that sense of identity while learning how to merge with another person. This individual is also struggling with differentiating from the
family-of-origin, the struggle between being someone's child versus being an
adult, along with seeking an identity in the workplace.

Then the individual becomes a member of a couple. This period can feel
exciting for individuals who are in love and enthralled with each other.
Becvar and Becvar (2006) refer to this time as the "honeymoon period," which
suggests a stage of bliss and unity. However, at this point the two individuals
are also likely to struggle with a variety of stressors, including adjusting their
expectations regarding existing family and peer relationships while forging
an identity as a couple. Changing from "I" thinking to "we" thinking can feel
daunting, especially for those who feel they are giving up individual freedom
in order to become part of a couple.

One example of a developmental crisis that occasionally emerges at this
point in the family life cycle is too much intrusion from the family-of-origin
into the couple coalition. For example, one or more of their parents may
intrude, offering too much help or advice, or act as if his or her child's new
commitment has been an act of disloyalty to the family-of-origin. Unless the
couple can establish a sufficient boundary around their relationship, such
family intrusion can even lead to their dissolution. Another form of intrusion
may be that either member of the couple may still be "acting single," such as
going out with friends rather than spending time to build a stronger couple
unit.

This process may involve another crisis as individuals change their
self-image so as to begin to feel more committed to the partner than to old
friends. The intensity that was experienced at the beginning of the relationship is also likely to begin to cool, and the couple may not be as attentive to
each other as they were at first. This could result in one or the other thinking
that since the strong passion of the "romance" has waned, they must be falling

out of love. At this point, the relationship may become vulnerable to an extra-marital affair or a separation.

If the couple stays together, they are likely to eventually drop much of the pretense that existed during the courting and honeymoon period. Initially, when each was attempting to manage the impression the other had of them, they were not completely genuine with each other. For example, she may have acted as if she liked football, and he may have led her to believe that he liked shopping for antiques, but gradually they have given up trying to get the other to see them as a "great catch."

At this stage, each will begin to reveal their true likes and dislikes; they may belch and flatulate in each other's presence and sit around the house with "bad hair" while munching on snacks and dropping crumbs into the couch. When she wants to go out dancing, he wants to stay home and watch TV. Although these types of concerns are common for couples, they do present potential crisis points. Each individual may feel as if he or she has been betrayed by the other and may ask, "Who are you? You are not the person you were when I promised to be with you for life!" To complicate matters even further, at this point many couples consider having children.

The Influence of Children on the Family Life Cycle

If the couple has not yet readjusted their commitment to, and expectations of, their relationship, the addition of a child may create an additional crisis. Sometimes, if the couple feels as though the marriage is drifting apart, they may mistakenly think that having a child will cement their union. Furthermore, unless the couple has established themselves well enough to make the transition to becoming a "parental coalition," the birth of a child may tend to separate them even more. Sometimes, the wife/mother will withdraw some of her affection from the husband while lavishing her love on the baby. The husband/father's reaction to this may be to spend more time at work or with friends. This scenario tends to set up a situation in which the mother and child (or children) develop their own coalition and the father becomes a stranger in the household.

Couples with children face further stressors as they attempt to respond to the needs of their children, manage their own lifestyle and career concerns, and keep their intimate relationship alive. Children are demanding and time-consuming. From the moment they are born, they require tremendous amounts of care and vigilance on the part of the caregiver. The couple unit therefore often struggles to realign their expectations of parenthood with the reality of care giving. This stage of the family life cycle can be further complicated by the couple's need to provide for children with special needs, cope with insufficient access to resources, or deal with financial constraints.

For many couples, these concerns evolve and change as children begin to attend school. During this period, the child is beginning to establish relationships outside the family. It may be a time for "sleepovers," going to camp, and extracurricular activities, and the child may be devoting a great deal of attention to peer relationships and offering affection to idealized surrogate parent figures. Our expectations for fathers or male caregivers during this time are less clear than those for the mother. Unfortunately, because of socialization and societal expectations, some fathers have been almost absent in our conceptualizations of parental responsibility. Mothers, however, are often expected to take on the role of the "soccer mom" who drives children to games, dance or voice lessons, attends PTA meetings, and helps with homework. How the parents work out their parenting roles will strongly influence the strength of the family and couple unit during this time.

According to Carter and McGoldrick (1999), as children reach adolescence the focus of the family shifts yet again. At this point the adolescent is allowed greater responsibility, and the couple may begin to reexamine their personal and career concerns. Their time for self-reflection may be limited, however, as they are called to deal with the phenomenon of adolescence. In most states the child will get a driver's license at age sixteen and begin to demand much more autonomy. Being mobile will make it possible for the teenager to spend more time away from the family. Family outings and vacations, "special" occasions, and family rituals now tend to be of less interest to the teenager, time spent at friends' houses increases, the child becomes more circumspect when asked about his or her day, and mood swings are par for the course as the child suffers the ambivalence that comes with wishing to remain dependent while craving independence. Interest in sex, music that mystifies the parents, and a culture that seems to be anti-establishment with a coded language that parents don't comprehend, all tend to further separate the teenager from the family. The child may suffer being "dumped" or ignored by someone whom he or she loves, will have fights and "fallings-out" with close friends, may not be chosen in competitions or elections, and will likely hate his or her nose, hair, face, body, etc.

The difficulties for teenagers at Erikson's "identity" stage are legion. The parents suffer feelings of helplessness as they become less able to intervene and make things better for their child. These crises are quite disruptive for the family, since this stage may represent the first truly major accommodation since the birth of the child that the family has had to make. Of course, all these difficulties are normal and expected to some degree, but that knowledge doesn't make it any easier to live through. In addition, this teenage stage sometimes brings on unexpected crises along with the normal developmental problems, such as drug experimentation, unwanted pregnancy, automobile accidents, decline in school performance, or suicidal threats. The child's respect for parental authority appears to be in decline during this time as he or she seeks greater independence, and the parents must begin to negotiate with the teenager, where before they simply "laid down the law." Parents at this stage must be sustained by the faith that once through the teenage years their relationship with their child will likely improve. Mark Twain is supposed to have said that when he was seventeen, his father was someone who knew nothing, but later, when Twain was in his early twenties, he was amazed at how much his father had learned.

In an informal poll of community counselors who work with families with adolescents, we asked a few counselors we know to identify the concerns they have heard in the past week. Three counselors provided the following: sixteen-year-old with a sexually transmitted disease; thirteen-year-old runaway who returned home unexpectedly and refuses to speak; thirteen-year-old girl who has been sexually abused by her stepfather; seventeen-year-old boy accused of sexually abusing an eight-year-old neighbor; several instances of boys suspended from school for offenses such as fighting, drug possession, and gun possession; and several instances of truancy. While these issues may seem challenging in and of themselves, they are all complicated by the fact that they are experienced within the context of a family. The families consist of numerous individuals, each with his or her own needs, and all existing within broader societal contexts that include challenges such as poverty, inadequate access to resources, parental stress, and the general demands of daily living. Clearly, working with families requires a thoughtful and thorough conceptualization, as well as courage, on the part of the counselor.

Later Stages of the Family Life Cycle

As children mature, the family will eventually begin to focus on launching children into the adult world. Most parents hope that the child will become sufficiently well-educated, socially appropriate, mature, confident, and skilled, so as to begin a life that is truly independent of the family. Marcia's (1980) investigations into the "moratorium" period during the "identity crisis" (mentioned earlier in this chapter) suggested that children these days are taking much longer to resolve their identity concerns than Erikson had reported. This means that the family must sometimes be prepared to welcome the child back after an aborted launch.

Because of this extended moratorium, young adults are often uncertain of their ability to cope with the "real" world. Their struggles with the "Who am I?" question extend well into adulthood; thus there is a growing tendency for children to return home after college, a failed marriage, or because of their lack of readiness to assume the responsibilities of a full-fledged adult. So if the family has accommodated to the child being gone, but then needs to, once again, redefine itself as the child returns, the parents and siblings still at home may feel "jerked around." Furthermore, the returning child may feel that he or she is a failure for not being able to cope with the demands of adulthood. Everyone feels as if he or she has not done a good job of launching or being launched.

Another crisis that sometimes occurs after all the children have been launched is the redefinition of the parents' marriage. First, they were lovers, then they were a married couple, then they became parents. Now, for years, they have seen themselves simply as "mother" and "father." If the mother has devoted her life to child rearing, to the exclusion of other interests, she may now experience what is popularly known as the "empty nest syndrome." If her husband has been less in evidence around the house during the child-rearing years, she may look at him one day and wonder what she ever saw in him. He may, in return, wonder whether he will be able to rekindle a relationship with the woman he has come to view only as the mother of his children. If they both see the launching period as the end of their work together, they may discover that the attraction that originally brought them together has been eclipsed by years of parenting. They now have a new "identity crisis" when it comes to their relationship. Their question becomes "Who are *we*?" Their parental coalition must change into a couple coalition once again if they are to sustain their marriage.

As society changes and women and men are freer to accept more diverse roles in society, the crisis of redefinition of marriage may eventually look very different. For example, if both the woman and the man in the family have been able to experiment with their desired roles in their family and society, they may be better able to adjust to changes after children leave. Even so, however, counselors can expect the launching of children to create systemic ripples that may be significant.

Another crisis that seems to be occurring with increasing frequency in American culture is what has been termed the "sandwich generation." This phenomenon exists in families where the children have returned home, or are still heavily dependent on the parents after they have ostensibly been launched. At the same time, the parents' parents have become old enough to be unable to adequately manage their own affairs, or they have become ill or senile. The couple who are attempting to rekindle their former relationship are now faced with the task of continuing to parent their children, while, at the same time, parenting their parents. They are "sandwiched" between the younger and the older generations.

Eventually, the children will be launched, and they will likely begin their own developmental journey if they marry, have children, and face the prospect of all the aforementioned crises. Their parents will usually work out

EXPERIENTIAL LEARNING

In addition to the growing body of excellent texts regarding family development and therapy, we encourage you to mine one of the most powerful and available resources you have—your own family.

- Recall your childhood memories, for better or worse.
- Create a comprehensive three-generation genogram, if possible, and use it to conceptualize yourself.
- Talk with family members who are available to you, and work to learn from your own experience.
- How did your history, culture, ethnicity, socioeconomic class, and childhood shape the person you are today?

an accommodation in their relationship, as well as handle the additional crises that come with their retirement from work, the death of their parents, becoming grandparents, and the possible illness and eventual death of one of them. To be a family is to be challenged at every developmental milestone along the way.

The family lifecycle is one of continual crisis points in which the members will experience anxiety, sadness, and anger. The developmental process of couples and families demands that the members must expect to deal with the agonies of conflict, change, and loss. So, what do you get for all this trouble? One of the authors of this book (JEM) observed the following: "In the span between your first breath and last, your family will account for 50 percent of your trouble and 75 percent of your joy. Not a bad return on your investment."

ETHICAL AND LEGAL ISSUES IN PRACTICE

The ethical standards of the American Counseling Association (2005) state that, as a counselor, you must actively attempt to understand the diverse cultural backgrounds of the clients with whom you will work. As we pointed out in Chapter 7, the way you see the world is not universal. Differences in worldviews are not only based on ethnicity, but are also associated with gender, sexual orientation, economic status, family background, and one's level of development in each of the areas discussed in this chapter. In truth, every single person is a "walking, talking culture" needing to be understood. You must suspend your own worldview and attempt to take the perspective of the other in order to gain true empathic understanding. Often, for instance, students come to our counselor training program stating that they wish to be a counselor based on some particular point of view, such as a "Christian" counselor or a "feminist" counselor. We have no fundamental objection to this. However, it is not your job as a counselor to indoctrinate clients to your way of thinking. You must instead come to know your client's way of thinking. Counselors are not missionaries.

Sarason, Sarason, and Pierce (1990) found that young people, less educated people, people with alternative lifestyles, and women are at greater risk than other groups to be diagnosed with mental disorders. It is important for you to remember that most of the theories of development contained in this chapter have been largely based on white, male, Western-oriented subjects. For this reason, you should be careful in assessing your client's level of development in a rigid or reified manner.

Furthermore, when dealing with families, it is important that you do not attempt to change them in the image of your own family-of-origin. Coming to know how your own family has influenced your attitudes and your ways of viewing the world may be the hardest task of all. Most of the influences on your belief system originated in your family and were unspoken, picked up by observation, and accepted as simply the way people do things. You learned what a family is by engaging in thousands of transactions with your parents, your siblings (provided you are not an only child), and other relatives with whom you were in contact.

A popular saying among family therapists is that "every transaction is a rule." You left your family possessing an unconscious rule for every type of transaction, without ever reflecting on most of these rules. Now, you will find that other families don't behave or believe as yours did. Your first reaction will be to think that this family needs to be "fixed." Of course, at such moments, you will be experiencing your own developmental crisis of "disequilibrium" and the need to move to a new level. Being a counselor is a lifelong developmental process.

The most relevant legal issues regarding lifespan development are the concerns related to child and elder abuse and neglect, as well as confidentiality and informed consent. These topics were presented in Chapter 3 but bear repeating here. The expectations for defining and reporting child and elder abuse vary by states, so it is imperative that you fully understand the legal expectations that govern your practice. Keep in mind as well that as a community counselor you are a frontline resource for individuals who are vulnerable due to age or disability. We can guarantee that at some point in your career, probably sooner rather than later, you will have to make treatment decisions based on legal expectations of practice.

CONCLUDING THOUGHTS

Knowledge of the various levels and domains of individual and family development should prove useful to you as you try to make sense of your clients and yourself. Ideally, you are functioning at the higher levels of development in most of these areas. It is certainly your job to continue to grow and develop as a person in order to be more helpful to others. As a community counseling graduate student, you can use your knowledge of human development to assess yourself. As a counselor, the most important instrument, or tool, with which you work is yourself. You should continually strive to fine tune and upgrade your capabilities as you continue your journey through your levels of development.

RECOMMENDED RESOURCES

Original sources as well as developmental and lifespan textbooks will be helpful to you as you begin your internships and first job. The following sources provide comprehensive information.

Bee, H., & Boyd, D. (2003). *Lifespan development* (3rd ed.). Boston: Allyn & Bacon.

Erikson, E. H. (1980). *Identity and the life cycle.* New York: Norton. (Originally published in 1959.)

Jordan, J. (Ed.). (1997). *Women's growth in diversity: More writings from the Stone Center.* New York: Guilford.

Jordan, J. V., Kaplan, A. G., Miller, G. M., Stiver, I. P., & Surrey, J. L. (1991). *Women's growth in connection: Writings from the Stone Center.* New York: Guilford.

McGoldrick, M. (Ed.). (1998). *Re-visioning family therapy: Race, culture, and gender in clinical practice.* New York: Guilford.

Miller, A. (1994). *The drama of the gifted child* (rev. ed.). New York: Basic.

We also recommend that you look into the International Association of Marriage and Family Counseling (IAMFC), a division of the American Counseling Association, which focuses on concerns very relevant to community counselors who work with families and couples.

Finally, numerous sources are available that suggest techniques and interventions for various age groups. As we mentioned earlier, children are not simply miniature adults. We have found the following to be particularly helpful.

Landreth, G. L. (2002). *Play therapy: The art of the relationship* (2nd ed.). New York: Brunner/Routledge.

Vernon, A. (2004). *Counseling children and adolescents* (3rd ed.). Denver, CO: Love.

Other Resources

Films such as *The Sweet Hereafter, In the Bedroom,* and *Antwone Fisher* provide challenging portrayals of individuals and families dealing with change and loss. The movie *Thirteen* is an intense look at the life of a young girl dealing with her own developing sense of self. The books *The Great Santini* and *The Prince of Tides,* both by Pat Conroy, also offer intriguing glimpses of the influence of family and environment over time. Mark Haddon's *The Curious Incident of the Dog in the Night-Time,* a novel told in the first person by an autistic adolescent, gives a fascinating picture of how life is for an autistic child, and what it's like for the child's parents and caregivers.

REFERENCES

American Counseling Association. (2005). *ACA Code of Ethics.* Retrieved August 22, 2005, from **http://www.counseling.org/Content/NavigationMenu/ RESOURCES/ETHICS/ACA_Code_of_Ethics.htm.**

Ainsworth, M. D. S., Bell, S. M. V., & Stayton, D. J. (1971). Individual differences in strange situation behavior of one-year-olds. In H. R. Schaffer (Ed.), *The origins of human social relationships* (pp. 17–57). London: Academic Press.

Aron, A., Aron, E. N., Tudor, M., & Nelson, G. (1991). Close relationships as including other in the self. *Journal of Personality and Social Psychology, 60,* 241–253.

Baron-Cohen, S. (1996). *Mindblindness: An essay on autism and theory of mind.* Cambridge, MA: MIT Press.

Becvar, D. S., & Becvar, R. J. (1999). *Systems theory and family therapy: A primer.* Washington, DC: University Press of America.

Becvar, D. S., & Becvar, R. J. (2006). *Family therapy: A systemic integration* (6th ed.). Boston: Allyn & Bacon.

Bee, H., & Boyd, D. (2003). *Lifespan development* (3rd ed.). Boston: Allyn & Bacon.

Benjafield, J. G. (1992). *Cognition.* Englewood Cliffs, NJ: Prentice Hall.

Bjorklund, D. F. (1989). *Children's thinking: Developmental function and individual differences.* Pacific Grove, CA: Brooks/Cole.

Bowlby, J. (1973). *Attachment and loss: Vol. 2. Separation: Anxiety and anger.* New York: Basic Books.

Bowlby, J. (1977). The making and breaking of affectional bonds. *British Journal of Psychiatry, 130,* 201–210, 421–431.

Bowlby, J. (1980). *Attachment and loss: Vol. 3. Loss, sadness, and depression.* New York: Basic Books.

Bowlby, J. (1982). *Attachment and loss: Vol. 1. Attachment*. New York: Basic Books. (Originally published in 1969.)

Brown, D., & Srebalus, D. J. (2003). *Introduction to the counseling profession*. Boston: Allyn & Bacon.

Bruner, J. S., Goodnow, J. J., & Austin, G. A. (1956). *A study of thinking*. New York: Wiley.

Buck, R., & Ginsburg, B. (1997). Communicative genes and the evolution of empathy. In W. Ickes (Ed.), *Empathic accuracy* (pp. 17–43). New York: Guilford.

Carter, B., & McGoldrick, M. (1999). Overview: The expanded family life cycle: Individual, family and social perspectives. In B. Carter & M. McGoldrick (Eds.), *The expanded family life cycle: Individual, family and social perspectives* (3rd ed., pp. 1–24). Boston: Allyn & Bacon.

Carter, E. A., & McGoldrick, M. (Eds.). (1980). *The family life cycle: A framework for family therapy*. New York: Gardner Press.

Ceasar, P. T., & Miranti, J. G. (2001). Counseling and spirituality. In D. Capuzzi & D. R. Gross (Eds.), *Introduction to the counseling profession* (pp. 208–223). Boston: Allyn & Bacon.

Davis, M. H. (1994). *Empathy: A social psychological approach*. Madison, WI: Brown & Benchmark.

Darwin, C. (1872/1955). *The expression of the emotions in man and animals*. New York: Philosophical Library.

Dennett, D. (1991). *Consciousness explained*. Boston: Little, Brown.

Echterling, L. G., Presbury, J. H., & McKee, J. E. (2005). *Crisis intervention: Promoting resilience and resolution in troubled times*. Upper Saddle River, NJ: Pearson/Merrill-Prentice Hall.

Eisenberg, N., Murphy, B. C., & Shepard, S. (1997). The development of empathic accuracy. In W. Ickes (Ed.), *Empathic accuracy* (pp. 73–115). New York: Guilford.

Erikson, E. H. (1963). *Childhood and society*. New York: W. W. Norton.

Erikson, E. (1975). *Life history and the historical movement*. New York: W. W. Norton.

Erikson, E. H. (1980). *Identity and the life cycle*. New York: W. W. Norton. (Originally published in 1959.)

Feldman, R. S. (2000). *Development across the life span* (2nd ed.). Upper Saddle River, NJ: Prentice Hall.

Flavell, J. H. (1992). Perspectives on perspective taking. In H. Berlin & P. Pufall (Eds.), *Piaget's theory: Prospects and possibilities* (pp. 107–139). Hillsdale, NJ: Erlbaum.

Fowler, J. (1995). *Stages of faith: The psychology of human development and the quest for meaning*. New York: Harper & Row. (Originally published in 1981.)

Fox, M., Fitzgerald, T., Erricker, J. L., Logan, J., Logan, O., & Ota, C. (1995). The question for meaning: James Fowler, faith development theory, and adult religious education. *Journal of Beliefs and Values*, *16,* 2, 27–30.

Gardner, H. (1982). *Art, mind, and brain: A cognitive approach to creativity.* New York: Basic Books.

Gardner, H. (1991). *The unschooled child: How children think and how schools should teach*. New York: Basic Books.

Gilligan, C. (1982). *In a different voice*. Cambridge, MA: Harvard University Press.

Hill, R. (1970). *Family development in three generations.* Cambridge, MA: Schenkman.

Hoffman, M. L. (1984). Interaction of affect and cognition in empathy. In C. E. Izard, J. Kagan, & R. B. Zajonc (Eds.), *Emotions, cognition, and behavior* (pp. 103–131). Cambridge, Eng.: Cambridge University Press.

Ivey, A., Ivey, M., Myers, J., & Sweeney, T. (2005). *Developmental counseling and therapy: Promoting wellness over the lifespan.* Boston: Lahaska.

Janoff-Bulman, R. (1992). *Shattered assumptions: Towards a new psychology of trauma*. New York: The Free Press.

Jordan, J. (Ed.). (1997). *Women's growth in diversity: More writings from the Stone Center.* New York: Guilford.

Jordan, J. V., Kaplan, A. G., Miller, G. M., Stiver, I. P., & Surrey, J. L. (1991). *Women's growth in connection: Writings from the Stone Center.* New York: Guilford.

Josselson, R. (1987). *Finding herself: Pathways to identity development in women*. San Francisco: Jossey-Bass.

Kagan, J. (1980). Influencing human interaction: Eighteen years with IPR. In A. I. Hess (Ed.), *Psychotherapy supervision: Theory, research, and practice* (pp. 262–283). New York: Wiley.

Kegan, R. (1982). *The evolving self*. Cambridge, MA: Harvard University Press.

Kohlberg, L. (1984). *The psychology of moral development: The nature and validity of moral stages*. San Francisco: Harper & Row.

Labouvie-Vief, G. (1980). Beyond formal operations: Uses and limits of pure logic in life-span development. *Human Development, 23,* 141–161.

Laing, R. D. (1970). *Knots*. New York: Vintage Books.

Leslie, A. (1994). ToMM, ToBy, and agency: Core architecture and domain specificity. In L. Hirschfeld & S. Gelman (Eds.), *Mapping the mind: Domain specificity in cognition and culture* (pp. 119–148). Cambridge, Eng: Cambridge University Press.

Marcia, J. E. (1966). Development and validation of ego identity status. *Journal of Personality and Social Psychology, 3,* 551-558.

Marcia, J. E. (1980). Identity in adolescence. In J. Adelson (Ed.), *Handbook of adolescent psychology* (pp. 159-187). New York: John Wiley & Sons.

Maslow, A. H. (1970). *Motivation and personality* (2nd ed.). New York: Harper.

McGoldrick, M. (Ed.). (1998). *Re-visioning family therapy: Race, culture, and gender in clinical practice.* New York: Guilford.

Miller, A. (1994). *The drama of the gifted child* (rev. ed.). New York: Basic.

Patterson, S. J., Sochting, I., & Marcia, J. E. (1992). The inner space and beyond: Women and identity. In G. R. Adams, T. P. Gullotta, and R. Montemayor (Eds.), *Adolescent identity formation* (pp. 9-24). Newbury Park, CA: Sage.

Perry, W. G. (1970). *Forms of intellectual and ethical development in the college years.* New York: Holt.

Piaget, J. (1926). *The language and thought of the child.* New York: Harcourt.

Piaget, J. (1963). *The origins of intelligence in children.* New York: W. W. Norton.

Pinker, S. (2003). No title. In J. Brockman (Ed.), *The new humanists: Science at the Edge* (pp. 34-51). New York: Barnes & Noble.

Piper, E. (2002). Faith development: A critique of Fowler's model and a proposed alternative. *Journal of Liberal Religion: An Online Theological Journal Devoted to the Study of Liberal Religion, 3,* 1, Winter.

Premack, D., & Woodruff, G. (1978). Does a chimpanzee have a theory of mind? *Behavioral and Brain Sciences, 1,* 515-526.

Presbury, J. H., Benson, A. J., Fitch, J., & Torrance, E. P. (1991). What can children's writing tell us about their cognitive development? *The Journal of Creative Behavior, 25,* 3, 244-249.

Rice, J. K. (1994). Reconsidering research on divorce, family life cycle, and the meaning of family. *Psychology of Women Quarterly, 18,* 559-584.

Sarason, B. R., Sarason, I. G., & Pierce, G. R. (1990). *Social support: An interactional view.* New York: John Wiley & Sons.

Schultz, D. P., & Schultz, E. S. (2000). *A history of modern psychology* (7th ed.). Fort Worth, TX: Harcourt College Publishers.

Sroufe, L. A., Cooper, R. G., DeHart, G. B., & Marshall, M. E. (1996). *Child development: Its nature and course* (3rd ed.). New York: McGraw-Hill.

Steere, D. A. (1997). *Spiritual presence in psychotherapy.* New York: Bruner/Mazel.

Taylor, M. (1996). A theory of mind perspective on social cognitive development. In R. Gelman & T. Kit-Fong Au (Eds.), *Perceptual and cognitive development* (pp. 283-329). San Diego: Academic Press.

Vernon, A. (2004). *Counseling children and adolescents* (3rd ed.). Denver, CO: Love.

Watson, J. D. (1999). Re-directing the course of human evolution. In S. Griffiths (Ed.), *Predictions* (pp. 296–298). New York: Oxford University Press.

Weiss, A. S. (1991). The measurement of self-actualization: The quest for the test may be as challenging as the search for the self. *Journal of Social Behavior and Personality, 6,* 265–290.

West, M. L., & Sheldon-Keller, A. E. (1997). *Patterns of relating: An adult attachment perspective.* New York: The Guilford Press.

Wolfe, T. (1934). *You can't go home again.* New York: Harper and Brothers.

Chapter 9

Building on Strengths: Working with Groups

We must learn to live together as brothers [and sisters] or perish together as fools.

Martin Luther King, Jr.

GOALS

Reading and exploring the ideas in this chapter will help you

- Understand the curative factors of groups
- Understand types of counseling groups
- Determine stages in the group counseling process
- Explore group leadership skills

OVERVIEW

This chapter presents information on principles of group dynamics, group leadership styles, group counseling methods, and ethical and legal considerations in group work. Group counseling can be defined as clients interacting to increase awareness of themselves as individuals and as group members, to examine possibilities for change, and to take action based on changes experienced within the group (Haney & Leibsohn, 2001). Patterns of interaction in other groups, such as families or peer groups, will provide valuable insight into your understanding of yourself and your clients as members of a counseling group.

As you are introduced to the concepts and practices associated with group work, remember that learning to work with groups in a counseling setting is a process that takes time and practice. Many students completing their counseling internship still have fears and concerns about working with groups. Many would rather stick to individual clients and leave the groups to "more experienced" counselors. Keep in mind, though, that as a community counselor you will use many of the same skills with groups that you rely on in individual counseling. Whether you're working with individuals or groups, you'll need to be present with your clients, validate their experiences, and help facilitate growth and change.

Contrary to the common misconception, group counseling is not "watered down" individual counseling. In comparing individual versus group modalities of helping, many researchers have found that both are equally effective for most clients (Srebalus & Brown, 2001). In fact, the group format can intensify the counseling experience and inspire some surprising personal discoveries. It can also be a complex encounter. The Council for the Accreditation of Counseling and Related Programs (CACREP) conceptualizes group work as a multifaceted discipline, including group theory, group counseling methods and skills, group roles and leadership styles, approaches to and types of groups, and ethical and legal concerns. This chapter will introduce you to many of these concepts in the context of community counseling. You will find more extensive exploration of all of these topics in a comprehensive group counseling book (i.e., Corey, 2004; Yalom, 1995).

Leading groups and facilitating the group process can feel especially daunting. Therefore, in order to be effective as a counselor in a group setting, you need to understand some important concepts and skills. It is also essential that you examine yourself as a group participant so that you can recognize your impact on others as well as understand multiple perspectives of clients.

KELLY'S DEFINING MOMENT: Sink or Swim

Kelly, a licensed professional counselor who has worked in community agencies for several years, is a confident group facilitator. She has offered divorcing parents groups, recovery groups, and court-mandated anger management groups. She has led therapy groups for dually diagnosed clients and facilitated personal exploration groups for adolescents with chronic illnesses. She has truly enjoyed each experience, even though she usually begins each session thinking, *Maybe I shouldn't do this. What if I am in over my head and don't have what it takes to work with this group?* However, as the groups take on a healing power of their own, she has been amazed by the energy of the group process. To her credit, groups that Kelly started over five years ago are still being facilitated by other counselors and are touching the lives of many individuals. Through her varied, taxing, and rewarding experiences with groups, Kelly has truly witnessed the power of the group experience.

It wasn't always this way. Kelly cringes when she remembered her first group experience. As a master's student, she had facilitated a single-parent support group that she started in response to a need articulated by local agencies. Upon hearing about Kelly's plan to start the group, one of Kelly's peers said, "What do you know about being a single parent? How can you possibly understand the needs of the group and be the kind of leader they need?"

Kelly's supervisor was more encouraging. She agreed to support Kelly's venture, but reminded Kelly to let the supervisor know immediately if she felt over her head. Kelly quickly found that the group experience was much more challenging than she had anticipated. After the second session, she went home feeling drained and shaky. *Now I know what it feels like when people are thrown in the water and told to swim,* she thought. She wrestled with intense feelings of self-doubt and incompetence. *What if the group takes control? What if I can't help them, or worse yet, what if the group process actually hurts them?* Kelly realized she did feel as though she were floundering, so she called her supervisor that evening.

After several hours of focused supervision, Kelly developed a plan. She realized that she had to exhibit appropriate skills to deal with group member issues, such as monopolizing and self-defeating behavior. She had to recognize how each member of the group played out "real-life" issues with other members of the group. She had to use immediacy to help group members change some of their relational patterns. She also had to realize that she was not the expert who needed to heal individual group members. Finally, she had to trust herself and the group process. "You knew when you needed help," her supervisor reminded her. "You can do this. You need to keep on your toes, and you need to trust your gut. Don't worry about these people liking you. Just do your job."

Kelly approached her third group session with a new attitude. She made some mistakes with the group, and the group members struggled at times to work cohesively. Soon, though, Kelly became comfortable enough to talk with the group about how they perceived the group process and her leadership. She pushed herself to quit focusing on herself and her insecurities and focus instead on the group and its movement. As a result, she saw firsthand that the group was itself a profound change agent for most participants. She realized her job was to learn how to best facilitate the process among group members, who had the capacity to heal themselves as well as others.

Questions for Reflection

1. What stereotypes do you hold regarding group counseling?
2. What fears, if any, do you have about facilitating groups?

3. Based on what you know now about counseling in general, for what types of concerns do you believe group counseling would be most helpful? Why these concerns?

THE CURATIVE FACTORS OF GROUP COUNSELING

According to Irving Yalom (1995), a leading theorist and practitioner of group counseling, eleven major factors can make groups a healing process for participants. Yalom named these components the Curative Factors of Group Therapy. After reviewing these factors, read "Sal's Opening" on page 305 and answer the questions.

- *Instillation of hope* occurs when members gain hope by becoming inspired or encouraged by each other, directly or indirectly, throughout the course of therapy.

- *Universality* is one of the most powerful curative factors as participants realize that they are not alone in their struggles and that fellow humans have similar experiences, feelings, needs, and concerns. The concept that "I am not alone" oftentimes is a welcome one after long periods of dealing with a difficult problem such as an addiction, a sexual identity issue, a major loss, or a relationship difficulty.

- *Imparting information* by the therapist or group members provides educational resources to group members. For example, group members may be exposed to several models of grief and loss or taught the "Twelve Steps" of overcoming addiction.

- *Altruism* connotes giving of oneself for the greater good of others. Groups provide many opportunities for members to provide each other with resources, support, encouragement, or challenges. As they help each other, group members are better able to transcend tendencies toward self-absorption. They can begin to see themselves as worthy individuals who have something to contribute to others.

- *Corrective recapitulation of the primary family group,* also provided by the group, involves providing an arena in which family-of-origin issues can be addressed through interactions with group members.

- *Development of socializing techniques* occurs as group members learn healthy and mutually beneficial ways of communicating with others in a social setting.

- *Imitative behavior* can be a positive development when members learn from the modeling of each other or the group leader.

Sal's Opening

Sal's wife died of breast cancer a year ago. Since then, Sal had been very depressed and had not wanted to leave his house. His friend suggested that he participate in a grief group through the local hospice, so Sal decided to try it.

Throughout the twelve-week group experience, Sal was confronted by group members on his lack of willingness to share his feelings about his wife's death. He learned from others' disclosures that expressing his feelings through crying, art, or writing could be very healing, so he decided to keep a journal. He wrote about his anger toward himself for not making better use of his time with his wife, as well as his anger at her for dying before he could retire and spend his golden years with her.

Sal found that not sharing his experiences was putting up barriers between himself and others, so he began to talk about the course of his wife's cancer, his anger, and how he felt holding her in his arms when she died.

Sal thanked the group for challenging and inviting him to come out from his hiding place. Once he was able to share his grief, Sal was able to address the questions surrounding the purpose and direction of his "future" life. He also invited a woman from his synagogue, who had recently lost her partner, to join the group.

Questions for Reflection

1. Name the curative factors you think Sal experienced as a result of the group process.

2. As group facilitator, what goals would you have in mind for Sal at the beginning of the group?

3. How could you integrate Sal's journal writing into his group experience?

4. How might Sal's invitation to the woman from his synagogue to join the group help or hinder his progress?

- *Interpersonal learning* happens as a result of the sharing, listening, giving feedback, and challenging that occurs in a group. Sharing on a deep level allows individuals to learn about the "shadow" aspects of themselves and thus practice changing negative relational patterns with each other.

- *Group cohesiveness* is often developed in groups and can be especially healing for individuals who have had difficulty with relationships or belonging. Belonging to a group contributes to a sense of well-being.

- *Catharsis,* the expression of pent-up feelings, may be healing for some individuals if facilitated non-destructively by a skilled counselor.

- *Existential factors*, such as meaning, meaninglessness, life purpose, and mortality, are addressed in groups and can contribute to healing by potentially providing members with resolution of troubling life questions.

A BRIEF HISTORY OF COUNSELING GROUPS

The idea that group work is a powerful way of intervening with people was a realization that dawned very slowly during the twentieth century. At first, groups were used simply because it was not possible to work with each person individually. The prevailing thought was that group work was a trade-off that at least provided an efficient way of seeing all who needed to be seen. However, the belief that group work was a less effective approach began to fade as positive results were increasingly noted. For example, Pratt (1907) began treating tuberculosis patients in groups because of the overwhelming number of people who were afflicted with the disease at the time. Surprisingly, what started as an efficient way of dealing with patients turned out to be quite effective as well. Patients who attended weekly meetings remained in good spirits, and 75 percent of them recovered, even though many had been given no hope of recovery (Kline, 2003).

Likewise, Burrow (1928) found that working with psychiatric patients in groups seemed to increase their social skills. Burrow concluded that the effects of isolation and poor interpersonal relationships played a major part in the development of psychopathology. Having people work together in a group tended to mitigate some aspects of their disorders. Later, in response to the overwhelming needs of the military during World War II, groups were set up to handle the psychiatric problems of returning soldiers. Although the group therapists during this time were relatively unsophisticated, they recognized that something powerful was taking place in their groups (Kline, 2003, p. 9).

During the initial stages of group work, groups were used for practical purposes such as teaching self-care. The first major theorist of group counseling, J. L. Moreno, surfaced in the 1930s under the leadership of Kurt Lewin. This proved to be an active time for the development of training and theory in the group movement. In the 1950s, group counseling distinguished itself from other counseling specializations such as individual, marriage, and family counseling (Gladding, 2003).

Through the 1950s and 1960s, the group movement continued to accelerate. In 1973, the Association for Specialists in Group Work (ASGW) was established through the American Counseling Association, and several journals devoted to group work began to publish around that time. Task groups or work groups arose during the 1970s, and psychoeducational groups were popular during the 1980s and 1990s (Gladding, 2003). Today, psychoeducational groups remain popular, and counseling groups are offered in settings such as community mental health centers, college counseling centers, hospitals, drug and alcohol treatment centers, veteran's organizations, and public schools (Srebalus & Brown, 2001). You may find yourself providing group counseling in any of these venues.

GROUP CONCEPTS

As you prepare to work with groups, you should understand issues such as types of counseling groups, leadership skills for group counselors, roles assumed by group members, and stages in the group counseling process. If you're going to truly endorse group counseling as an effective modality, you should also understand the factors of effectiveness in group counseling as well as the advantages and disadvantages of group counseling. As you learn about each of these concepts, you will be asked some questions about yourself. Awareness and exploration of the self as you learn about working with groups are critical factors in your development as an effective group counselor.

Elements, Conditions, and Processes

As everyone knows, water is made up of the elements hydrogen and oxygen. But the behavior of these elements varies according to the conditions in which they are placed. Put these elements into a condition of minus 32 degrees Fahrenheit and you get ice. Put them into a condition of plus 212 degrees Fahrenheit and you get steam. In between there is water, warm or cool, depending on the temperature of its condition. Alter the condition, and the processes that take place among the elements will alter accordingly.

So it is with people in group conditions. People, with their individual personalities, are the elements. The design or context of the group in which people find themselves is their condition. And the processes—behaviors and experiences—that take place among the people are the result of an interaction between individual personalities and the group condition. The way in which you as a counselor design the group condition will determine whether you get a process that is closer to ice or to steam.

Social psychologists have shown that context is a powerful influence on the behaviors of individuals, regardless of their personalities. Although their inherent character is the same, regardless of where they are, the same person will behave somewhat differently in a church, at a party, at work, or on vacation. Each of these conditions calls for different behaviors, and we all find ourselves affected by the behavioral norms of these various locations.

Furthermore, this change in behavior will result in an alteration of the way this person experiences himself or herself.

Group conditions are generally designed to accomplish an intended goal. Thus, as a facilitator you need to understand group processes in light of a desired outcome. The type of group you are organizing will make a difference in how you design the condition. For example, if you were a military general or a CEO of a large corporation, you might wish to design a setting in which the process is formal, cool, and deliberate—closer to ice than to steam. This is because the processes within such groups are generally carried out rationally and without great displays of emotion. The people—or elements—in such a group are functionaries. They have membership in the group because they can contribute to the ultimate goal of the group. The military exists to defeat their enemies in war. The corporation exists to make money. If group members do not contribute to these goals, they are usually replaced. The welfare of the members is not the primary concern of the group. It is not that such groups are heartless; they simply need to have group processes that contribute to their efficiency. Their organizations need to operate like well-oiled machinery.

Counseling groups, on the other hand, are designed to operate closer to the other end of the spectrum between ice and steam. The goal of a counseling group *is* the welfare of the individual group members. Members are not viewed as functionaries of some greater task, but as the focus of the group itself. The group process should be decidedly warmer than that of a corporate board meeting and may occasionally erupt into heated discussions if it is functioning successfully. Blowing off steam is encouraged in a counseling group.

In your training to become a facilitator of counseling groups, you will acquire the skills to create the necessary condition for such processes to take place. You will learn how to intervene in the process when it becomes either too icy or too steamy. Unlike the military or the corporation, your goal will be to establish a process that is focused internally, and one through which individual members begin to experience themselves and others in new ways. Your hope is that these people will leave your group having been enhanced as individuals and with greater social skills. People who begin the group as strangers will become more intimate with each other, will practice new behaviors together, and will take what they have learned back with them to their lives outside the group.

TYPES OF GROUPS

Groups can take many forms in community settings. Throughout your journey as a practicum student, intern, and practitioner, you will probably be a member of, as well as facilitator of, many different types of groups. At this point in your life, from what kind of group do you think you would most benefit? Would it be a peer support group where you could share common everyday concerns with people in a life situation similar to yours? Would it be a psychoeducational group in which you'd learn particular skills such as stress management or relationship building? Perhaps you would rather participate in a counseling group in which you could work on deeper issues you have uncovered in your training experience so far. You may discover that the type of group that would be most beneficial to you now might be different a year from now.

As counselors, we should be prepared to provide effective services through offering different types of groups to meet our clients' needs. We also should be aware of existing, ongoing groups in the community to which we can refer clients when appropriate. Ways to find out about groups being offered in the community include looking in the local newspaper and contacting other agencies such as substance abuse agencies, hospices, religious nonprofits, and community or women's centers. Most community counselors keep a list of community agencies that offer specific groups for various issues as a helpful resource for linking clients with services that are most appropriate for them.

Therapy Groups

Typically, therapy groups are intended to help clients struggling with problems likely to interfere with their daily functioning. These groups require the counselor to have a thorough understanding of abnormal as well as normal development, and to be prepared to help clients remediate deeply ingrained patterns of ineffective behavior (Association for Specialists in Group Work, 2000).

Although this type of group work may require the counselor to attend to pathology first and wellness second—thus prevention is more secondary than primary in nature—therapy groups, like all groups, emphasize helping members develop more effective ways of interacting with others while dealing with mental illness or other maladjustment.

Most community counselors who work in outpatient and inpatient settings are likely to have the opportunity to facilitate therapy groups. Stacy, for example, was a counseling student completing her internship in a hospital setting. She was assigned to work with outpatient clients who were dealing with depression. After meeting with her supervisor and reviewing some books and notes from her training, Stacy chose to utilize cognitive-behavioral therapy because of its usefulness with individuals dealing with depression. She established a warm and respectful relationship with the group members that enabled her to begin challenging their self-defeating thoughts and behavior. Gradually, the members began to focus more on possibilities rather than failures. Soon, the group members began to challenge and support each other's efforts to make active decisions to better their own lives. The members became mutual change agents, and Stacy found success by drawing upon her knowledge of the significant issues her clients were dealing with.

Counseling Groups

Counseling groups focus on self-awareness, growth, prevention, and actualization of one's potential. As opposed to therapy groups, counseling groups tend to emphasize normal developmental issues rather than pathology. Community counselors who lead counseling groups often utilize a specific theoretical approach, such as cognitive-behavioral, Adlerian, person-centered, or existential as a basis for the therapeutic process. Counseling groups can be offered in many settings, such as mental health centers, private practices, college campuses, K–12 schools, hospitals, and treatment centers. Some groups are centered on specific issues, such as recovery from substance abuse, self-esteem, divorce, grief, or anxiety. On the other hand, many counseling groups do not have specific topics and focus generally on understanding the self in relation to others and reaching one's potential for greater well-being.

As a practitioner, you may be involved in leading a variety of counseling groups in different community settings. For example, one community counselor may lead anger management groups at a nonprofit agency for at-risk youth and another counselor may run several groups on substance abuse at a treatment center. Yet another may be leading grief groups for families, adults, and children at a community hospice while another community counselor could be facilitating groups for male batterers or court-ordered parents in need of parenting skills at a family services center.

Self-Help Groups/Support Groups

Self-help groups, also known as support groups, have become increasingly popular in the past twenty years. Self-help groups are usually led by the members themselves and typically do not involve a trained leader. Self-help or support groups may meet in various places in the community, including community centers, libraries, and places of worship. Such groups focus more on inspiration and encouragement rather than personal and interpersonal growth (Corey, 2004). Most self-help or support groups focus on a particular issue such as obesity, divorce, single-parenting, sexual identity, or career changes. These groups often provide emotional support and encouragement for members confronting the same issue. Oftentimes self-help or support groups become politically active in order to effect social change and policy to advocate for persons dealing with a particular concern.

Ray, for example, decided to join Alcoholics Anonymous® (AA) after hearing about this well-known support group from a friend. The "About AA" section on the website for AA (**www.AA.com**) explains, "Alcoholics Anonymous® is a fellowship of men and women who share their experience, strength and hope with each other that they may solve their common problem and help others to recover from alcoholism. The only requirement for membership is a desire to stop drinking."

Ray believed that joining a group of people with problems similar to his own would be the most effective way to honestly confront the drinking problem that had caused so much pain in his life and division in his family. Ray did not want an "expert leader" who might not be able to relate to the complex issues that he was facing, such as his problem keeping a job and maintaining his marriage while struggling with his addiction.

Washington and Moxley (2003) note that group work can be especially effective with addicted persons as new behaviors and coping skills are learned, modeled, and practiced. Further, information sharing and support in groups help combat a sense of deep isolation. Many individuals can benefit from connecting with others who can relate to the complexities of a common issue. For instance, Blye and Fisher (1999) provided an example of support groups for gay men. They noted that support groups for gay men may be especially helpful by providing information, decreasing feelings of loneliness and despair, and helping members deal with fears about being identified as gay.

Psychoeducational Groups

Psychoeducational groups are groups with the purpose of educating members on specific issues. The group leader is usually a content expert who provides valuable information. These groups are geared toward educating specific populations, such as children or victims of sexual assault, and address topics such as safe sex, recovery from abuse, and building healthy relationships. The focus of psychoeducational groups is more on the content and curriculum of what is being conveyed than the therapeutic process of the group. Such groups are offered in many settings, such as college campuses, K–12 schools, community centers, or places of worship.

Christa, for instance, joined a psychoeducational group designed to educate women on reentering the workforce. Christa was a single mother raising two children, and she wanted to achieve a higher-paying, more satisfying job. She signed up at the local resource center for women for the *Women-to-Work* program. The group leader instructed participants on career exploration, résumé building, computer use, job searching, personal finance management, and interviewing skills. Another group member, Chevonne, inspired Christa to take additional computer courses with her at a community college, and Christa was able to build her skills while building a new friendship. The women exchanged childcare and called each other weekly to check on each other's progress.

By the time the group was over, Christa had some tangible skills with which to secure and maintain a job that fit her interests and talents and had begun to build a network of support that could help her meet her new goals.

Psychoeducational groups offered by community counselors often take a preventive focus. Frieman (1994–1995) described a group experience for divorcing parents designed to help them refrain from hurting their children unnecessarily during the divorce process. In this group experience, leaders teach non-adversarial approaches to separation and divorce during two three-hour sessions which are one week apart. Parents learn proactive measures for dealing with stress, developmentally appropriate methods of communicating with their children about the divorce, and ways of creating a businesslike parenting partnership. The second part of the group process involves family therapy sessions, which would fall under the therapeutic/counseling group category. The groups Frieman referred to are run by the Children of Separation and Divorce Center, a nonprofit community agency in Maryland.

Personal Growth Groups

Personal growth groups are not designed for people who feel they are currently facing difficult personal struggles. Rather, these groups are for people who feel that their lives are going relatively smoothly, but who want to enhance their well-being by improving relationships. Most community agencies do not have sufficient time or resources to offer personal growth groups, but many community counselors facilitate these groups in private practice.

People who participate in personal growth groups may be interested in exploring influences of gender or race, engaging in spiritual growth experiences, or expanding their creative abilities. For example, in the 1980s, poet and writer Robert Bly conducted workshops for men who wanted to explore parts of themselves previously squelched by societal expectations. During this time, many men took part in personal growth group experiences, much like women had already been doing as part of the women's liberation movement.

In addition, today many people take part in spiritual growth groups. Meg, a successful professional in a committed relationship, felt like she was managing her life well. However, she felt that a deeper connection to her spiritual self would help her become a more centered person. She became a part of a spiritual growth group at her local life enrichment center. There, she discovered that engaging in meditation and rituals in a group setting enhanced her already satisfying life.

Structured Versus Unstructured Groups

The best type of group for a specific client depends on the client's life circumstances and current needs. Counselors and clients alike need to

EXPERIENTIAL LEARNING

Take some time to think about what you would want to work on if given the opportunity to participate in a group counseling experience right now.

1. What outcomes would you hope to achieve as a result of your group work?

2. What type of group would you prefer—therapy, self-help, psychoeducational, or personal growth? Why?

3. If you were asked to facilitate a group right now, which type of group would be most appealing to you? Why?

4. You may be working with clients now, or observing faculty or peers as they work with clients. If so, what types of groups might be most appropriate for the clients you've seen? Why?

determine whether a structured or unstructured group experience would be most effective in dealing with a particular presenting concern or issue.

Structured groups usually involve a planned sequence of sessions around a specific topic. Such groups have beginning and ending dates, as well as therapeutic and educational goals. Structured groups may include a pre- and post-measure to determine the effectiveness of the group experience. These groups can center on topics such as anxiety management, adjustment to college, family changes, living with a substance abuser, or self-esteem. Mathis and Tanner (2000) noted that structured groups are particularly helpful when dealing with family-of-origin issues. Structured activities with such groups can include family script reenactment, guided questions about family of origin concepts, goal-setting for future interactions, and psychoeducational content (Mathis & Tanner, 2000). Moore and Freeman (1995) asserted that structured groups for survivors of suicide give the highest level of help.

Unstructured groups usually take the form of therapy or personal growth group experiences in which self-awareness, relationships within the group, and actualization of one's potential are the ultimate goals. There is no specific plan or timetable for realizing those goals. Unstructured groups do not have an agenda per se, and such groups tend to last as long as the members and facilitator believe the group is needed. Unstructured groups tend to be less popular in the community setting due to limitations of time and resources and the demands of managed care. In addition, unstructured groups may lack the direction and planning needed to address issues relevant for community counseling work.

EXPERIENTIAL LEARNING

Read the following scenarios and determine which kind of group you think each person might benefit from most. Specifically, decide whether each client should be referred to a counseling or therapy group, a self-help group, a psychoeducational group, or a personal growth group. Then decide whether a structured or unstructured group experience would be a better fit. Discuss your rationale with your classmates.

1. Marla has recently been divorced from her spouse of fifteen years. She has two children and wants to find a way to start a new career. She also would like to focus on building her self-esteem so she does not end up in another abusive relationship like her recent marriage.

2. Charles is a junior in college who has come to terms with his sexual identity as a gay man. Charles is worried about telling his friends and especially his parents. He has already received individual counseling and is comfortable with his sexual orientation, but he is uncomfortable with the social consequences of coming out.

3. Antoine and Sharla have recently lost their five-year-old son to childhood leukemia. The stress of their son's illness has taken a toll on their marriage. They are devastated because of their loss and would like to gain support from others who have been through something similar.

4. Pam has struggled with anxiety for over ten years, since her twenties. She has recently moved to a new town and is starting a new career. Pam feels that it is time to get help for her anxiety, as it seems to be preventing her from living a happy life.

5. Kevin feels that his life is rather balanced. However, he would like to go deeper and become more aware of his inner life and experiences. Kevin would like to expand his own creativity and explore his spirituality through a group experience.

GROUP LEADERSHIP SKILLS FOR COMMUNITY COUNSELORS

Effective group counseling requires the same fundamental skills that allow counselors to build trusting, therapeutic relationships in individual counseling. Applying these skills to groups, though, feels different. More people are in the room. The interaction among the various personalities feels unpredictable. What if the group members stage the equivalent of a mutiny? What if the group leader can't keep up with the process? If you are feeling intimidated by the prospect of facilitating a group, remember that one effective way to gain competence is through taking risks and consulting with others as you do so. As you learn about the following skills used by group facilitators, try to think of other situations in which you have used each of the skills. Then, imagine applying these skills in a group setting.

Corey (2004) summarized Nolan's (1978) work on leadership interventions by providing an overview of group leadership skills. Here, we cover most of the skills highlighted by Corey, focusing on the most essential ones for community counselors. As each skill is reviewed, remember to try and think of a time when you implemented this skill, either with another individual or in a group setting. You will recognize some of the skills listed below as those we mentioned in Chapter 5.

- *Active listening* requires nonjudgmental attending to another's verbal and nonverbal communications in order to promote trust and self-disclosure.

- *Restating* is a method of paraphrasing what a participant has said in order to clarify and check for meaning.

- *Summarizing* requires pulling out the essential information and repeating it to the client to enhance continuity.

- *Asking open-ended questions* can stimulate thinking, discussion, self-exploration, and group focus.

- *Confronting* is an important technique because it challenges members to examine contradictions and conflicting messages that hinder self-awareness and effective relationships.

Also, the LUV Triangle of Listening, Understanding, and Validating is essential for group work. The basic counseling skills of *reflecting feelings* (communicating an understanding of members' feelings), *using supportive responses* (providing encouragement), and *empathizing* (identifying with clients to demonstrate understanding and promote self-exploration) help create an environment of trust and understanding among group members and between group members and the facilitator.

Additional skills include:

- *Goal-setting* allows the group to maintain some structure while working toward specific, meaningful goals that promote a sense of efficacy among members.

- *Evaluating* includes appraising the group process in order to assess its effectiveness and make necessary changes along the way.

- *Giving feedback* involves honestly sharing observations about the behaviors of individual members and the interactions among the group.

This process helps members to understand how they affect others and to address personal strengths and weaknesses with each other.

- *Protecting* group members may be important at times when the psychological or emotional well-being of a member is threatened by another member or by the group process. The facilitator must step in when ethical boundaries are being crossed and also warn members of the consequences of various actions.

- *Blocking* is a protective measure to stop unproductive group behavior such as monopolizing by a group member.

- *Self-disclosure,* just as in individual counseling, can be used therapeutically when it is offered in the best interest of group members to increase trust and self-understanding and possibly promote understanding and hope.

- *Modeling* involves inspiring group members by promoting desired behaviors through setting an example.

- *Linking* allows the facilitator to illuminate common themes emerging in the group in order to increase group cohesion.

- *Terminating* includes preparing the group members for the end of the group experience and helping members integrate understanding and insight from the group experience into their everyday lives.

Not all counseling groups feel as ambiguous as the one described in "Like Night and Day" (see page 317). Providing structure and sharing expectations prior to beginning the group will reduce ambiguity. You will find group counseling as a community counselor quite different from leading groups for psychologically minded counseling graduate students. However, we have found that in all types of counseling, the counselor must learn to trust the process and take risks.

What Members Can Do to Contribute to the Group Process

Here is a list of suggestions we often give to counseling group members during the first session.

1. Be open. Challenge yourself to take risks by disclosing to others.
2. Ask for feedback about yourself.
3. Give honest and helpful feedback to others.
4. Speak directly to the person you're addressing.
5. Speak for yourself by using "I" statements.
6. Share aloud any reactions that you notice.
7. Stay "in the room," focusing on here and now experiences.

Like Night and Day

Angel and Norma were graduate students beginning their group practicum experience. Both students were asked to facilitate a personal growth group for first-year students enrolled in the master's counseling program. "You can structure your groups in any way you like," their supervisor told them. "I prefer, though, that you allow the process to unfold as it will. Your group members are counseling students. They should be able to handle the ambiguity of the counseling process. You'll each have eight students in your group." Angel and Norma were excited and a little nervous about beginning their groups. They agreed to meet for supervision immediately after their first group sessions.

Angel's first session felt surreal to her. She took literally her supervisor's suggestion to let the process unfold. She began the first session with no real agenda other than a desire to hear from each person and to help them determine what they wanted from the group. She expected the group members to jump in eagerly. Instead, they looked at her with a mixture of hesitance, confusion, and in one case, outright hostility.

"But what are we supposed to *talk* about?" Greer, an outspoken group member demanded. "You need to give us some more direction. We can't just flounder around in here week after week."

Some of the other group members expressed agreement, although one person, Scott, mumbled that he thought the group members should be willing to take responsibility for the group.

"How?!" Greer demanded.

"I don't know," Scott replied sheepishly.

When Angel went to supervision after the first group session, she felt like crying. As she entered her supervisor's office she heard Norma saying excitedly, "I love working with groups. I think I'm finding my niche! How was yours, Angel?"

That did it. Before she could even sit down Angel felt her eyes starting to fill with tears. "I think I stink at this," she said. "My group is ready to kick me out. They seemed completely dissatisfied with me, from beginning to end. One person was almost nasty."

Their supervisor helped Norma and Angel talk about their very different experiences and encouraged them both to write about their reactions. "Don't give up," the supervisor told Angel. "This is a learning experience. Think and write about what's going on for you, for them, and among all of you in your groups."

The next week, Angel's group again felt challenging. She reflected their feelings of discomfort and commented on the process she saw occurring. She observed out loud that Greer seemed dissatisfied, and she wondered what Greer wanted to offer to the group. She asked directly what some of the silent members were thinking and feeling. *What the heck,* she thought. *I'm going to work hard in here, even if some of the members aren't going to.*

At the end of the session, Angel felt tired, but less disheartened. "I'm trying," she told her supervisor. "I'm not sure they are, but I am."

(continued)

(Like Night and Day, continued)

As they met in supervision, Angel and Norma realized that their styles were drastically different. Norma's group, early on, had agreed that they would talk about a different group member each week. The person would discuss his or her history, how he or she chose to enter the counseling profession, and what she or he wanted out of life.

"No confrontations?" Angel asked. "No challenges? No awkward silences or demands on you as the leader?!"

"Nope," Norma replied. "It's all really civilized. They agree at the end of each session who's going to be in the spotlight next week." When Angel described what had happened in her group, Norma listened with a mixture of vicarious fear and surprise.

After a few weeks, Norma said tentatively, "You know, your group experience sounds a little crazy. It seems slightly out of control, and I think it would feel scary for me as a leader. What I'm realizing, though, is that your group members are learning things about themselves. Some of them are taking risks. *You're* taking risks. I don't feel exhausted after my group, and I don't feel in over my head. But I'm not sure my group is really a group. I think we're a collection of people telling stories. We have no real problems, but we have no real process either."

"Finally!" their supervisor said. "I was wondering when you all would get to this. Let's talk about what's really going on in these groups. Let's talk about what's really going on with you as leaders."

Questions for Reflection

1. If you were given the same instructions as Norma and Angel, how would you prepare for your first group sessions?

2. How do you think you will respond if you feel a group member is expressing hostility to you as group leader?

3. If you were Norma and realized that your group was "a collection of people telling stories," what would you do?

4. If you were Angel facing the reluctance to participate on the part of a number of group members, what would you do?

---

8. Take responsibility for the group process, rather than letting others do it.

9. Make sure someone is finished with his or her thought before changing the subject.

10. Be concrete, rather than abstract.

11. Call others on "out-of-bounds" behaviors.

12. Be sure to take your air time, but don't monopolize.

13. Share your perceptions, rather than asserting "facts."

14. Offer your personal sentiments or reactions, rather than speaking for the group.

15. Follow up on what others have said, rather than remaining silent.

16. Describe, rather than interpret, the actions of other members.

17. Look around the room and study other people's faces and body language, rather than averting your eyes or staring at the floor.

You may want to develop your own list for group members, remembering to revise the list as you offer groups for different needs and client issues. For instance, when offering groups for court-ordered clients, we sometimes include in our lists statements such as "Violence is not permitted and is immediate grounds for rejection from the group" and "Weapons are not permitted in the counseling rooms." When working with children and adolescents, we adjust our language and simply remind group members to respect each others' rights, share, take turns, and listen. Then, as the group leaders, we attempt to model and reinforce appropriate member behavior.

LEADER RESPONSES TO MEMBER BEHAVIORS

Initially, because of uncertainty, the ambiguity of the group process, and the presence of other group members, your group clients will likely experience some difficulty with the group process. As you respond to their behaviors in the group, you will ideally teach your group clients how to connect in ways that will increase the interaction among the members and create conditions for authentic responding.

Below are some brief scenarios that illustrate what you might do in response to certain member behaviors.

- *A member looks only at the leader when talking.* You may want to respond nonverbally at first by not keeping eye contact with the speaker. Instead, you can shift your gaze to the other members to model that behavior to the speaker. If the speaker continues to look only at you, then you might say, "You seem to be talking only to me. How about directing your conversation to other members of the group?"

- *A member talks in generalities while not making eye contact with anyone in particular.* You can say something like, "You seem to be talking to the group as a whole. Can you be more specific and pick someone in the group to speak to about this issue?"

- *One member speaks of another member in the third person.* You might respond to this by making eye contact with the speaker and suggesting, "How about saying that to [the person being talked about]." At that point, you can turn your gaze to the other person to communicate your expectation that the speaker will now engage directly with that member.

- *A member couches individual feelings or opinions in "we" terms.* For example, if a member says, "I think the group is feeling a little nervous right now," you can ask the speaker, "Would you be willing to speak for yourself, by saying 'I' instead of 'the group'?" Or you may want to check with the entire group by saying, "Susan is saying that the group feels nervous. Is that true of all of you?"

- *A member of the group may distance him- or herself from the process by responding more as a counselor than a member.* If one member says to another, "How long have you been bothered by this feeling?" then you may suggest to the speaker, "Instead of asking Jenny about *her* feeling, would you say something about yourself in regard to what she has disclosed?" Or you may want to ask the speaker, "How did it make *you* feel when Jenny was talking about her situation?"

The following are other scenarios potentially calling for counselor response.

- *No one responds when a member discloses something.* You can offer the question, "I wonder if anyone else feels the same way that John does?" Or you may want to focus on the member who disclosed by asking, "What's it like for you to reveal something like that and then have everyone sit in silence?"

- *The group seems reluctant or stuck.* You might ask the group as a whole, "It seems like we were rolling along pretty well and then suddenly hit a wall. What's going on with you?" When you finish, you can look directly at several members while letting the silence build.

- *A member talks directly to another member who does not respond.* You can say to the speaker, "It seems that you would really like to make a connection with Jerry. What's it like for you to extend to him and get nothing back?" Or you may turn to the other member and ask, "What do you think it is like for Harriet to talk to you and get nothing back?"

- *One member "name-calls" another.* For example, if one member says to another, "I can't believe you're being such a bitch about this!" then you could respond quickly with, "Instead of calling Nell a name, could you please tell her how you are feeling at this moment?" If the member then responds by saying, "Well, I feel that *she* is . . .," you can interrupt with the request, "Could you please talk about *you*?"

- *A member "story-tells" to the point where others show signs of losing interest.* You can ask the speaker, "What kind of a reaction do you think you are getting from the group?" Or you could ask, "In what way would you like the group to help you regarding this problem?"

- *A group member shows signs of having an idea or a strong feeling, but says nothing.* You might offer a brief observation and an invitation

EXPERIENTIAL LEARNING

Read the following and determine how best to help Lei.

Lei is the leader of an anger management group. Six adolescent males from group homes in the area have been referred to Lei's community mental health center for supplemental services. By the third session of an eight-session group, Lei has found that one group member, Todd, consistently dominates the group with sensationalized stories about his conflictual encounters with one of the staff members in his home. Lei has noticed that when Todd takes over, the other group members seem to shut down. Some roll their eyes and comment among themselves. Lei grew up in foster care and remembers how angry he felt at times with people who did not seem to understand his circumstances or the intense pain he felt.

1. Decide which leadership skills Lei most needs to implement. How can he use each skill?

2. What, specifically, might Lei say to Todd? How could Lei follow up to ensure that Todd has not felt humiliated or rejected?

3. How might Lei's personal experiences affect his ability to assess and then intervene in this situation?

by saying, "Looks like something is going on with you. Would you tell us about it?"

- *A member looks at another expectantly for a relatively long time.* Try directing your gaze from the person being looked at to the expectant one, saying, "I noticed you looking at Ted. It seems like you are trying to make a connection with him."

ROLES ASSUMED BY GROUP MEMBERS

In addition to the various skills and techniques of group leadership discussed above, you will also need to recognize and respond to a variety of roles that group members often assume. As early as 1948, Benne and Sheats analyzed the roles people tend to play in groups. Expecting the emergence of predictable role behavior in groups will help you understand how the group process is being affected. It will also help you anticipate how you will deal with roles that become problematic in your groups.

People bring their typical styles to a group. If the group organization either calls for, or permits, a role with which a group member is familiar, then the member may begin to act in that familiar way. A group is, after all, individuals acting through roles to produce an amalgam of group process. MacKenzie (1990) suggested that group role behaviors fall into roughly four categories: sociable, structural, divergent, and cautionary. Each of these roles carries with it the possibility for both positive and negative effects on the group interaction.

People who tend to develop warm interpersonal relationships are likely to take on *sociable roles*. By communicating concern and involving others in the conversation, they help to create a positive condition for the group. These behaviors serve to help make the group members feel safe in a comfortable group climate. However, according to Kline (2003), too much of this behavior in a group may "block the expression of anger, confrontation, and discussion of member conflicts" (p. 24). People in sociable roles may rescue others from their discomfort or prevent the authentic expression of differences. Extreme sociability may limit the nature of the group interaction to "warm and fuzzy" norms in which people are only allowed to say positive things to each other.

Members who assume *structural roles* are those who work to organize the group so that it can accomplish certain goals. These members attempt to clarify group procedures and establish guidelines for group interactions and boundaries. Such behaviors can help to reduce the tension produced by a general uncertainty as to how to proceed as well as ease the sense of ambiguity surrounding the group's purpose. On the downside, these organizing behaviors may tend to reduce the group's level of emotional expression by turning it into an organization of people pursuing a certain task according to a fixed agenda. Kline (2003) suggested that such groups could become rigid or formal in their interactions and lack spontaneity.

Members who challenge the group norms and who differ with the consensus are taking on *divergent roles*. The positive aspects of such behaviors are that these members keep the group norms in question and allow for the group process to evolve flexibly rather than reaching premature closure about the norms and purpose of the group. Keeping the process open allows for a diversity of input and prevents what some have called "group think." In the extreme, however, such divergent behaviors can be disruptive to the group's attempts to negotiate goals and may be seen as motivated by hostile intent, attempts at deliberate sabotage, or negative resistance to accepting membership in the group. The group members may then engage in "wolf pack" attacks in which they gang up on the divergent member. Such an event would reduce the level of risk that individuals may be willing to show. As the saying goes, the nail that sticks up is hammered down.

"Hold-outs" are members who take on *cautionary roles*. They seem unwilling to fully involve themselves in interactions or to become full-fledged participants in the group process. They appear self-protective and reluctant. They may decline invitations to speak or resist attempts on the part of other members to actively engage with them. Kline (2003) suggested that this behavior may force other members to "examine their commitment to the group and willingness to self-disclose" (p. 25). Such introspection could be helpful to the group process. In the extreme, however, cautionary member behaviors lower the group norms for self-disclosure. Most groups tacitly establish a rule that all members must disclose and contribute at roughly the same level. If, for example, some people risk revealing personal information, while others seem only to act as voyeurs, the self-disclosing members begin to feel overexposed and will begin to withdraw. If the interventions of group members, or the group leader, do not succeed in drawing out cautionary members, the group cohesion may be threatened. While the cautionary member may be privately thinking, *I'm just protecting myself; you all can go on without me,* the group will nevertheless be negatively affected. Sometimes, silence and nonparticipation will more profoundly influence the group process than will overt hostility.

Another way of conceptualizing member roles was developed by Capuzzi and Gross (1992). They noted that group roles function in three ways. One is to facilitate or build, another is to maintain, and a third is to block.

Facilitators/builders keep the group moving in a positive and productive manner. They especially help during the formation of the group by seeking input from others, managing conflict, initiating interactions, and taking into account all perspectives. *Maintainers* focus on the social and emotional aspects of the group and encourage honest expression and acceptance of all types of feelings from other members. Maintainers may encourage, harmonize, compromise, or even follow as they work to keep the group healthy. Finally, *blockers* are group members who sabotage the group's progress by doing things like manipulating, dominating, seeking excessive attention and recognition, and critically judging others in the group. They may see themselves as outsiders and thus divert the group's progress toward cohesion.

As you begin to think about your role as a leader of a counseling group, you can expect to see most of the member role behaviors described above appearing in varying degrees in your future groups. As a community counselor you'll need to think about how to influence the group process in order to achieve the blend of these behaviors that will produce a therapeutic end for all the members. How people behave in groups is a combination of the roles they habitually enact in their lives and the way they perceive the condition of the group. While all of the above roles are predictable, you can never know exactly how they will combine in your group. You cannot fully design the group so that your ends will be achieved precisely. In many ways, a group takes on its own life, and the best you can do as the leader is to throw a saddle on it and ride. But you can take the reins and guide it, attempting to head it in the right direction.

EXPERIENTIAL LEARNING

Think back to your participation in various groups. Recall the most fulfilling and challenging times you experienced in these groups. Explore what it is about *you* that affected these group experiences. Identify a time when you were a facilitator/builder, a maintainer, or a blocker.

1. With which role are you most comfortable, and how does this role usually affect the other members of the groups you are a part of?

2. What are the benefits and costs associated with the role you typically assume?

3. How would you like to build upon or alter your "typical" mode of interacting?

4. If—or, more likely, when—you are asked to participate in groups with your student peers, how will you manage your personal relationships both inside and outside the group setting?

STAGES OF GROUP COUNSELING

In addition to expecting to encounter various member roles, group leaders can expect their groups to process through various stages (Corey, 2004; Tuckman & Jensen, 1977). Following a pregroup stage, the phases of counseling groups are: forming, storming, norming, performing, and transforming. Many group counselors refer to this final stage as "adjourning," but we have never been fully satisfied with that term. First of all, it doesn't rhyme with the other stages of a group. Second, the term implies that groups simply end by saying "goodbye." We prefer "transforming" because it indicates that the individuals in the group have changed due to the experience they have had together, and that each member will take something of the group interaction away that will make for a richer life.

To explore these stages further, let's use an example of a counseling group facilitated by Andrea, a community mental health counselor. Andrea was asked to provide a group for adolescents whose families were facing transitions. The adolescents were referred to her family services community agency by school counselors who determined that they were at risk academically and emotionally. Their families were not able to provide transportation or pay for counseling so the agency was able to use some of its grant funding to transport the group members and waive the fees.

In the *pregroup* stage, it was important for Andrea, as it is for all counselors, to go through several steps before actually beginning the group. First,

Andrea needed to decide for whom the group was appropriate. She decided to include only high-school-aged adolescents because they would be at similar developmental stages. She realized that a heterogeneous group (a group involving members with diverse backgrounds and experiences as opposed to a group with as much in common as possible) would be most beneficial because students already had family struggles in common. She believed they could benefit from diversity of background and experience as they worked together. Andrea also needed to decide on the structure and timeline of the group. Andrea decided to offer a structured group and limit the group to eight one-hour sessions. Finally, the task of recruiting and screening group members remained. To recruit group members, Andrea first used the referrals from school counselors and asked permission to post signs in the school counselors' offices to advertise the group. Andrea was working with minors, so all of her invitations to students were first approved in writing by the students' parents or guardians.

After she received about eight names and two self-referrals and gained permission, Andrea began screening group members. Because this is an important part of the group process, she made sure she had enough time to talk with each potential group member and explain confidentiality. She also discussed the goals of the group. She screened members to see if they were going to be able to actively participate without dominating or sabotaging the group. When she determined that each member was committed to maintaining confidentiality, actively participating in the group, and not in immediate need of other services such as individual therapy or psychiatric services, Andrea invited him or her to attend.

Andrea had to screen out Jeremy because he would be moving in the next four weeks and could not commit to active participation in the group. She also screened out Emily, who confided that her father was kicked out of the home for sexually abusing her and her little sister, but that her mother had not reported it. Andrea felt that Emily needed one-on-one counseling, in addition to confidential support for the report to Child Protective Services that Andrea had to make, before Emily was ready for a group.

At the end of the screening process, Andrea had a number of students who showed promise for success. Maya's parents had been divorced for three years, and her mother was getting remarried to someone Maya liked. Maya wasn't sure, though, how she felt about her stepsister who would also be moving in. Another member was Jim, whose parents had told him only a week ago, to his surprise, that they were splitting up. Jim said it wouldn't make much difference anyway because both of his parents worked second-shift so he didn't see much of them and he basically took care of himself. Cameron's entire family had suffered from emotional abuse related to the alcoholism of her stepfather who left a year ago. Jamal, who lived with one parent every other week, had a mother and father who amicably divorced last year but were under great financial strain. Chantal had been living with her father and his girlfriend and her two teenage sons since her mother left a few months ago to live with a female partner. The last member was Evan, who was still angry over his parents' divorce, which happened two years ago after one of his parents found out the other one was having an affair. Evan was depressed and would not talk to anyone at school.

During the *forming* stage, Andrea followed Srebalus and Brown's (2001) guidelines by reiterating the group rules and clarifying expectations for group members. She also facilitated self-disclosure by inviting members to share their genuine reactions and feelings to her, the group process, and other group members. Andrea reminded the group members of the rules of confidentiality and consistent participation; group members were free to add any additional rules by consensus. All of the group members wanted to add the rules that group members would not interrupt each other, would not provide quick-fix solutions to each other's problems, and would not make critical statements about each other's families. Finally, Andrea invited self-disclosure by providing verbal and nonverbal validation, reflection of feelings, and encouraging other group members to respond directly to the person who shared.

The *storming* stage of the group process involved working through group tensions, issues of power, relational difficulties, and expectations for participation. This stage can consume energy as well as create frustration and confusion. However, working through difficult power issues and relational tensions can provide group members with newfound skills as well as a sense of connectedness to the fellow group members. In the group Andrea was facilitating, storming took the form of competing for "whose situation was worse." The group tended to shut each other out by devaluing the power of each other's experiences. Evan and Chantal especially tended to gang up on other group members by saying they could not possibly understand what betrayal is like. As a result, the group members who were more accepting of their own family situation, such as Maya and Jamal, would shut down and not participate. Jim continued to act like nothing was bothering him. Andrea had to work hard to establish equal power and comfortable sharing in the group. She gave all members feedback on their style of relating and used immediacy to gauge group members' reactions. Finally, members started to share their perceptions of what was happening in the group. Maya and Jamal agreed to participate more while Evan and Chantal practiced showing more empathy for other members. Jim was invited to share but was never forced to participate.

Throughout the *norming stage,* the group adopted some informal rules and patterns and began to establish a sense of cohesiveness and trust. First, the group members agreed to validate each other when a feeling or experience was shared. They tried to replace judgment with empathy. Also, the group elected to have "rounds" at the beginning and end of the group through which all members could share how they were that day, what they hoped to get out of group, and finally, what their experience of the group was like that day. Group members agreed to be emotionally present so these goals could be accomplished. After the group began to trust each other with emotional concerns, the quieter members like Cameron and Jim were able to share the grief they felt over losing families they thought would always be intact.

The *performing* or *working* stage built upon the norming process and helped group members maintain their momentum through actively working on problems presented in the group. Andrea noticed that although group members were now comfortable sharing their feelings and experiences with the group, they were not so open with their family members. Group members also tended to get stuck in the "poor me" syndrome. Thus, Andrea encouraged role-plays to explore family dynamics. She began using a solution-focused approach by helping group members note progress and find hope in each other's stories.

Finally, the *transforming* stage of this group was crucial for all group members. Because the group was predetermined to have eight sessions, group members were aware of the ending date. Andrea was careful to remind group members at the end of every group how many sessions they had left. Andrea wanted to make sure that the group had a positive closure experience, unlike the endings many members had with their families. She asked the group to plan their last session.

The group members decided to have a ceremony in which each member would bring a symbol of the person they were becoming in their new families. After each member shared, group members would state one wish they had for that person as they left the group. Then, Andrea talked about next steps for each group member, providing resources they could draw upon and facilitating a discussion about future directions as members left the group. Because all members were students in the same school, they decided to exchange phone numbers and e-mail addresses to keep supporting each other as time went on. Andrea scheduled one follow-up group for two months after the group ended to check each member's progress and assess any needs for further referral.

ARE GROUPS REALLY EFFECTIVE?

In many ways, working with people in groups offers advantages over one-to-one contact. People can experience feelings of belonging and affiliation with others who share their concerns. They have the opportunity to exchange ideas and personal stories and to discover that their reactions to situations outside the group are not abnormal. They can practice social skills and receive feedback on how they affect each other. Further, they can share their meanings while producing a mutual narrative of their individually lived events.

A number of outcome studies were conducted on the efficacy of group therapy that yielded encouraging conclusions. Yalom (1995) wrote that "the answer is very clear: there is considerable evidence that group therapy is at least as efficacious as individual therapy" (p. 218). Dies (1993) reached the same conclusion after conducting a meta-analysis of forty years of group studies. We humans are a gregarious species. It should therefore be no surprise that we desire group contact and that being with others who are perceived to be like ourselves is growth producing. Whether it is called a process of therapy or simply referred to as nourishment for the human spirit, the practice of people sharing their concerns with each other in group situations has been found to be productive for each involved individual. We now know that working with people in groups is not only an efficient method, but it is effective as well. Groups can have the power to heal.

IMPORTANT CONSIDERATIONS FOR GROUP COUNSELING

As you learn more about group work and group counseling in your training, you will encounter many considerations you'll need to explore. The reality of group counseling for community counselors is that groups are often formed on an ad hoc basis in an attempt to meet immediate needs. Group members are sometimes chosen based on convenience rather than through meticulous screening. Group members often come and go, and many group members will choose to miss that last, vitally important group session rather than be present and attempt to work through the closure process. Providing group counseling can therefore be frustrating as well as exhilarating for community counselors.

However, group counseling works, is efficient, and can be a powerful, transformational experience. It is likely here to stay. As you begin your work facilitating groups, you can expect to encounter several pertinent issues: developmental considerations, multiculturalism, technology, and, of course, ethical concerns.

Developmental Issues

Developmental considerations are essential to your success as a group counselor. A counselor who works with children and adolescents must make suitable modifications to the process. For example, research indicates that confrontation is not productive with children and that the curative factor known as catharsis is usually not therapeutic for children or adolescents (Shechtman, 2002). Also, children tend to self-disclose quickly and are not able to self-introspect as well as adults; thus, play techniques may be especially helpful. Groups with elderly clients will deal with very different life tasks and concerns than groups with clients in youth or middle-age. The group counselor must tailor interventions and approaches to the developmental concerns at hand, including demonstrating competence and sensitivity with developmentally delayed clients. Creative interventions are often helpful. Interactive journal writing, used to communicate with group leaders and other members (Parr, Haberstroh, & Kottler, 2000), and art therapy, used to express emotions and facilitate healing in cases such as tragedies and life crises (Gonzalez-Dolginko, 2002; Stiles & Mermer-Welly, 1998), are examples of interventions that can be used to break down barriers with clients of all ages.

Multiculturalism

Just as in any other form of counseling, as a group counselor you need to be keenly aware of multicultural considerations in the group process. You will have clients from diverse backgrounds and will need to be informed about issues related to factors such as culture, race, gender, socioeconomic status, and sexual orientation and identity. The diverse backgrounds of your clients will influence the way they interact with you and each other. Issues such as respect, awareness, power, and trust will arise as diverse clients come together in a group setting.

Group counselors must be educated and skilled at working with diverse populations and understanding issues unique to different groups of people. For example, if a white counselor from a middle-class background is facilitating a racially and economically diverse group of individuals dealing with issues of sexual identity, multiple layers of awareness have to be considered and addressed within the counselor, among group members, and between group members and the counselor.

The Association for Specialists in Group Work (1998) has adopted *Principles for Diversity-Competent Group Workers,* a statement of multicultural competencies that define basic skills for group counselors. These principles are a helpful starting place for community counselors who want to ensure that they have sufficient self-knowledge and commitment to practice effectively with diverse clients. The principles are available at **http://www.asgw.org/diversity/htm.**

Technology

The development of technology has influenced the group counseling process in that many online groups are now taking place. Online groups require specific counseling skills and interventions, and individuals facilitating such groups should receive professional training. Although software to help online groups run smoothly is available (Jacobs, Masson, & Harvill, 2002), currently the benefits of online groups are unclear and more research is needed. Imagine what an online group might look like, and you can see that the group process could become chaotic and unpredictable very quickly.

For now, group counselors can be reasonably safe in using online resources from credible sources and in using e-mail to convey messages to group members. However, in both cases, group leaders should remind clients that confidentiality can never be assured in Internet communication. Furthermore, any time counselors use e-mail to communicate with clients they should clearly identify their expectations regarding electronic communication. For instance, counselors may want to remind clients not to "reply all" to e-mail messages unless they really want everyone in the group to read their message. Counselors should clearly explain the limits of their own use of e-mail, such as letting clients know that they only check e-mail occasionally and therefore cannot be expected to respond to emergencies via the Internet. The process of using e-mail and other electronic communication with clients can open a floodgate of questions and concerns, so we caution counselors to anticipate possible outcomes as much as possible prior to using this type of technology to communicate with group members.

ETHICAL AND LEGAL ISSUES IN PRACTICE

As a community counselor you need to be familiar with the ethical considerations that abound in group work. Confidentiality is a major concern with groups; you need to inform and remind group members that a breach of confidentiality has serious consequences for all group members. However, you cannot guarantee confidentiality because you cannot control what members may do outside of the group session.

Just as you would in individual counseling, you also need to inform people of the risks, such as the emotional toll of self-disclosing and the pain of recalling memories, they may encounter in groups. Dual relationships are likely to arise, and it falls to you to ensure that the group process and therapeutic relationship are not jeopardized (Jacobs, Masson, & Harvill, 2002). Also, you must be an advocate for the profession by leading groups only for which you are qualified to facilitate.

The ASGW's Best Practice Guidelines, available at **www.asgw.org/best.htm,** is a helpful resource, as is the ACA Code of Ethics. The Best Practice Guidelines specify that group counselors are ethically obligated to screen members so as to include only those whose goals are compatible with the group mission and who are not likely to jeopardize other members. Group leaders also are expected to protect members from physical or psychological harm by taking "reasonable precautions." As you encounter ethical dilemmas presented by group members or the process itself, it is always wise to seek consultation from an experienced group counselor. At this point in your training, you are not expected to be an expert on group counseling. However, it is important to begin now to explore the array of potential ethical and legal questions that will arise for you as you work with groups.

When thinking about the legal implications of group work, consider that any ethical breach on your part could make you vulnerable to legal action. In particular, we encourage you to be vigilant in safeguarding the welfare of your clients, remembering your obligations to protect confidentiality, and not practicing outside the scope of your competence. Similarly, legal expectations regarding your duty to warn and to report abuse are just as important in group counseling as they are in individual counseling. Therefore, as always, be as well-prepared for your work as possible, and when faced with questions, consult.

CONCLUDING THOUGHTS

As you have examined yourself as an individual throughout this chapter, ideally you have come to recognize your own patterns as a group member. You also may be more confident about your own ability to carry out the roles and responsibilities as a group leader. As you progress through your training to become a community counselor, you will learn first-hand the complexities of evolving into a competent, ethical, and skilled group facilitator. Remember that developing into such a facilitator means taking appropriate risks under good supervision as you develop your skills. As long as you are willing to do what it takes to become a competent group leader, including deeply examining your own self, you will be able to witness positive changes in the lives of the group members with whom you'll work.

RECOMMENDED RESOURCES

Irving Yalom has provided what many consider to be the definitive guide to group counseling: Yalom, I. D. (1995). *The theory and practice of group psychotherapy* (4th ed.). New York: Basic Books.

We also recommend that you become familiar with the following organizations, which provide excellent support and resources to counselors who work with groups:

Association for Specialists in Group Work

www.asgw.org

The International Association of Group Psychotherapy

www.iagpweb.org

Other Resources

Several novels have offered richly textured accounts of group dynamics. *The Divine Secrets of the YaYa Sisterhood,* by Rebecca Wells, for example, which is much better than its film version, describes the evolution of friend and family dynamics over time. *The Lord of the Flies* by William Goldman is also considered by many to provide a fascinating and disturbing view of group process and roles.

There are two versions of the film *Twelve Angry Men,* which is an interesting portrayal of the dynamics of a jury. As you watch either of these movies, you can practice your skills at identifying different member roles and group stages. Two documentaries, *The Color of Fear* (which we mentioned in Chapter 7) and *Walking Each Other Home: The Color of Fear II,* are powerful accounts of a group of diverse men who form a marathon group to deal with the issue of racism. Of course, you can watch these documentaries for the content, but you can also observe the process of group dynamics.

Just for fun, you can watch *The Color of Night,* a Hollywood-produced movie that features Bruce Willis as a group therapist. It offers one of the most ridiculous portrayals of a therapy group session in the history of movies. See how many instances you can find of stereotypes, myths, and misconceptions about group counseling clients and procedures.

Finally, some other movies worth looking at that involve intense group dynamics include *One Flew over the Cuckoo's Nest, Anger Management,* and *28 Days* (which depicts a recovery group experience).

REFERENCES

About AA. (n.d.). Retrieved July 8, 2004, from **http://www.aa.org/default/ en_about.cfm.**

Association for Specialists in Group Work (1998). *Principles for diversity-competent group workers.* Retrieved August 9, 2005, from **http://www.asgw.org/diversity.htm.**

Association for Specialists in Group Work (2000). *Professional standards for the training of group workers.* Retrieved August 29, 2005, from **http://www.asgw.org/training_standards.htm.**

Benne, K. D., & Sheats, P. (1948). Functional roles of group members. *Journal of Social Issues, 2,* 42-47.

Blye, F., & Fisher, A. (1999). Searching for support and community: Experiences in a gay men's psychoeducational group. *Canadian Journal of Counseling, 33,* 127-141.

Burrow, T. (1928). The basis of group analysis, or the analysis of the reactions of normal and neurotic individuals. *British Journal of Medical Psychology, 8,* 198-206.

Capuzzi, D., & Gross, D. R. (1992). Group counseling: Elements off effective leadership. In D. Capuzzi & D. R. Gross (Eds.), *Introduction to group counseling* (pp. 39–57). Denver, CO: Love.

Corey, G. (2004). *Theory and practice of group counseling* (4th ed.). Belmont, CA: Wadsworth.

Dies, R. R. (1993). Research on group psychotherapy: Overview and clinical applications. In A. Alonso & H. I. Swiller (Eds.), *Group therapy in clinical practice* (pp. 473–518). Washington, DC: American Psychiatric Press.

Frieman, B. B. (1994–1995). Parenting seminars for divorcing parents. *Parenting Today, 23,* 18–19.

Gladding, S. T. (2003). *Group work: A counseling specialty* (3rd ed.). Upper Saddle River, NJ: Merrill/Prentice Hall.

Gonzalez-Dolginko, B. (2002). In the shadows of terror: A community neighboring the World Trade Center disaster uses art therapy to process trauma. *Art Therapy: Journal of the American Art Therapy Association, 19,* 120–122.

Haney, H., & Leibsohn, J. (2001). *Basic counseling responses in groups.* Belmont, CA: Wadsworth.

Jacobs, E., Masson, B., & Harvill, R. (2002). *Group counseling strategies and skills* (4th ed.). Pacific Grove, CA: Brooks/Cole.

Kline, W. B. (2003). *Interactive group counseling and therapy.* Upper Saddle River, NJ: Merrill/Prentice Hall.

MacKenzie, K. R. (1990). *Introduction to time limited group therapy.* Washington, DC: American Psychiatric Press.

Mathis, R. D., & Tanner, Z. (2000). Structured group activities with family-of-origin themes. *Journal for Specialists in Group Work, 25,* 89–103.

Moore, M. M., & Freeman, S. J. (1995). Counseling survivors of suicide: Implications for group postvention. *Journal for Specialists in Group Work, 20,* 40–47.

Nolan, E. J. (1978). Leadership interventions for promoting personal mastery. *Journal for Specialists in Group Work, 3,* 132–138.

Parr, G., Haberstroh, S., & Kottler, J. (2000). Interactive journal writing as an adjunct in group work. *Journal for Specialists in Group Work, 25,* 229–242.

Pratt, J. H. (1907). The class method of treating consumption in the homes of the poor. *Journal of the American Medical Association, 49,* 755–759.

Shechtman, Z. (2002). Child group psychotherapy in the schools at the threshold of a new millennium. *Journal of Counseling & Development, 80,* 293–299.

Srebalus, D. J., & Brown, D. (2001). *A guide to the helping professions.* Boston: Allyn & Bacon.

Stiles, G. J., & Mermer-Welly, M. J. (1998). Children having children: Art therapy in a community-based early adolescent pregnancy program. *Art Therapy: Journal of the American Art Therapy Association, 15,* 165–176.

Tuckman, B. W., & Jensen, M. A. (1977). Stages in small group development revisited. *Group and Organizational Studies, 2,* 419–427.

Washington, O. G. M., & Moxley, D. P. (2003). Group interventions with low-income African-American women recovering from chemical dependency. *Health & Social Work, 28,* 146–156.

Yalom, I. D. (1995). *The theory and practice of group psychotherapy* (4th ed.). New York: Basic Books.

Chapter 10

Discovering Options: Career Counseling

If you do not feel yourself growing in your work and your life broadening and deepening, if your task is not a perpetual tonic to you, you have not found your place.

Orison Swett Marden

It is a great gift to have skills and abilities that meet critical needs in the world.

Bessie Parker

Far and away the best prize that life offers is the chance to work hard at work worth doing.

Theodore Roosevelt

GOALS

Reading and exploring the ideas in this chapter will help you:

- Appreciate the influence of work in the lives of people and the importance of career counseling

- Gain knowledge of the history and current trends in career development, career counseling, and career information

- Understand different types of interventions with people who are in the attaining, maintaining, and sustaining modes of career development

- Begin to grapple with the issues that interfere with people's job attainment and satisfaction with work

---

OVERVIEW

This chapter presents information on career development theories, career counseling, and the interrelationships among work and other life roles. You'll also have the opportunity to discover some of your own career development processes. The existing literature related to career development is immense, so we'll just scratch the surface here. You'll explore these topics in much greater depth and detail in your career development course. For now, just get a feel for the scope of career development and career counseling and consider how these interface with your future work as a community counselor.

The positive correlation between career development exploration and personal and professional health is well documented (Krumboltz, 1979; 1994). The American Counseling Association's (ACA) accrediting body, the Council for the Accreditation of Counseling and Related Educational Programs (CACREP), believes a clear understanding of career issues is critical for the development of professional counselors. No decision is more personally relevant than the work to which someone will commit a life. Work and lifestyle issues will undoubtedly influence your adult clients, regardless of their primary presenting concern.

ALEX'S DEFINING MOMENT: Anasthasios/Arisen

Alex, a community counselor with over thirty years of experience, provided the following story regarding his own career journey. *The name Anasthasios means "arisen" in Greek. In Greek mythology a Phoenix-like bird struggles, eventually raises itself from its parental surroundings, and finally soars to the temple of the sun.*

"I was born in the United States and christened Anasthasios Alexiou. My parents had come to America in the midst of the Great Depression. As a youngster I played in my parents' leather shop and had no real friends outside my immediate family. By the time I was old enough to attend school I could add and subtract columns of figures, sew a straight seam on a peddle-driven machine, prepare skins, and do all manner of difficult tasks necessary in making fine coats and hats. I could not, however, speak very much English. In those days, much as it is now, it was not uncommon for children from outside the prevailing social culture to be taunted and bullied, especially when they had to leave the safety of their homes and extended families to attend school.

"Mother was very concerned about my fitting in at school so she changed my name to Alex, a shortened form of our last name. I was forced to learn some survival strategies early on. I sequestered myself behind a large boy on the first day of school and the teacher didn't find me for awhile, but when she did, it may have been a turning point in my young life. The first time she called on me, I panicked and pretended that my eyes were bothering me. A few more steps in this dance of deception finally led me to an optometrist and a pair of very thick glasses which I didn't need and which my family could ill afford.

"Soon, after responding with silence and looks of confusion whenever called on by the teacher, I was required to take the Stanford Binet Intelligence Test. Before I was placed in special education, however, my mother, armed with an interpreter from our neighborhood, was able to convince the principal and my teacher that I wasn't in need of special services—I just needed to learn the language of the country where I was born. My parents could not afford tutors, so on Saturdays and after school they used bilingual babysitters who were instructed to teach me to speak English. I stayed in school, but largely because of my horrendous start in school, I was never a star pupil.

"After graduation, my father became ill, and I was forced to work at any job I could find in order to support my parents and younger brothers and sisters. In my twenties I worked at a cemetery digging graves and doing maintenance work for eight hours each day and then worked four more hours, six days a week doing odd jobs at a public library. I was befriended by a librarian and she urged me to go to college. After much coaxing I finally did decide to go to college to become a teacher. My first education course was "The Psychology of Children with Special Needs," which required us to volunteer at a school for handicapped children. I felt an immediate connection to the children and they seemed to respond to me as a kindred soul. I had found my calling.

"I worked first as a special education teacher, but soon realized that I wanted to work more closely in a therapeutic manner with children and their families. Years later, still supporting my family, working, and going to school part-time, I finally finished a Master's Degree in Community Counseling. Over the years I worked for several community agencies as a counselor and eventually became a regional supervisor for community service boards in the Midwest.

"Now I'm retired after a thirty-year career and looking back, it never seemed like work. It was what I should have been doing all along with my life. I was drawn to the field because of the compassion I felt for children with special needs. They reminded me of a little boy back in Brooklyn who hated the thought of going to school and facing the shame, ridicule, and bullying. These children inspired me to keep doing what I had to do, day after day and year after year, as if I were being pulled along by the force of an invisible magnet. Regardless of the hardships and no matter how tired I was, I just had to keep on going.

"When he was old enough to understand, I told my son Michael about my struggle to learn English and get an education while supporting a family. He thought about it for awhile and finally said that he wanted to change his name to Anathasios. At that point I felt a cycle had been successfully completed in my life."

Questions for Reflection

1. What people have been significant influences on your career path?

2. How do you see your childhood interests manifest in your choice to be a counselor, or in your current lifestyle?

3. Are there interests that you have not yet pursued? If so, how might you engage with those areas of your life either now during your training or later in your work as a community counselor?

SHOULD YOU BE INTERESTED IN CAREER COUNSELING?

Looking at the title of this chapter, you may have been tempted to read no further. Perhaps you were saying to yourself, "I am training to be a Community Counselor. I'm not interested in 'career guidance.' I am going to assist people toward achieving better mental health." Heppner, O'Brien, Hinkelman, and Flores (1996) found that most graduate students and beginning counselors share this attitude regarding career counseling. If you number yourself among this group, you are certainly not alone in the mistaken belief that career counseling is nothing more than an endless process of advising, testing, and providing reference material in order to assist a somewhat helpless person find the right job. Who would want to spend his or her day doing work of this nature?

But a moment of reflection should reveal to you that work is the centerpiece of most people's lives. Any time you meet someone new, after exchanging names, often the next thing that you ask each other is, "What do you do?" A work role is much more than what one does for a living; it is a major part of most people's identity. Sigmund Freud, when asked to sum up the criteria for mental health, is reported to have succinctly replied, "Love and *work*" (Schouten, 2004). As Kottler (2004) put it, "Everyone, and I mean everyone, is engaged in some purposeful, productive activity" (p. 273). We call such activity "work."

Furthermore, the term *career* may be misleading, because it seems to imply a distinction between one's job and the rest of life. The current training standards of our profession in this area focus mainly on theories of career development and decision making, sources of information, career and educational planning, and assessment techniques for helping people find work that best fits their personalities and levels of development. Perhaps it is this seemingly narrow focus that has kept career development from enjoying the prestige of other forms of counseling and psychotherapy.

The profession of counseling began with "vocational guidance" as its principal domain (Kottler, 2004). Since that time, people have sought to broaden the connotation of such work by calling it "career counseling" instead of vocational counseling (Brown & Strebalus, 2003). However, we have been acquainted with several Catholic nuns and priests who describe their life's work as "vocation." And some of them have given over their lives to service with a pledge of poverty. Their vocation is not pursued for financial gain. When asked about their meaning of this word, they have all stated that vocation is the work to which one dedicates his or her complete self; it is an act of total love. In this view, perhaps "vocation" is the proper term; but no matter what we call it, one's dedication to productive activity is the centerpiece of a meaningful life.

In the Tennessee Williams (1955) play *Cat on a Hot Tin Roof,* the character "Big Mama" tells "Maggie the Cat" that if her marriage is on the rocks, the rocks are in the bed. Viewed this way, it would seem that Freud's first criterion of mental health (love) has little to do with career counseling. However, we would claim that the second criterion—work—is very often responsible for the rocky times in life. When work is problematic, life becomes problematic. Kottler (2004) pointed out that when clients begin to deal with career-related issues, "you will likely end up exploring family, cultural, gender, and related issues that are part of the bigger picture" (p. 291). The realization of the importance of satisfactory work led Crites (1981) to claim that "The need for career counseling is greater than the need for psychotherapy" (p. 14). With our emphasis on work and attainment in the United States, there is no reason to believe that this need has changed.

Furthermore, understanding of the importance of mental health issues in the workplace has grown steadily in recent years (Schouten, 2004). For example, in 1998, the American Psychiatric Association formed the Committee on Psychiatry/Business Relations. That committee, in turn, gave rise to the National Partnership for Workplace Mental Health. There is a growing realization that providing mental health services in the workplace can prevent, or treat, those issues that affect job performance and can help people toward greater satisfaction with their lives in general.

Herr and Cramer (1996) identified several positive social and psychological factors, besides the obvious economic benefits, of being fulfilled in one's work. They stated that work is a place where many needs can be met, such as the need to be with others, to possibly make friends, to attain status, to feel valued, to achieve the satisfaction of a well-done job, to elevate self-esteem, to gain a sense of order, and to experience self-efficacy and responsibility. Obviously, being in the right job can enhance one's life in many ways.

On the other hand, people often experience personal issues that can seriously detract from their job performance and fulfillment in their work. Among the mental health issues that relate directly to work are job dissatisfaction; substance abuse and addictive behaviors such as gambling; inequity relating to women, gays, people of color, and the disabled; work addiction and burnout; job loss; physical injury, HIV/AIDS, or other illness; sexual harassment; family crises; wellness and nutrition; plus all the mental disorders normally seen in clinical practice, such as depression, anxiety, and personality disorders.

Many people, including many beginning graduate students, seem to believe that career counseling is primarily employment counseling—getting people jobs. Further, Kottler (2004) pointed out that many counselors still subscribe to the myth "that 'real' counseling is personal/emotional and that vocational/career counseling is somehow a second-class cousin that requires fewer skills and is more 'routine'" (p. 292). However, as you can see from the above discussion, assisting people in their career aspirations and their world-of-work is much more than simply fitting them into the proper job slot. Career counseling is aimed at helping people live productive, rewarding, and fulfilling lives. Isn't that what you hope to do when you become a community counselor?

THE CAREER COUNSELING PROCESS

Career counseling is a process in which the counselor and client are engaged together as a team. Clients are experts on their own history and can provide the counselor with information about their background, values, dreams, and real and/or perceived obstacles. Hansen (1997) described the career counseling process using a concept called *Integrative Life Planning* (ILP). "Integrative Life Planning is a complex, comprehensive process of examining critical themes influencing our lives and identifying patterns and strategies which can help us to understand, manage and perhaps even shape those influences" (p. 23). ILP promotes the integration of elements of mind and body with spiritual, physical, emotional, and career development. By exploring themes of the integration of work and family, diversity concerns, meaning in life, and personal and social change, clients will feel more connected to the process of career counseling because they will be seen as a "whole person" by the counselor, not just a compilation of traits and abilities.

In addition to the "whole person" approach, wellness is a relevant focus for community counselors. Wellness "incorporat[es] the 'total person' as the target of intervention. In wellness approaches, body, mind, and spirit are integrated in a purposeful manner by the individual, with a goal of living more fully within all spheres of functioning" (Smith, Myers, & Hensley, 2002, p. 91). A focus on wellness creates a more comprehensive view to life and career planning. Some questions counselors might explore with clients from a holistic/wellness perspective include:

- What are the values you hold most dear in your life? How do these values manifest themselves in your work life as well as other aspects of your life?
- What gives you a sense of meaning and how do you incorporate this into your work life?
- What does having a sense of balance mean to you and how might you strive for it in your life?
- What is a metaphor you would use to describe yourself as a person? How has this metaphor manifested itself in your career life?
- What careers seem to bring together who you are with what you do? How have you attempted to seek or avoid such careers?
- What obstacles have you encountered in your journey to career success? How can you overcome them? What kinds of assistance would you need to help you overcome them?

Gysbers and Moore (1987) also provided a specific model of the career counseling process. They believed that career counseling involves primarily two phases, (1) problem identification with the client and (2) satisfactory resolution of the identified problem. In phase one, they identified the following three substages:

- Establishing a working relationship and defining roles
- Developing an understanding of the client's characteristics and environment
- Making a diagnosis of the client's problem

    In phase two, Gysbers and Moore identified the following stages:

- Making an intervention
- Evaluating the impact of the intervention
- Terminating if the intervention is successful

In many ways, career counseling is like any other counseling, and often there will be multiple issues to work through with your clients. We recommend that counselors working with career concerns take adequate time to get to know their clients before initiating any work with formal career assessment instruments. Often it is tempting for counselors to jump to conclusions before fully understanding the client and their particular needs and issues. Listening, understanding, and validating your client may require several sessions.

Just Do It

One of Lania's first clients in her counseling practicum was Antony, a twenty-eight-year-old man struggling with career issues. Antony had been an athlete in college and now worked as a sales representative for a company that made athletic equipment. He told Lania that he found the job "boring and a little embarrassing." Lania was intrigued by Antony and felt optimistic about his ability to make sound career decisions. He was bright and eager to share his experiences with her. She believed the best way to proceed with Antony was to help him explore his interests and options, and then help him develop a plan for making career decisions.

After her second session with Antony, Lania began to feel slightly unsettled. Whenever she tried to help Antony become concrete, to identify goals and pinpoint interests, Antony seemed to become evasive. He would shift his focus to his past, or dwell instead on how unhappy he was in his current position. Lania had given Antony a homework assignment to write down his "ideal day," and Antony had failed to do the homework. What's going on with this guy? she wondered.

She met with her supervisor and complained, "My client won't really do anything. He just comes in and complains. I'm not sure he really wants to deal with his career issues at all."

"What do you think he wants to deal with?" asked her supervisor.

Lania was confused. "Well, he said he had career concerns. So that's how I've been treating it. I've been following a model of exploring interests, exploring options, and then taking action."

"I know you've been listening, but I'm wondering if you've really heard him."

Lania was silent. She understood what her supervisor was asking. Had Lania really been hearing Antony's struggle? In her mind, she had created a career counseling situation that was discreet and unconnected with Antony's personal concerns. As she reflected in supervision, Lania realized that Antony did want to deal with his career issues, but he also wanted to tell his story. She suspected that he felt disappointed, perhaps even like a failure, because he had not yet been able to translate his athletic talent into a rewarding career. He needed his concerns to be heard and understood. He wanted his experience to be validated. Then, perhaps, he could move on to explore his interests, explore his options, and take action.

Questions for Reflection

1. What are your expectations for the career counseling process?

2. What do you feel will be most challenging for you as you help people work through their career concerns?

Specific intervention strategies usually then emerge from the therapeutic relationship by getting to know your client well, gaining specific information that emerges from assessment instruments, and from noting the client's reactions to their assessment results. These clients may also need specific help with job interviewing skills, résumé and letter writing, and job search strategies, as well as building self-esteem and a sense of confidence and competence along the way. Finally, we recommend that you check in with your clients to see if the strategies are meeting their needs and goals. For instance, consider Lania's experience with Antony in "Just Do It" on the previous page.

Before delving further into the practice of career counseling, it's important to present a brief overview of some of the theories of career development that have achieved status in the field. These theories will inform your practice and guide you as you interpret the information gleaned from interventions and assessments.

CAREER THEORIES

Career theories seek to describe and explain why individuals choose specific careers and attempt to explain the various career adjustments people make across the lifespan. The following brief overview of theories serves as a sample of historical and modern theories still in use today. According to Brown (2000), changes from one career to another are common in the early years of employment, but radical job changes also occur in midlife as well, especially in today's changing society. One study found that almost half of working adults in a particular sample were considering changing careers, and one in four were expecting to make a major career change within a year (Dolliver, 1999).

Another trend indicates that as many as 50 to 60 percent of newly hired employees quit their jobs within the first seven months (Schlossberg, 1997). Such frequent and rapid job changes are quite different from the "old school" notion of remaining true to one's employer while the employer reciprocated with loyalty to the employee. Changes in the employment landscape require that we see the following theories as a compass, or road map, to help us understand where people have been, where they are now, and where they might be going in the future.

Parsons' Trait and Factor Theory

Frank Parsons (1909) is considered the "father" of the modern career development movement in America. Parsons asserted that each person is unique and each has certain characteristics, or "traits," comprising this uniqueness. Corresponding to these traits of each person, Parsons also believed that every workplace environment also had unique characteristics, or "factors," that need to be considered. The goal of the career development professional or counselor, then, was to know the individual, know the workplace environment, and seek to make a good match between the two.

This theory may sound rather basic. However, consider the first postulate of Parsons—each individual is unique with various traits that can be discovered, understood, and measured. Understanding the uniqueness of each person is not an easy task, because so many variables are involved in the makeup of each person. A considerable amount of knowledge and experience is required to understand the essence of a person's nature. Consider also that each work environment is unique. With literally thousands of careers to track and research, it is nearly impossible to know all the details involved in each career field. However, the trait and factor approach is still considered viable by many career counselors today. Many other theories have emerged in the last fifty years as either clarifications or extensions of Parsons' theory, while others emerged as counterpoint to this theory. Perhaps the most well-known embellishment of the Parson trait and factor approach in use today is the theory of John Holland.

Holland's Typology Approach

John Holland (1973) created the typology approach which, similar to Parsons, states that every person and workplace environment is unique. Holland categorized each career and each person as one of six types: Realistic, Investigative, Artistic, Social, Enterprising, or Conventional. Again the goal is to make the best match possible between the person and the workplace. According to Gottfredson (1981), there are varying levels of prestige associated with each type, with investigative ranking highest, followed by enterprising, artistic, and social types. The lowest prestige types would then be realistic and conventional.

The best possible scenario would be when a good match occurs between personality type and career type. This fit requires much self-knowledge, as well as understanding of the world of work. The career counselor would attempt to help the client with the process of self-discovery, as well as facilitate discovery of various careers well matched to the personality type. In other words, Holland believed that it is equally important for individuals to become self-aware and to become knowledgeable about occupational requirements so that people can make educated career decisions.

Following years of research, Holland created an instrument to measure these variables. Today, the current version of the Self-Directed Search (SDS) is used to sort individual interests and the corresponding workplace environment. The SDS will provide the individual with a three-letter code, with each letter referring to one of the six types (e.g., Artistic, Conventional). A person with a three letter code of SEA, for example, would have the strongest preference for social environments followed by an interest in enterprising and artistic environments.

As previously mentioned, counselors are cautioned against oversimplifying this process since individual development is a complex and multifaceted process, and fully understanding the world of work is also a daunting task. The Holland code may be an ideal starting place for counselors to begin discussing client preferences and aspirations. Ideally, clients will then be active in investigating further what they discover about themselves as a result of the Self-Directed Search. One benefit of the Self-Directed Search for community counseling use is the ease with which it can be administered and explained to clients. The general idea that different work environments exist seems logical and is intuitively appealing. The process of talking about work environments and preferences can help clients to explore their desires and abilities.

Ginzberg and Associates

Ginzberg (1972) also saw the uniqueness of each person, but viewed this unfolding human drama from a developmental perspective. Ginzberg believed there were three distinct stages or phases in career development: (1) the fantasy stage, from birth until around age eleven; (2) the exploration phase, from about age twelve until twenty; and (3) the reality stage, from about age twenty on. Take a moment to remember the fantasy careers you've dreamed about, and the various careers you've actually explored or pursued. Then, consider the actual jobs you've held and the careers for which you've trained.

While the stages may seem rather static, remember that human development is a dynamic process. Even in adulthood, whenever individuals become disillusioned or dissatisfied with their career, the developmental stages may be revisited. For instance, if John, a factory worker, were to become unhappy in his current career, the first thing that may happen is that he might begin to fantasize about other career options. Eventually, he may shorten the list of options down to a few jobs he will explore or research in more detail. This activity, in turn, may lead him to seek a new realistic career choice.

Donald Super's Model

Super also approached the career journey from a developmental perspective (1957, 1976). His theory outlines several primary stages: growth (birth to age fourteen), exploration (ages fourteen to twenty-four), establishment (ages twenty-four to forty-four), maintenance (ages forty-four to sixty-four), and decline (age sixty-five to death), with most primary stages including several substages. Later Super (1990) adapted and envisioned several key developmental transition points, one in early adolescence, and others during early, middle, and later adulthood. Following each transition, the development cycle begins anew, from growth through decline. His theory is often called the "cycle-recycle" theory. Super saw the importance of discovering the unique attributes of each person, yet he saw this process as a lifelong drama. Self-concept is an important part of Super's theory. Super's approach is therefore appealing to many counselors, because it begins to capture the complexity and dynamic nature of career and life choices.

Ann Roe's Theory

Ann Roe's theory is psychodynamic and developmental in nature (1956). Roe believed that early childhood experiences significantly shape each person, and therefore the career development process. Of particular interest to Roe was the parent-child interaction. She believed that different relationship styles led to different (met or unmet) needs, and the motivation for a particular career is to meet, express, and satisfy that particular need in adulthood. For example, an overprotecting parent would encourage dependency, a need that might be addressed in a career choice through service-oriented fields. The over-demanding parent might lead the individual toward an achievement-oriented career. Neglectful or rejecting parenting, according to Roe, might lead one toward a career with scientific or mechanical interest. An accepting parental style could lead one toward relational careers like teaching or counseling. Although much research has been conducted, little has resulted to support Roe's thinking. However, many do believe there is a powerful connection between family dynamics and career choice. The career genogram is an exercise promoted by McGoldrick and Gerson (1999) to enable counselor and client alike to discover this powerful connection.

Roe also utilized Maslow's theory regarding the human hierarchy of needs to describe the various motivations toward particular careers. She stated that persons primarily motivated by survival and safety needs generally gravitate toward more non-person-oriented career fields, while those motivated more by such needs as self-esteem, social connectedness, or self-actualization tend to gravitate toward more person-oriented careers. This position also has held much interest among career developmentalists, yet has not been validated by research.

HELPING PEOPLE ATTAIN, MAINTAIN, AND SUSTAIN A CAREER

There are three main areas or modes of career counseling in which you are likely to find yourself intervening as a community counselor. These modes represent aspects of your clients' lives that are affected by their careers. First,

EXPERIENTIAL LEARNING

Duane Brown (1996) espoused a career development theory primarily based upon the concept of values, or what each person holds to be most important in life. Brown believed that our values drive all our important decisions, so it is necessary to study our values, where they came from, and how they affect our current career choices.

A Values Auction

This exercise works best in a group. Get together with your classmates and identify ten to fifteen values that are dear to you. For many, these values include love, health, loving family relationships, career satisfaction, money, etc. Your list may be very different, of course, so try to find some consensus with your classmates. When you've completed your list, give each person the equivalent of $500. (Play money will do fine or pieces of paper identified as $100 and $50 dollar bills.) Then, begin a values auction. Ask one person to refrain from bidding and serve as auctioneer. The auctioneer should go down the list, one by one, and ask who will bid how much for each value. As you play the values auction, pay attention to what values seem non-negotiable for you. For instance, will you spend your entire $500 to make sure you can have love? Some people experience much anxiety when they participate in the values auction. The idea of giving up one important value, such as family, for another important value, such as health, is too stressful to contemplate. Thankfully, our lives do not necessarily dictate that we make such extreme sacrifices. Most of us will, however, reach a point in our lives when we have to choose between two very compelling options. Helping people through these decision points in their lives may be a crucial part of your counseling practice.

you may be involved in helping them *attain* a career. To *attain* means to gain or achieve, or to come into possession of something. In this mode, you will be helping people to dream, explore, and obtain work which might become their life's career. You may be helping them gain certain interpersonal skills that will enhance their chances for advancement in their work setting. You might be assisting people toward understanding their interests and aptitudes relative to the world of work and in gaining employment that will be adequate to their financial needs, as well as fulfilling to their spirit.

Next, you will be helping them *maintain* a career. To *maintain* means to support an existing state, to repair, or make something more efficient. Problems on the job such as substance abuse, sexual harassment, or difficulties with coworkers may be the subject of your work with clients. Your interventions in this mode will be designed to help people do well in their careers and to aid them in overcoming issues that might detract from their efficiency or fulfillment in their work.

And finally, you may be helping them *sustain* themselves through transitions in their career and their lives in general. To *sustain* means to give support or relief, or to help someone "bear up" under difficulties. Many issues, such as job change or loss, family and parenting problems, and retirement and the preservation of one's identity, will be brought to you as a community counselor. Being a community counselor means that you will be involved in every aspect of people's lives—their inner life, their interpersonal processes, their life pursuits, and the community in which they exist.

Attaining

The first step toward helping people with their careers is to help them realize what they desire and value in life, and how this relates to work. As a community counselor, it is likely that the clients with whom you work will present first with issues that confound their career development process. For example, clients may be undereducated, abusing substances, struggling with lack of access to resources, or experiencing mental or emotional problems that interfere with their ability to live fulfilling lives. Your job will be to thoroughly assess and respond to these concerns while ensuring that you do not overlook the preventive focus of community counseling work. Preparing clients to explore productive and fulfilling career and life choices is thus often a critical concern for community counselors.

Kottler (2004) suggested that in addition to your general assessment procedures, you might begin by asking your client to rank-order, according to personal preference, work-related items such as flexibility, high income, security, power, collegiality among coworkers, opportunity to help others, status, independence, responsibility, and opportunities for creativity.

If, for example, people rank "security" high, and "responsibility" low, it is unlikely that they would be comfortable in starting their own business. If they were to rank "opportunity to help others" high, and "high income" low, they might be comfortable with the work of a community counselor. The ranking task would give you some initial talking points to begin your exploration during the *attaining* mode of career development.

Community counselors are also encouraged to help clients explore the influence of their families and their own community and environmental contexts on their career desires and paths. For instance, in the Defining Moment at the beginning of the chapter, Alex identified early experiences that influenced his career path. Clients may be asked to identify how childhood experiences, parents' or caregivers' careers, and other messages have affected the client's view of work and career issues. Factors such as socioeconomic status, educational attainment, and emotional and cognitive development are also relevant. This type of information may be vital in helping you assess your clients' interests and readiness regarding their own career development.

Many counselors also find that assessment instruments such as the Kuder Occupational Interest Survey, the Holland Self-Directed Search (SDS), the Campbell Interest and Skills Survey, and the Career Assessment Inventory can be helpful in the first stages of clients' efforts toward attainment. You can find information on these and other instruments online at **www.dantes.doded.mil/dantes_web/distribution/guide4-text.htm.**

Depending on your clients' abilities and needs, you can also direct your clients to sources of information regarding occupations to enhance their understanding of the world of work in general. One of the best sources we know is a website called Virginia View. This site has existed for many years and was created by the faculty in the counselor education program at Virginia Tech University. The site can be accessed at **www.vaview.vt.edu/index.htm.** Virginia View includes suggestions for career development for clients at various levels of development and has valuable links to other sources. In addition to the above, you can suggest that clients arrange to interview people who occupy positions to which they aspire, or shadow these people at work. You can also direct them to literature on the career paths they are thinking about.

Maintaining

After they attain a career and begin to understand the role of their work in the broader contexts of their lives, many people need assistance in maintaining commitment to and productivity in their work. People run into many obstacles on the job, and in their personal lives, that interfere with their performance, advancement, or the retention of their positions. As a community counselor you are likely to be called upon to assist clients to overcome such roadblocks. Many problems that people need to deal with stem from their behaviors on and off the job. For example, people who are struggling with addictions, who are having trouble controlling their anger, or who are distracted by family issues, will not perform optimally in their work. In addition, people often find themselves in areas of work for which they lack certain skills. For example, people who are promoted on the job sometimes find that they lack the necessary reading, writing, mathematical, or language and presentation skills that are required of their new position. On an even more elementary level, people sometimes need to learn the fundamental behaviors necessary to keep a job, such as arriving on time, engaging in certain deference behaviors with supervisors, or interaction rituals with customers. In such cases, your work is remedial. You are attempting to change the client's behaviors so that they fit the career choice that the person has made.

Roadblocks are also encountered by people through no fault of their own. For example, women, ethnic minorities, gays, and people with disabilities often find themselves trapped in careers that call for knowledge and skills that are far below their abilities. They chafe in dead-end jobs and find their work life unfulfilling. They may be overlooked for promotion, they may experience harassment or downright hostility from coworkers, or, in the case of people who are disabled, they may find that areas of their work site are inaccessible to them or that they are limited in their opportunities by low expectations of supervisors.

The *maintaining* mode of counseling requires that you see your work as doing whatever is necessary to help people retain their careers and to advance within them. Your interventions will range from basic education to intensive personal counseling. As Richardson (1996) suggested, in order for us to view our work in perspective, we should probably change the name of career counseling to counseling/psychotherapy regarding work, job, and careers. Within the broad area of maintaining, we present four primary areas of interest: Employee Assistance Programs, job adjustment, substance abuse counseling, and burnout.

Employee Assistance Programs

Employee Assistance Programs (EAPs) are designed to work with employees in both preventive and therapeutic modes in order to avoid or remediate problems they are experiencing that negatively affect their job performance. Such programs are usually associated with the company's department of human resources (sometimes known as the personnel department). Community counselors can be hired as in-house counselors for businesses' and institutions' EAPs, and counselors in private practice can sometimes expand their work by consulting with business and industry and obtaining contracts with companies that do not have their own on-site employee assistance programs.

EAP work can be especially enjoyable because counselors can be involved in a variety of activities. For example, you might be designing wellness programs or creating workshops on money management, effective parenting, and nutrition. You may be engaging in individual and group counseling, crisis intervention, family counseling, and substance abuse counseling. In other words, any activity that is likely to improve employees' productivity on the job by remedying the distracting aspects of their lives is viewed as valuable by the employers who would be contracting for your services. In some organizations, EAPs are the first referral option for people who have emotional and/or mental issues. Although it may not "look" like community counseling at first glance, community counselors are actually quite at home in these positions, because they offer primary and secondary prevention activities within the community of the employing organization.

Job Adjustment Counseling

Sometimes your work will involve helping people make a better adjustment to their current job. They may report feeling uncomfortable or dissatisfied with their own performance, their work setting, or their relationships with coworkers or supervisors. Perhaps dissatisfaction with work has exacerbated personal issues, or perhaps personal issues have led to problems at work, and the combination of the two has brought the client to your door. In these cases, you'll need to assess what your clients want for their lives, including how they see work fitting into their overall lifestyle. Therefore, you will find it helpful to explore your clients' expectations and values relative to their jobs.

Dawis and Lofquist (1984) suggested the use of the Minnesota Importance Questionnaire (MIQ) as a method for making your clients' values more explicit as the content of your counseling sessions. While this instrument would have obvious utility for the attaining mode, you may also find the constructs helpful as you work with job adjustment in the maintaining mode. The MIQ assesses six major values that people may have regarding their jobs. Each value contains certain needs that your clients may express. The six values are Achievement, Comfort, Status, Altruism, Safety, and Autonomy. People vary according to the degree of each value they seek to satisfy through their work.

- *Achievement* includes the need to feel that one's work is something that makes full use of the person's abilities, as well as the need for a feeling of accomplishment in the assigned tasks. People have a greater sense of achievement or accomplishment when they can take pride in the product that results from their work. People who work on assembly lines often fail to have a sense of how their contribution results in the final product. (An interesting similarity: Counselors often have little knowledge of the results of their efforts with clients. If you do your job well, your clients will often credit themselves for the accomplishment.)

- *Comfort* may be achieved by being busy all the time, having a sense of independence, engaging in a variety of tasks, feeling fairly compensated for one's work, and having good working conditions. Specific working conditions, such as lighting, heating, amount of work space, employee benefits, and the promise of steady employment will all contribute to the feeling of comfort on the job (Sharf, 1992).

- *Status* means that there is the opportunity for advancement, recognition for a job well done, some level of authority, and the feeling of being "somebody" at work. Sometimes people initially enjoy a job, but later lose interest in it when they realize that it is "dead-end" without much opportunity to rise in the company, or to be valued by superiors as an individual.

- *Altruism* can be satisfied by having coworkers who are easy to work with, not feeling morally wrong in the completion of tasks, and being able to do things for others. People who highly value altruism, for instance, may have difficulty in a sales job that offers products that are either worthless or harmful.

- *Safety* comes about when the person feels that company policies are administered fairly, that one's immediate superior will back up the employee with top management, and that supervisors are competent to train and evaluate employees. Arbitrary hiring and firing practices, poor attention to worker safety, or the lack of adequate training of employees who do hazardous work, can all threaten one's sense of safety on the job.

- *Autonomy* means that one has the freedom to try out new ideas and to make one's own decisions. Creative people like to be able to come up with novel approaches to their work and to be able to independently implement them without supervisors "micromanaging" their efforts.

While all the above values and needs are required for everyone's job satisfaction, you will find that each individual will desire some of these aspects of work more than others. If you think about your own hopes and desires for a career as a community counselor, some of the values and needs listed will stand out as very important to you, while others will be less so. Keeping these criteria in mind will help you to assist people to talk about their job dissatisfaction, and will provide you with clues as to what needs to be done. When you are dealing with people who complain that their work is not fulfilling, then assessing their values and needs relative to the work they are doing is a good way of ascertaining the "fit" between the employee and the job.

Sometimes, job maladjustment comes about when someone's abilities do not match the requirements of the work demanded of them. Assuming that the problem is not lack of intelligence, or major deficiencies in essential skills (such as poor writing ability in a journalism job, inadequate oral communication skills in a job that demands many presentations before an audience, or lack of basic mathematical ability in a scientific job), you may be able to help your client think about ways to deal with some aspects of the work that are unfulfilling. No job will completely satisfy every value and need that the person has.

Furthermore, sometimes a cost-benefit analysis is required when thinking about aspects of the job. The authors of this book have all had jobs that generally were satisfying, and to which we were able to make adequate adjustments, but we have found that even the most rewarding of these jobs required us to participate in activities for which we felt inadequate, or which we found onerous. It is unreasonable to think that somewhere out there exists the perfect job. Satisfactory job adjustment means that most aspects of the work will prove rewarding, while those that are not must be dealt with through compensating strategies.

While helping clients with job adjustment issues you will also be helping them deal with important aspects of their lives. Therefore, you may find that you need to help clients make realistic appraisals of their jobs, their skills, and their options. The only way you can do this effectively is to ensure that you have adequately conceptualized the client in his or her own unique context.

Substance Abuse Counseling

As you work with clients who are experiencing career transitions, welfare-to-work concerns, or basic career exploration, you are likely to encounter clients who are simultaneously struggling with powerful addictions. The number of clients who are struggling with substance abuse appears to be growing. Imagine the challenge of holding down a full-time job and carrying out additional life responsibilities while battling an addiction. This section is designed to give you an overview of basic substance abuse issues so that you will take care to address this critical concern in order for true progress to be made with career interventions.

Alcohol abuse remains epidemic and is responsible for both employee absences from work and employee illness, both physical and psychological. You will find that many of your clients may be "dually diagnosed," meaning that in addition to a DSM diagnosis for their presenting problem, they also have difficulties with substance abuse. This problem is underreported because denial is prevalent among substance abusers; they tend to minimize the contribution that their use of substances plays in their other concerns. In extreme cases they may lose jobs, drivers' licenses, and eventually, their families through divorce. Still, they may continue to blame other circumstances for their problems. As you attempt to help substance abusers, you may find yourself becoming discouraged by their lack of progress. The key to successfully working with such clients is to keep your expectations reasonable and to refrain from believing that these clients are always giving you the full story regarding their behaviors. A healthy skepticism on your part will keep you from getting discouraged and burning out.

In the United States today we live in a drug culture. Pharmaceutical companies constantly assail us with ads on television that promise a better life if we will simply ask our doctor for a prescription for their medications. We cannot avoid advertising that extols the social advantage of alcohol consumption, or the sophistication one attains by drinking designer caffeine products. Magazine ads show happy people using tobacco products, and movies are replete with characters who are involved in illegal drug use. The general message is that drugs are part of the fabric of the good life. Nystul (2003) reported that alcohol and drug use (not including tobacco) accounts for approximately 40 percent of hospital admissions and 25 percent of deaths in the United States, "costing society an excess of $300 billion a year in addition to human suffering and lack of productivity" (p. 423).

So, why do people use drugs? Kottler (2004) pointed out that people experience positive short-term effects from the use of various substances. They provide a sense of euphoria, suppress pain, lubricate social interactions, reduce stress, alleviate boredom, qualify people for membership in peer groups, and provide entertainment by altering states of consciousness. Drug use is commonplace, and drug abuse (misuse) is problematic. It will be important for you to remember that because drug use has been incorporated into our way of life and because it delivers positive psychological effects, people are reluctant to give it up.

When you are dealing with someone who has a drug problem, you may find it useful to think about the stage of change in which the person is operating. Prochaska, DiClemente, and Norcross (1992) have offered a useful model of the way people change in their response to their own substance use and abuse. Motivational Interviewing and the Stages of Change Model begins with a stage in which people do not see themselves as having a problem, and it progresses to a stage in which they will take action to alter their behavior. Each of the stages, described below, will have implications for your intervention.

Precontemplation: In this stage, your clients will have no plans to change their behaviors. They may be referred to you by others who think they have a problem or need help, but their resistance and denial prevent them from agreeing with this view. Difficulties in their lives and their work are minimized and they will likely decline your invitations for counseling regarding the issue. The most you can do is attempt to establish a nonjudgmental and cordial relationship with these clients, and state your availability if they should wish to return at a later time.

Contemplation: In this stage, your clients will admit to a problem and state that they are considering a change, but they are not quite ready to make a commitment to actively engage in the change process. They are weighing the pros and cons of making the change. It is important that you respond by using the "LUV Triangle" (Presbury, Echterling, & McKee, 2002). You will carefully listen, communicate your understanding, and validate their worldview. You must remember that substance use has many positive effects for these clients; asking people to give up something without replacing it with something else that is rewarding will seem like a poor exchange to them. Do not push for change at this stage.

Preparation: At this stage clients have usually tried unsuccessfully to change their behavior and plan to try again within the next thirty days. You may, at this stage, begin to help clients explore the costs and benefits of changing. For example, if alcohol is the problem, quitting drinking may mean that regular nights out with friends at the local bar will be seriously threatened. If this means giving up a circle of friends as well as the alcohol, clients may not consider this to be something worth doing. As Becvar and Becvar (2003) put it, "You can't just do one thing" (p. 363). Changing one aspect of a person's life has a ripple effect. The client has good reason to proceed cautiously, and you must respect this reluctance.

Action: At this stage, clients have taken steps to address the problem. In the case of substance addiction, they may have entered a "detox" program to make sure that the effects of the substance have been physically removed from their system. This is only the beginning of a sequence of actions they must take. Sometimes, they can enter a "rehab" program for thirty days to begin to alter their habits and attitudes. This plan can sometimes put their job at risk if the employer is not supportive. Also, they may lose their salary for this period of time. If clients can keep in contact with you by phone or e-mail, you may be able to continue to provide support during this difficult time.

Considerable debate exists as to whether the goal of alcohol-abuse counseling should be abstinence or controlled drinking. Organizations such as Alcoholics Anonymous® (AA) consider alcohol abuse to be a disease and state that abstinence is the only path to a cure. Others consider abuse to be a behavior problem that can be modified so that it does not affect one's family, job, finances, or friendships. Obviously, given the choice, most clients would rather try controlled drinking. However, controlled drinking is unlikely to be a viable option if the degree of alcoholism is severe (Peele, 1992; Rosenberg, 1993).

Maintenance: Once clients arrive at this stage, they are well into the process of change and your job is to help them stay on track so that they do not "backslide." Sometimes, people have to rehearse new behaviors many times before they are completely successful. You can help them retain their self-esteem in spite of relapses by pointing this out. Substance abuse counseling requires a great deal of patience on your part. You must control your need to "fix" clients. Perhaps this desire is a "rescue fantasy" on your part; the danger is that you will become angry with clients and communicate your disappointment if they fail after you have put so much effort into helping them. You will probably have the opportunity to take a course in substance abuse counseling during your training so that you become familiar with the various treatment modalities for these clients. Substance abuse is definitely a career issue, because it affects so many workers. But even if you, as a community counselor, are not directly involved in work-related interventions, you will need to develop your skills for working with substance abuse. It is a ubiquitous concern in our country.

Burnout

We have mentioned burnout several times in this text, so by now you probably have a sense of how relevant this issue may be for community counselors and their clients. According to Carroll and White (1982), any number of stressors can lead to burnout. They see burnout as a psychobiological phenomenon in which symptoms may occur suddenly and persist over long periods of time. People are not always aware that they are in a burnout condition, either because of denial or a symptomatic general numbness. They may view their lack of performance on the job as laziness, and others may see it as malingering. People who are "addicted" to their work are probably most at risk for burnout. They tend to see the job as their life, and they work many more hours than are required, without adequate time spent in leisure activities. They may be "control freaks" who believe in the old adage that "if you want a job done right, you must do it yourself." When they observe a decline in their performances, they tend to feel immense guilt and punish themselves.

Edelwich and Brodsky (1982) identified four stages in the burnout process as follows:

- Stage one is *enthusiasm*. In this stage, workers enter the job or task with unrealistic expectations regarding the outcome. They expect to accomplish far more than is reasonable because of their hopeful, rose-colored view of the situation. New counselors are often at risk for burnout, because they tend to enter the profession with something we've mentioned before, the "rescue fantasy," the belief that if they try hard enough their clients will all be "cured."

- Stage two, *stagnation,* begins when the worker starts to feel that personal, financial, or career needs are not being met, and that the personal effort he or she has expended is not being met with sufficient results.

- Stage three, *frustration,* begins when the worker begins to question his or her effectiveness, thinking "Maybe I really can't do this!" If, at this stage, the supervisor or counselor can help the employee reassess expectations and recognize his or her limits, the person can usually be turned away from the final stage, *apathy*.

- Stage four, the *apathy* stage, represents full burnout. The worker is in a state of disequilibrium and immobility. There is little awareness of what is happening, and she or he may defy any attempts at intervention (Gilliland & James, 1988). At this stage the person will likely exhibit a myriad of symptoms: job performance and efficiency are reduced; substance use may increase; absenteeism increases; the person may become a "clockwatcher" or chronic complainer; there may be a dread of coming to work; irritability increases; physical symptoms such as fatigue, ulcers, gastrointestinal problems, or poor coordination emerge; and depression, cynicism, or paranoia may be prevalent in the person's attitude.

"'Burnout' is not simply a sympathy-eliciting term to use when one has had a hard day at the office. It is a very real malady that strikes people and may have extremely severe consequences" (Gilliland & James, 1988, p. 473). The irony involved in this situation is that the more people are committed to their work, the more susceptible they are to burnout. Human service workers are greatly at risk for burnout. We encourage you to learn as much as you can about the symptoms of burnout and some of the interventions that have been successful in preventing or treating this condition. Because you will be in a profession in which burnout is rampant, you need to understand your own reactions to situations at work and learn to recognize when you need to pull back from too much involvement by finding more meaning and balance in your life away from your job.

Sustaining—Crises and Transitions

At some point in their work most community counselors are called on to help their clients sustain their commitment and sense of purpose as they face life and career transitions. According to Sharf (1992), there are four types of transitions or crises that people experience in their lives that affect their jobs: "anticipated, unanticipated, 'chronic hassles,' and events that don't happen (nonevents)" (p. 201). *Anticipated events,* such as graduating from high school or college, marriage, the birth of a child, starting a job, or changing jobs do not usually take us by surprise. Nevertheless, all change presents us with a crisis, because all of life's turning points are crises. *Unanticipated events* tend to hit us harder, because we are usually unprepared for them. The death of a family member, being fired or laid-off from a job, suffering an injury, or being diagnosed with a major illness are all examples of unanticipated crises. *Chronic hassles* may include long commutes to work in heavy traffic, a difficult supervisor, deadline pressures, discrimination at work, or dealing with a disability. *Nonevents* are things that we expect to happen but that fail to be realized. Applying for a desired job but not being hired; expecting, but not getting, a raise or a promotion; being denied an application for a change in position or a transfer to a new community; or wishing to spend more time with family but feeling trapped by financial considerations are examples of nonevents. All these situations are crises that pose difficulties for people in their careers.

There is a Chinese symbol that can be interpreted to mean crisis, danger, or difficulty, but it can also mean *opportunity*. Unfortunately, when people are in crisis, being able to envision new and positive possibilities resulting from the situation at hand is not their usual reaction (Echterling, Presbury, & McKee, 2005). Your job, when dealing with people in any form of crisis, is to help them toward this vision. Erikson (1963) used the concept of crisis as the foundation of his stages of human development—a crisis is a turning point in our lives, a brief but crucial time in which people suffer pain, confusion, and heartache. We have all experienced crises in our lives, and we have survived them. However, it is important to remember that not only do people survive, they may also have the opportunity to *thrive* as a result of these turning points (Echterling, Presbury, & McKee, 2005). *Webster's New World Dictionary* states that the experience of thriving is: "to prosper or flourish; be successful; to grow vigorously." When we are attempting to help people *sustain* during these crises, we are trying to foster growth—to help them *thrive* in spite of events that are largely unwelcome in their lives.

Helping People with Job Loss

In our culture, much of who you are is what you do; our identities are sometimes heavily invested in our jobs. What happens, then, to someone whose job is eliminated by organizational restructuring, forced retirement, "downsizing," "outsourcing," or when the work to which people formerly dedicated themselves is taken over by a computer? The answer is that they suffer a loss, and this loss involves more than just a job. Shutz (1967) stated that the three basic interpersonal human needs are inclusion (the need to associate and belong), control (the need to master situations and avoid helplessness), and affection (the desire to be positively regarded by others). These human needs are often satisfied through our involvement in the workplace. The loss of our job is a life crisis because our identity, our feeling of control, our self-esteem, and our sense of belonging may all become threatened by this situation. The crisis literature is very clear as to what happens when we encounter loss.

John Schneider (1984) suggested that with any loss, however severe, people go through predictable stages of a grieving process. If we are sensitive to this process, it is possible to provide support that will mitigate against the possibility that someone will become stuck in any of Schneider's stages. While many people might appear unaffected by alterations in their job roles, hundreds of investigations have shown that any significant change in a person's life produces stressful reactions.

Over thirty years ago Ruch and Holmes (1971) conducted studies of the life-changing events that create stress, from which they developed their well-known scale of stressors, each with an assigned value. In this list of forty-three stressors, seven were directly job-related. "Loss of a job" was very high on the list, and "Change to a different line of work" made the top twenty, ranking only one point behind "Death of a close friend" and three points behind "Sex difficulties" (p. 15). Unless they are dealt with, stress reactions can show up as chronic diminished productivity, burnout, lack of creativity, and/or social isolation, not to mention potential translation to an unlimited array of physical ailments. As you attempt to help people who are experiencing life-changing events relating to their career, you may find it helpful to consider Schneider's (1984) grief stages in order to understand where your client may be in the process.

- Stage one is the initial awareness of loss. In many cases, the employee will be called to the job superior's office or work-station and given the bad news. Other times, a "pink slip" in the pay envelope is the employee's notice of termination. In other situations, such as a plant closing or a company's relocation, the employee may be involved in an "outplacement" program designed to help him or her seek new employment. In any of these cases, you can expect the person to experience the first stage of loss. These reactions may include shock, confusion, numbness, detachment, disbelief, and disorientation. Someone at this stage is not yet ready to consider options or to be optimistic regarding new employment. Once again the most helpful intervention at this stage is the "LUV Triangle"—carefully listen, communicate your understanding, and validate the person's story about the job loss (Echterling, Presbury, & McKee, 2005). Do not reassure or attempt to get the person to "look on the bright side." The ability to see positive aspects of the situation will come at a later stage. "Communicate your faith in the individual by expressing neither skepticism nor the desire to debate. . . . Your quiet and accepting manner can promote a sense of validation that the person is lacking during this time of crisis" (p. 20).

- Stage two is characterized by an attempt to limit awareness by "holding on." This is, to a degree, a denial phase in which the person attempts to place a positive "spin" on the event. A casual observer may mistake this for a recovery and believe that the grieving is complete. However, Schneider states that this phase includes muscular tension, sleep disturbance, a desire to leave, ruminations, and guilt. Still, in this stage, the person is attempting to marshal resources and deal with the situation. "Holding on" is the attempt to mobilize inner resources or hopes in order to stave off immobility and disequilibrium, and to get back in touch with coping strategies that have worked in the past (Gilliland & James, 1988). It is important that you do not try to get the person to "face the facts" because this stage represents an important attempt to limit feelings of helplessness and despair. "Convey your confidence in the person's resilience by refraining from giving glib advice. . . . [Communicating] your belief in someone's resourcefulness sends a powerful message of validation" (Echterling, Presbury, & McKee, 2005, p. 20).

• Schneider's stages three and four are characterized first by "letting go" in order to limit awareness, followed by the dawning awareness of the extent of the loss. In these stages the person attempts to withdraw from the situation, but then realizes the feelings of grief. What first may be the experiences of depression, shame, cynicism, self-destructive ideation, or loss of memory, may give way to exhaustion, pain, preoccupation, loneliness, hopelessness, and lack of a future orientation. Intervention at this point may help to reorient the person toward a more hopeful view. In the transition between stages three and four, the person is already engaged in the active process of surviving the crisis of the job loss. Asking "getting through" questions about the ways that someone has been able to cope with the situation to this point is a way of focusing your intervention on what is working, instead of what was broken (Echterling, Presbury, & McKee, 2005). "Some common 'getting through' questions are: 'How did you get yourself to do that?' 'How did you manage to handle the crisis the way that you did?' 'What did you draw from inside yourself to make it through that experience?'" (p. 24).

• In stages five and six, the person begins to gain perspective and resolve the loss. The person now can mourn what is permanently gone, but can also begin to see possibilities for growth in the situation. At this time, the person becomes more open to experience, accepts things as they are, and feels more secure or at peace with the situation. Now, the future will open up and plans can begin for the next step, whatever that may be. You must take care not to rush the person into making choices at this stage. The future is still too uncertain and the person's motivation is still weak. You need to help the person sustain the optimism that has emerged, but realize that he or she is back at the attainment mode of development. Everything is new and unknown, which makes any movement a step into unknown territory. As the counselor, you are now the fellow traveler in the person's new quest.

• Stages seven and eight represent the ideal stages of recovery from the loss. Schneider refers to these as reformulating loss in the context of growth and transforming loss into new levels of attachment. At these levels, people begin to rediscover resources within themselves and come to view their situation as a challenge. Obviously, this ideal, which is stated in somewhat rhapsodic, self-actualizing terms by Schneider, may be out of reach for many people. What may be more likely is that people who are deeply grieving may continue to do so, despite the fact that they may be able to carry on and find new employment. It would seem, however, that for them to regain a sense of safety and self-confidence, they must approach these latter stages.

As the counselor, you should applaud whatever steps the person is willing to make. Focus should be on the successes the person has achieved, however small. While you can also offer information and assistance characteristic of the attainment mode, you must take care not to get ahead of the client's progress. This may cause a regression to a former stage. For example, offering employment information before the person is ready to seek a new position may increase his or her anxiety level. At the time of the loss of the job, self-esteem and self-confidence were likely lost along with it. Staying in rhythm with the client's progress is your best technique. Any time he or she seems to "backslide," that is your signal that you have not offered enough of the LUV Triangle. Go back to listening, communicating your understanding, and validating whatever stage the person seems to be in. Providing a forum in which people can voice their concerns in an accepting atmosphere helps make their confusing emotions clearer and less daunting. Sometimes group discussions can assist individuals in feeling less alone, because they learn that their emotions are shared by others and are not weird or "crazy."

CAREER COUNSELING WITH DIVERSE POPULATIONS

In order to effectively serve your clients, you will need to attend to their unique characteristics and concerns that can affect the career counseling and career development processes. In addition to their struggles with mental illness, concerns of living, and career and work problems, some clients face particular challenges that influence their work—and therefore their personal—lives. We focus specifically here on clients with disabilities, women, and minorities.

Disability Issues and Career Counseling

Whether or not you find yourself specializing in rehabilitation counseling, you will certainly be dealing with many clients whose disabilities are a hindrance to their emotional, social, and vocational lives. According to Clarke and Crowe (2000), "individuals with disabilities as a group may have the highest rate of unemployment and underemployment in the United States" (p. 58). Underemployment means that the person is employed in a job the demands of which are far below his or her set of abilities. For example, someone who formerly functioned as the chief executive officer of a large company may now be employed as a grocery clerk.

The 1990 Americans with Disabilities Act (ADA) defines disabilities as impairments that substantially limit a major life activity, that are of importance to most people's lives, and that are permanent or long-term. Disabilities include emotional, cognitive, behavioral, and physical impairments that can be congenital or can occur as the result of illness or accident. Over forty million people in the United States have some sort of disability. While your program may not offer a specialization in Rehabilitation Counseling, you can see from this statistic that you will be working with many clients who have disabilities.

In some ways, these clients' needs will not be so different than those of other clients. Enright (1997) pointed out that people with disabilities suffer from low self-esteem, lack of self-confidence or self-efficacy, and indecision or poor decision-making skills. These are familiar issues to all counselors. However, people with disabilities may have the additional burden of social stigma, lack of adequate role models or social support, and a restricted range of occupational opportunity. According to Bolton (2001), the goals of rehabilitation counseling are gainful employment, independence in living, and greater participation in the community. These are achievements we would wish for all our clients. Depending on your work setting, you will likely encounter clients with a range of disabilities that affect their work and career options. We encourage you to become familiar with the responsibilities involved in rehabilitation-oriented counseling by exploring the American Rehabilitation Counseling Association, a division of the American Counseling Association. The website address is **www.arcaweb.org.**

Gender Issues and Career Counseling

Career counseling often demands that you, as a community counselor, help your clients balance their career fantasies with the reality of their life experiences. Can a woman, for instance, be a successful airplane pilot? Can a man be a successful day care provider? In this age of androgyny, are there still such categories as "women's work" and "men's work?" If career choice existed on a "level playing field," meaning that women had equal access to all careers and there were no glass ceilings preventing their advancement in careers of their choice, would there then be no difference in the types of work preferred by men and women? Perhaps not.

As we all know, in most cultures, men and women are socialized differently. Biologically, men and women differ in their sexual characteristics. Some neuroscientists even claim to have found structural brain differences between the sexes that would account for differences in cognitive and emotional functioning. While this latter assertion remains controversial, it seems clear that, in general, there are differences between men and women. So the question is: Do men and women naturally gravitate to different kinds of work?

We are assuming that as you read this you are currently involved in a training program, studying to become a counselor. As you reflect on the composition of your peer group, what is the ratio of men to women in your program? If this ratio is typical, there will be more women than men. Counseling, because it has historically been founded on a nurturing, helping relationship, seems to be stereotypically women's work. With some exceptions, being a counselor requires that the person possess a strong empathic sense and a good intuition. Research conducted by O'Neil (1982) suggested that women may be often guided by emotions and intuitions and are more likely to make decisions "on the basis of feelings rather than careful analysis" (p. 22). Men, on the other hand, tend to prize such things as power, control, competition, toughness, and "logical and analytical thought" (p. 21). "The mental processes that are involved in considering the abstract and the impersonal have been labeled 'thinking' and are attributed primarily to men, while those which deal with the personal and interpersonal fall under the rubric of 'emotions' and are largely relegated to women" (Belenky, Clinchy, Goldberger, & Tarule, 1986, p. 7).

The power imbalance between men and women in society is very relevant to this picture. Thinking and logical reasoning, for instance, are valued more highly than feelings and connection in our society, regardless of the relative contributions and efficacy of these different modes of experiencing. Skovholt (1990), who researched gender differences in self-disclosure, found that many men characteristically avoid emotional intimacy and that women are far more likely than men to self-disclose to intimates. Zunker (1998) asserted that men generally have what he called a "fear of femininity" (p. 392) and they tend to stay away from traditionally female occupations, such as social work, nursing, elementary school teaching, and secretarial work. He stated that "there continues to be prejudice, ridicule, and negative perceptions of the men who choose them[;] . . . gender typing of careers is still prevalent in our society, and those who deviate experience the scorn of those whose thinking is dominated by gender-role stereotyping" (p. 397).

As you consider this information, reflect upon how your gender has influenced your career path so far. How has it opened doors for you, and how has it limited you? These are questions that are very relevant as you conceptualize and try to help your clients make personally relevant career and life choices. If you haven't already done so, we recommend that you investigate some of the core writings regarding feminist theory and therapy. Regardless of your theoretical orientation as a community counselor, feminist theory and feminist approaches to therapy provide provocative and often compelling suggestions for responding to societal limitations placed on clients because of their gender (May, 2001; Worell & Remer, 2003). These types of resources also suggest ways in which counselors can appropriately respond to clients who are choosing to limit themselves because of narrow or rigid gender stereotypes.

Women and Work

As of the year 1991, nearly half of the work force in the United States was female, the average education levels of men and women were approximately equal, and the percentage of women in executive and managerial jobs had risen dramatically (Seligman, 1994). So it would seem that we have entered an enlightened age in which women are gaining equity and that gender differences in the workplace are largely ignored in favor of ability. As we've mentioned, counseling, for example, appears to be largely a female career, since the work seems to call for stereotypically feminine talents: caring, nurturing, and establishing relationships. But Seligman pointed out that while women held 59 percent of the counseling positions in 1994, they were earning 19 percent less than men in similar positions.

While being female is not technically a minority status, women are continuing to experience the discrimination and constraints on salary and advancement in the workplace that people in minority groups also suffer. Spokane and Hawks (1990) found similarities in work settings that are endured by both women and minorities. These include limits on career options, stereotyping of work roles, lower expectations for achieving aspirations, and factors outside of work that interfere with career advancement. Sharf (1992) stated that women face certain situations in the workplace that are usually not experienced by men. "Women are much more likely than men to experience discrimination, make decisions based on child-raising and family issues, and face sexual harassment" (p. 211).

As you work with women clients who are dealing with career issues, you will find that while things are changing in the marketplace, women still, on average, carry a heavier burden when it comes to work. Many are working two jobs: one for economic gain and one to keep the family functioning. During World War II, the famous image of women as "Rosie the Riveter" showed the country that "man's work" and "woman's work" were not that different. Women went into the factories to build the tanks, planes, and bombs that helped win that war. Then, when the men came home from the fighting, women had to give up their jobs to these returning military men.

By then, the notion that men were workers and women were housewives had been shattered by the experiences of women in the workplace. The Women's Movement and a changing economy led more women to work outside the home. By 1988, 65 percent of women with school-aged children, and 56 percent of women with children under the age of six were employed outside the home (Seligman, 1994). Today in the United States, women are marrying later in life and having fewer children; however, they are still often juggling two careers. Some have put off having children in favor of a career, but, as the age of menopause approaches, many face a crisis of having to choose between children and career. The lack of adequate leave policies in their workplaces and few good childcare facilities make this decision seem crucial.

As a counselor, part of your job will be to advocate for better conditions for all your clients. You should be active politically and attempt to influence local policies that tend to unfairly restrict any of your clients. However, it is also important for you to recognize the limit of your ability to change systems that have been in place for ages. Therefore, when working with an individual client, you can help raise her consciousness as to how these systems work so as to avoid self-blame on the client's part. One particularly obvious difficulty you will be dealing with is when your client has been sexually harassed. Although men can be sexually harassed at work as well, we focus here on women, who are the primary targets of this type of behavior.

Sharf (1992) cited the work of Till (1980) who listed the increasing levels of severity of harassment experienced by women in the workplace.

Level one is *gender harassment*. This refers to verbal remarks or any non-physical behaviors that are sexist in nature. Sexist stories or comments made in an atmosphere in which the woman will obviously overhear them is harassment at the lowest level of offense.

Level two is *seductive behavior*. Unwanted sexual advances, such as asking about the woman's sexual life or expressing sexual interest in her are examples of behaviors at this level.

Level three is *sexual liberty*. At this stage, the offer of a sexual encounter in exchange for some reward takes place. A supervisor offers a raise in pay or a promotion, or a teacher offers a good grade.

Level four is *sexual coercion*. This is a threatening situation in which the woman experiences the possibility of loss or injury if she does not respond favorably.

Level five is *sexual assault*. In this case, the woman has experienced a forceful attempt to kiss, touch, or fondle her. Obviously, attempted rape is also included in this category, but would be such a blatant violation that no person hearing of it should doubt that it goes well beyond sexual harassment.

The problem with the lower levels of harassment is that they are more ambiguous in meaning. The perpetrator could claim that the woman simply misunderstood the perpetrator's statements or gestures. This ambiguity can cause the woman to doubt herself or minimize the violation. Your job as a counselor is to help her sort through what she believes to be the intention of those who have made her feel uncomfortable on the job. Of course, once the behavior reaches level five, the meaning becomes clear, but still if she complains to

EXPERIENTIAL LEARNING

As you think about gender and career issues in your own life, broaden your conceptualization to include cultures such as ethnicity and class. Then, create a career genogram for yourself (mentioned earlier in the chapter), and consider in particular the lessons you have learned from your family regarding career and work.

1. How do those lessons reflect your socioeconomic class and culture?

2. What limits and privileges have been placed on you as a result of your gender, class, and culture?

3. How might those experiences enhance and/or hinder your work with clients who have had drastically different experiences than yours?

superiors or legal authorities, it can become a "he said, she said" situation in which the cost may seem to exceed the possible benefit.

For this reason, many women consider harassment simply the price they must pay to be successful in a career. Sexual harassment is illegal. As you work with a woman who is experiencing such behavior, your job is not necessarily to simply get her to go to the authorities. In that case, you would be engaging her in the classic game of "Let's you and him fight" (Berne, 1964). As it is with your work with people on all other issues, your job is to help your client explore options, gain confidence, and make her own decisions as to what is to be done.

Cultural Issues and Career Counseling

There are two myths in American culture that are imbedded in the assumptions of most of us. The first is the myth of "rugged individualism." We tend to see people as separate agents who work alone and reap the rewards of their efforts. People's talent, their intellect, and their drive to succeed will combine to ensure their success in the workplace. The second myth, existing as a close corollary, is the "American Dream." The belief in the American Dream goes something like this: "Work hard, save your money, and you can rise from the lowest to the highest strata of society." This myth implies that every American citizen, given his or her desire to do so, can find success and happiness in this land of opportunity. Stories of people who began their careers working in the mailroom and then ended up as president of the company abound. Of course, it does not take much reflection to realize that such stories are inspirational but do not accurately portray the average experience of most people in our country.

If your client is gay, rural poor, African American, Latino, Native American, disabled, or female, the likelihood is that he or she will face barriers in the workplace that do not exist for many white males. Furthermore, cultural expectations may also affect your client's aspirations and sense of efficacy.

When you read the theories of career counseling, they seem to imply that each individual has free choice in an arena of unlimited opportunities. They appear to suggest that as a counselor, you simply match the client's interests and abilities to a job category, and the rest will take care of itself. As we have said, barriers exist in the workplace for some groups of people, but what is less obvious are the cultural inhibitions that sometimes "keep people in their place." Matsumoto (1996) identified some cultural values that may be somewhat at odds with the dominant culture, and which will affect people's attitudes toward work and career. For instance, in some cultures it is important to minimize uncertainty in many aspects of life. In the workplace, this attitude results in "fear of failure, less risk taking, higher job stress, more worry about the future, and higher anxiety" (Zunker, 1998, p. 423). Also, because of their cultural backgrounds and their life experiences before entering the workplace, many people view security and "9 to 5" working hours as the most desirable aspects of a good job. Such attitudes may tend to limit advancement in their careers. Still other cultures prize collectivism over individualism. People from such cultures are more dependent on the companies they work for, are less likely to display individual initiative, tend to rely more on group decisions than their own intuitions, and are more likely to conform than to display their creativity.

You are undergoing graduate training in order to become a professional community counselor. You have been well-educated, and it is possible that you have unconsciously adopted much of the "rugged individualism" and "American Dream" myths. Your attitudes toward work may be aligned pretty well with those of the dominant culture. If so, it is important that you realize that not everyone views work and career as you do. Learn about other cultures. Share the story or your career journey, and ask others who are different from you to tell you about theirs. Seek to know what people who are culturally different than you must deal with when making decisions about their careers. If you keep in mind that career counseling, like psychotherapeutic counseling, must be tailored to the person you are attempting to help, then you will be more effective as you counsel people toward coming to grips with work and career. Adopt that nonexpert "I'm not from around here" attitude when you are counseling anyone regarding his or her career. Investigate the beliefs, prejudices, and assumptions that you bring to the counseling situation. As you increase your consciousness and understanding of cultural differences, you will become a better counselor in every aspect of your work.

ETHICAL AND LEGAL ISSUES IN PRACTICE

Ethical standards for career counseling have been developed by the National Board for Certified Counselors (NBCC) and the National Career Development Association (NCDA). Ethical issues relevant for career counseling are also covered in the ACA Code of Ethics. When you are using assessment inventories or tests in the process of helping clients attain personal career information or screening for employment, you must inform clients of the purpose for doing so. You must select instruments that are appropriate to the client's cultural background and administer them under standardized conditions. It is incumbent upon you to be properly prepared to use and interpret the instruments you will use with clients. If you are reporting the results of testing to a third party, you must remember that the person you are working with is your primary client and must be fully informed of how the results will be used.

As in all other forms of counseling, your primary responsibility is to respect the integrity and promote the welfare of the client. You are obligated to continue to self-explore and become more conscious of your own biases and prejudices regarding gender, people of color, socioeconomic stats, and cultural differences when attempting to help clients. This self-awareness will allow you to maintain an objective and neutral stance when engaging in evaluation procedures and to communicate your positive regard to clients (Kottler, 2004). Finally, because the world of work is constantly changing, you must attempt to keep up to date on trends in education, business, industry, and professional fields.

Since 1964, many laws have been passed to protect people's right to work and to shield them against discrimination. You will occasionally have a client who is complaining of maltreatment on the job, so it is in your best interest to know what recourse is available for that person. We will offer a brief listing of some of these laws, but we also suggest that you familiarize yourself with them in greater depth. You can access more information about these laws on the Internet by using a search engine such as **www.google.com.** Here is a brief listing of some laws that may be helpful to your clients who have been mistreated by training institutions or employers.

Title VII and *Title IX* are sections of the 1964 Civil Rights Act and the Education Amendments of 1972 that prohibit discrimination against women and minorities in all areas of employment. Title VII also sets standards for the use of tests in career counseling and employment screening so that they do not discriminate against culturally diverse populations.

The Rehabilitation Act of 1973 provided for access to rehabilitation services for adults who were physically or mentally disabled and when such disabilities interfered with the ability to obtain or maintain a job.

The Americans with Disabilities Act of 1992 prohibits discrimination against people with disabilities in the areas of job application, hiring and firing, advancement on the job, wages and fringe benefits, training, and work conditions.

PL 93-112 is a law that requires colleges to provide career services to people with disabilities, such as visual or auditory impairment.

These laws, and others not mentioned here, are designed to provide a "level playing field" for all citizens who participate in the world of work. Sometimes, as a community counselor, your most effective intervention for clients is providing them with information or putting them in touch with legal assistance when their rights have been violated.

Despite the Civil Rights Act and other protective legislation, some gaps still exist for some people who wish to maintain their employment. One glaring example is the military policy known as "Don't Ask, Don't Tell," in which military employees' sexual orientation is addressed. More recently, this policy was expanded to, "Don't Ask, Don't Tell, Don't Pursue, Don't Harass" (DADTDPDH). This is "the only law in the land that authorizes the firing of an American for being gay. There is no other federal, state, or local law like it" (www.sldn.org, p. 1).

While this law put an end to questions about sexual orientation upon induction into the service and decreased the "witch-hunts" in the military, still, people can be investigated and administratively discharged if they (1) overtly state that they are lesbian, gay, or bisexual; (2) engage in physical contact with a person of the same sex for sexual gratification; or (3) marry, or attempt to marry, someone of the same sex. Behaviors such as having a gay friend, going to a gay bar, attending a gay pride event, or reading gay magazines or books are never to be considered sufficient evidence for initiating proceedings against someone in the military. If you should have a client who is experiencing pressure to confess a sexual preference, or is being harassed because of suspected homosexuality, you can direct him or her to the website for the Servicemembers Legal Defense Network at **www.sldn.org.** The site advises people who are under duress to "say nothing, sign nothing, and get legal help."

CONCLUDING THOUGHTS

If you haven't already taken our advice to interview community counselors, then now's the time. Make sure the counselors you interview have been in the field for at least five years. That way, the career "honeymoon" period will

Career and Life Case Study: Bringing It All Together

Kim is thirty-one years old, a first generation Korean-American woman, and the single mother of a five-year-old son. Kim has been working full-time as a financial advisor for a large firm since her mid-twenties. She is successful, and the firm is talking about making her a partner. However, Kim is beginning to question her career path. She chose her career because she felt it would be a rewarding and stable path full of opportunities for success. Financial success was important to her because her parents struggled to make ends meet after immigrating to the United States.

However, Kim often thinks of pursuing a more meaningful and flexible career that allows her to provide international services for nonprofit groups who deal with underserved clients. Kim is afraid of what her family might think because they are so proud of her success, and she wonders if she will be able to support her son adequately if she takes this step. Kim also does not want to be seen as someone who is opting for a more flexible job because she could not "handle" her responsibilities as a single mother.

Questions for Reflection

1. What are the personal issues Kim is struggling with? What are the professional issues Kim is struggling with? How are these issues interrelated? Which issues would you focus on first with Kim?

2. Try to apply each of the career theories mentioned in this chapter to Kim's situation. Which theory seems relevant for Kim? Why or why not? Could you modify any of the theories in your work with Kim?

3. Consider elements of multiculturalism (i.e., race, culture, gender, socioeconomic status) and their impact on Kim's situation. How do these elements impact Kim's situation and how are they relevant to your counseling relationship with her?

4. Finally, try to identify any pertinent legal and/or ethical issues that you would take into consideration with Kim.

---

have passed, and they will give you a more realistic picture of the pros and cons of their jobs. Ask them how they arrived at their career choice. Inquire about their educational and career journeys. How did they arrive at their current positions? Question them about the aspects of their jobs they enjoy the most, as well as the parts they dislike the most. If you have the luxury of time, ask them about future trends in the field. Note the level of passion for their career. Then, after the interviews, reflect on the information received from these encounters. How has this affected your thoughts and feelings about your own career choice?

RECOMMENDED RESOURCES

We encourage you to regularly read the core journals in the field of career counseling, such as *The Career Development Quarterly* and *The Journal of Career Development.*

We also recommend the following websites:

www.counseling.org/jobs—This is the official website of the American Counseling Association, and current jobs are posted and updated regularly.

www.ajb.dni.us/—America's Job Bank is maintained by the New York State Department of Labor. This site regularly lists hundreds of thousands of jobs. Searching is by state or region and by type of position. Most jobs are full time and in the private sector.

www.jobhuntersbible.com—This is Richard Bolles' webpage for *What Color Is Your Parachute?* Bolles offers advice regarding career preparation, including practical tips on résumé writing, interviewing, networking, and starting well once you are selected for employment. This is an excellent launching pad for other quality career-related websites.

ncda.org—The National Career Development Association official website.

www.monster.com—This web portal is one of the most comprehensive sites for job searching and résumé posting as well as receiving practical help on building your résumé and preparing for interviews.

www.bls.gov/oco/—The *Occupational Outlook Handbook* is published biennially by the federal government. This handbook is one of the most important sources about careers.

www.access.gpo/gov/plumbook/toc.html—Known as the "Plum Book," this site is the Internet edition of *The U.S. Government Policy and Supporting Positions.* This is a database of over 9,000 civil service positions for the executive and legislative branches of government.

References such as the *Dictionary of Occupational Titles* and the *Occupational Outlook Handbook* provide detailed and current information about current and future trends in career development. Computer programs such as SIGI-Plus (System of Interactive Guidance and Information) and DISCOVER are two programs widely used in the United States to provide helpful career information. Many college and university career development centers will have these resources available for student use.

Other Resources

The movie *Working Girl* is a lighthearted view of one woman's struggle against patriarchy in the world of business. *Wall Street* provides a more intense depiction of work and its effects. Perhaps the most thought-provoking film to consider is *American Beauty,* which reveals the cumulative toll that career and life choices take on a man and his family.

REFERENCES

Becvar, D. S., & Becvar, R. J. (2003). *Family therapy: A systemic integration.* Boston: Allyn & Bacon.

Belenky, M. F., Clinchy, B. M., Goldberger, N. R., & Tarule, J. M. (1986). *Women's ways of knowing: The development of self, voice, and mind.* New York: Basic Books.

Berne, E. (1964). *Games people play: The psychology of human relationships.* New York: Grove Press.

Bolton, B. (2001). Measuring rehabilitation outcomes. *Rehabilitation Counseling Bulletin, 44,* 67–75.

Brown, B. B. (2000). *Changing career patterns.* Washington, DC: Office of Educational Research and Improvement. (ERIC Document Reproduction Service No. ED346082).

Brown, D. (1996). Brown's values-based, holistic model of career and life-role choices and satisfaction. In D. Brown, L. Brooks, & Associates (Eds.), *Career choice and development* (3rd ed., pp. 337–338). San Francisco: Jossey-Bass.

Brown, D., & Srebalus, D. J. (2003). *Introduction to the counseling profession.* Boston: Allyn & Bacon.

Carroll, J. F. X., & White, W. L. (1982). Theory building: Integrating individual and environmental factors within an ecological framework. In W. S. Paine (Ed.), *Job stress and burnout* (pp. 41–60). Beverly Hills, CA: Sage Publications.

Clarke, N. E., & Crowe, N. M. (2000). Stakeholder attitudes toward ADA Title I: Development of an indirect measurement method. *Rehabilitation Counseling Bulletin, 43,* 58–65.

Crites, J. O. (1981). *Career counseling: Models, methods, and materials.* New York: McGraw-Hill.

Dawis, R. V., & Lofquist, L. H. (1984). *A psychological theory of work adjustment.* Minneapolis: University of Minnesota Press.

Dolliver, M. (1999, September 6). Maybe it's not too late to become a fireman. *Adweek, 36,* 40.

Echterling, L. G., Presbury, J. H., & McKee, J. E. (2005). *Crisis intervention: Promoting resilience and resolution in troubled times.* Upper Saddle River, NJ: Merrill/Prentice Hall.

Edelwich, J., & Brodsky, A. (1982). Training guidelines: Linking the workshop experience to needs on and off the job. In W. S. Paine (Ed.), *Job stress and burnout* (pp. 133–154). Beverly Hills, CA: Sage Publications.

Enright, M. S. (1997). The impact of short-term career development programs on people with disabilities. *Rehabilitation Counseling Bulletin, 40,* 285–300.

Erikson, E. H. (1963). *Childhood and society.* New York: W. W. Norton.

Gilliland, B. E., & James, R. K. (1988). *Crisis intervention strategies*. Pacific Grove, CA: Brooks/Cole.

Ginzberg, E. (1972). Toward a theory of occupational choice: A restatement. *Vocational Guidance Quarterly, 20,* 169–176.

Gottfredson, L. S. (1981). Circumscription and compromise: A developmental theory of occupational aspirations. *Journal of Counseling Psychology, 28,* 6, 545–579.

Gysbers, N. C., & Moore, E. J. (1987). *Career counseling: Skills and techniques for practitioners*. Englewood Cliffs, NJ: Prentice Hall.

Hansen, L. S. (1997). ILP: Integrating our lives, shaping our society. In R. Feller & G. Walz (Eds.), *Career transitions in turbulent times* (pp. 21–30). Greensboro, NC: ERIC/CASS.

Heppner, M. J., O'Brien, K. M., Hinkelman, J. M., & Flores, L. Y. (1996). Training counseling psychologists in career development: Are we our own worst enemies? *The Counseling Psychologist, 24,* 1, 105–125.

Herr, E. L., & Cramer, S. H. (1996). *Career guidance and counseling through the life span: Systematic approaches* (5th ed.). Reading, MA: Addison-Wesley.

Holland, J. L. (1973). *Making vocational choices: A theory of career*. Englewood Cliffs, NJ: Prentice Hall.

Kottler, J. A. (2004). *Introduction to therapeutic counseling: Voices from the field* (5th ed.). Pacific Grove, CA: Thompson-Brooks/Cole.

Krumboltz, J. D. (1979). *Social learning and career decision-making*. New York: Carroll.

Krumboltz, J. D. (1994). Integrating career and personal counseling. *Career Development Quarterly, 42,* 143–148.

Matsumoto, D. (1996). *Culture and psychology*. Pacific Grove, CA: Brooks/Cole.

May, K. M. (Ed.). (2001). *Feminist family therapy*. Alexandria, VA: American Counseling Association.

McGoldrick, M. & Gerson, R. (1999). *Genograms: Assessment and intervention* (2nd ed.). New York: Norton.

Nystul, M. S. (2003). *Introduction to counseling: An art and science perspective*. Boston: Allyn & Bacon.

O'Neil, J. M. (1982). Gender role conflict and strain in men's lives: Implications for psychiatrists, psychologists, and other human-services providers. In K. Solomon & N. B. Levy (Eds.), *Men in transition* (pp. 5–40). New York: Plenum.

Parsons, F. (1909). *Choosing a vocation*. Boston: Houghton Mifflin.

Peele, S. (1992). Alcoholism, politics, and bureaucracy: The consensus against controlled-drinking therapy in America. *Addictive Behaviors, 17,* 49–61.

Prochaska, J. O., DiClemente, C. C., & Norcross, J. (1992). In search of how people change: Applications to addictive behaviors. *American Psychologist, 47,* 1102–1114.

Roe, A. (1956). *The psychology of occupations.* New York: Wiley.

Rosenberg, H. (1993). Prediction of controlled drinking by alcoholics and problem drinkers. *Psychological Bulletin, 113,* 129–139.

Richardson, M. S. (1996). From career counseling to counseling/psychotherapy and work, job, and career. In M. L. Savickas & W. B. Wash (Eds.), *Handbook of career counseling theory and practice* (pp. 347–360). Palo Alto, CA: Davies-Black.

Ruch, L. O. & Holmes, T. H. (1971). Scaling of life change: Comparison of direct and indirect methods. *Journal of Psychosomatic Research, 15.*

Schlossberg, N. K. (1997). A model for worklife transitions. In R. Feller & G. Walz (Eds.), *Career Transitions in Turbulent Times* (pp. 93–104). Greensboro, NC: ERIC/CASS.

Schouten, R. (2004). What is organizational and occupational psychiatry? *Psychiatric Times, 21,* 7.

Seligman, L. (1994). *Developmental career counseling and assessment* (2nd ed.). Thousand Oaks, CA: Sage Publications.

Schneider, J. (1984). *Stress, loss, and grief: Understanding their origins and growth potential.* Baltimore: University Park Press.

Sharf, R. S. (1992). *Applying career development theory to counseling.* Pacific Grove, CA: Brooks/Cole.

Shutz, W. C. (1973). *Elements of encounter.* Big Sur, CA: Joy Press.

Skovholt, T. M. (1990). Career themes in counseling and psychotherapy with men. In D. Brown, L. Brooks, & Associates (Eds.), *Career choice and development: Applying contemporary theories to practice* (2nd ed., pp. 197–261). San Francisco: Jossey-Bass.

Smith, S. L., Myers, J. E., & Hensley, L. G. (2002). Putting more into life career courses: The benefits of a holistic wellness model. *Journal of College Counseling, 5,* 90–95.

Spokane, A. R., & Hawks, B. K. (1990). Annual review: Practice and research in career counseling and development. *Career and Development Quarterly, 39,* 98–128.

Super, D. E. (1957). *The psychology of careers.* New York: Harpers.

Super, D. E. (1976). *Career education and the meaning of work* [Monograph]. Washington, DC: Office of Career Education, U.S. Office of Education.

Super, D. E. (1990). A life-span, life-space approach to career development. In D. Brown, L. Brooks, & Associates (Eds.), *Career choice and development: Applying contemporary theories to practice* (2nd ed., pp. 197–261). San Francisco: Jossey-Bass.

Till, F. (1980). *Sexual harassment: A report on the sexual harassment of students.* Washington, DC: National Advisory Council on Women's Educational Programs.

Whiston, S. C., & Brecheisen, B. K. (2002). Practice and research in career counseling and Development—2001. *Career Development Quarterly, 51,* 98–154.

Williams, T. (1955). *Cat on a hot tin roof.* New York: Signet.

Worell, J., & Remer, P. (2003). *Feminist perspectives in therapy: Empowering diverse women* (2nd ed.). Hoboken, NJ: Wiley & Sons.

Zunker, V. G. (1998). *Career counseling: Applied concepts of life planning.* Pacific Grove, CA: Brooks/Cole.

Chapter 11

Expanding Our Knowledge Base: Research and Evaluation

In order to be able to ask, one must want to know, and that means knowing that one does not know.

H.G. Gadamer

GOALS

Reading and exploring the ideas in this chapter will help you:

- Become aware of approaches to research and evaluation
- Appreciate the value of research in successful community counseling
- Understand the basic principles of program evaluation in community counseling

---

OVERVIEW

This chapter presents information on research methods, principles of program evaluation, and an explanation of their relevance to community counselors. Each of the chapters of this book has been inviting you to envision yourself in one of the many roles or tasks that community counselors can perform. Likewise, this chapter asks you to think of the counselor as using research and evaluation skills. Although we know that some counselors in training are interested in the topic of research, we also suspect that some are now thinking of skipping to the next chapter. "I never liked statistics," some of our students tell us, or "I don't see any way I'll ever need this stuff." If you're thinking along those lines, give us a chance to reframe your vision of research and evaluation.

LOU'S DEFINING MOMENT: Who's Guilty?

Lou was in the second year of his job as an outpatient counselor for a regional hospital. In addition to his work with hospital patients, Lou had a small caseload of clients through the hospital's Employee Assistance Program. He enjoyed the diversity of his caseload and often relished the relief that he felt when working with his EAP clients. They were less distressed than his other clients, and he often felt almost collegial in his work with them. Lou's casual attitude toward his clients changed, however, as a result of his work with Thomas.

Thomas was an x-ray technician at the hospital who came to see Lou for help in dealing with his high stress level. Thomas's daughter Alexis, who had autism, was experiencing an especially difficult transition to her new special education classroom. Thomas and his wife Lucinda, who was also employed at the hospital, were frequently called to Alexis' school to respond to Alexis' crises. Thomas was beginning to worry not only about his own work and life balance but about the long-term implications of Alexis' autism.

Lou and Thomas met several times, and Lou felt their therapeutic relationship was exceptionally strong. He empathized with Thomas' plight and understood the toll that disorders such as autism can take on families. At the end of one session Thomas asked Lou what he thought about "Facilitated Communication" for people with autism. He showed Lou a brochure that described a revolutionary technique which enabled people with autism to "unlock their imprisoned thoughts and feelings." With the help of a specially trained facilitator, children with autism were able to express themselves with heart-felt eloquence. According to the brochure, the facilitator supports the wrist of the person with autism, who then taps out words on a keyboard. The idea was that people with autism were simply imprisoned within their bodies. Inside, they were normal. If they could be supported physically so they could type, the incarcerated soul of the person would be released and genuine feelings could be displayed. "Sounds like an interesting possibility," Lou said. "Researchers are coming up with amazing interventions all the time. I'll look into it for you."

After that meeting Lou and Thomas didn't meet again for several weeks. Lou went on vacation, and Thomas changed work shifts in order to give himself more time with Alexis. Then, Lou received an emergency page. He assumed that one of his outpatient clients was experiencing a crisis, so he was surprised to find Thomas waiting for him. As they hurried to a counseling room Thomas explained that he and his wife had pursued Facilitated Communication for Alexis. They had initially been pleased with the results. Today, though, the facilitator told Thomas and Lucinda that she needed to report them to Child Protective Services. According to her report, Alexis revealed through her facilitated typing that Thomas had sexually abused her.

Lou was stunned as he listened to Thomas' story. Thomas was tearful and distraught as he denied the abuse had occurred. He told Lou he didn't know how much more stress he could handle. Lou spent an hour and a half with Thomas and eventually called Lucinda in to help them both talk about their reactions to the charges. After he ended the session with the plan to meet again tomorrow, Lou called a pediatrician at the hospital for consultation regarding autism and Facilitated Communication.

When he finally got to talk with the pediatrician, Lou was appalled to find that the physicians at the hospital, as well as several developmental specialists who consulted there, saw Facilitated Communication as a bogus intervention. "I'd caution any patient away from such a technique until there are legitimate outcome studies to support it. The last thing I'd want to do is build false hopes in a parent," the physician explained. Lou felt sick as he left the pediatrician and prepared to call Thomas. On one hand, he was hopeful that the Facilitated Communication was flawed and that the charges would be proven groundless. At the same time, though, he found himself trying desperately to remember whether he had actually recommended that Thomas and Lucinda try the technique. He realized with a jolt that he felt as though he were trying to prove his own innocence.

Postscript: This controversial procedure generated hundreds of studies concluding that Facilitated Communication had no scientific support for its efficacy (e.g., Bligh & Kupperman, 1993; Green, 1994; Hirshoren & Gregory, 1995). In fact, the American Psychological Association passed a resolution in 1994 stating that Facilitated Communication is not a scientifically valid technique and warned that information obtained through Facilitated Communication should not be used to confirm or deny allegations of abuse.

Questions for Reflection

1. In light of what you have just read, what policies and procedures would you recommend for promoting and using experimental intervention techniques?

2. How can you as a community counselor do your best to ensure that neither you nor your clients will be harmed by pseudo-scientific "breakthroughs" such as Facilitated Communication techniques?

WHY STUDY RESEARCH AND EVALUATION?

Evaluating interventions, measuring effectiveness, and researching issues are processes that are inextricably tied to counseling. Informally, you are already performing these tasks with every client that you see. Together, you and your client explore goals, discuss the progress of counseling in achieving these goals, and examine carefully the conditions that can lead your client to personal success. Research and evaluation as discussed in this chapter are merely more formal and intentional applications of these processes.

Research and evaluation also parallel the counseling process in that these activities take place in the context of a relationship—between you and your clients, between you and your funding sources, and between you and your professional colleagues. It is vital that your work be collaborative, open, and genuine. For example, to reflect this sense of collaboration in research, we use the term "participants," rather than "subjects," to refer to clients involved in a counseling study. Further, like counseling, research and evaluation in particular ideally focus on personal strengths and resources. For too long, the majority of studies in the field have focused on disorders, pathology, problems, and dysfunction. Finally, similar to counseling, research and evaluation should be integrated into the cultural tapestry of people's lives. When you undertake a community counseling study, you need to work together with members of the community, make certain that your project is respectful of their cultural perspective, and do your best to help community members to become more empowered.

Throughout your career as an ethically practicing counselor, you will continually be asking yourself about the effectiveness of your professional work. Your clients will be dependent upon you to keep abreast of new directions in counseling, being especially attuned to evidence of effectiveness. Your agency, center, or group practice will be expected to answer questions of accountability. Third-party payers will seek measures of effectiveness. You will need to communicate the condition of your clients to others in order to receive payments or make referrals. To answer these questions, you will not only have to have faith in your counseling skills and your approach, you will have to have a solid understanding of the basic principles informing counseling research and evaluation.

Research and Evaluation Defined

The twin concepts of research and evaluation tend to overlap considerably. *Research* is often considered an overarching term, especially when it is used to include basic and applied research. Classically, basic research is used to refer to the tightly controlled and strictly designed research intended to push back the frontiers of knowledge. This research can lead to new discoveries, new truths, and generalizable conclusions. Some people refer to basic research as "pure."

Applied research refers to research designed to solve a specific problem. Applied research often focuses on the "down and dirty" non-controllable aspects of working in the real world. *Evaluation* and *Assessment* may be considered forms of applied research. Evaluation measures programmatic effectiveness. Individual assessment, the evaluation of a client's case, deserves more focused attention because of its unique relevance to the work of community counselors. Individual assessment is described in Chapter 6. We have chosen to emphasize the differences between research and evaluation to help you toward seeing that these approaches, with similar methodology and tools, are both means of disciplined inquiry important to the counselor's practice.

RESEARCH

Stephen Isaac (Isaac & Michael, 1995) laid out a practical guide to thinking about research. He noted that research emphasizes control and manipulation of the variation among the participants involved in a study in an effort to establish a cause-effect relationship. General research design begins with a testable hypothesis. Then a researcher implements a research design that enhances internal and external validity, controls and manipulates variance among subjects, and seeks to draw inferences that are explanatory and predictive. The classic methodology paradigms in research are the experimental method and the correlational method. In an experiment, you would set up the situation in which you control your intervention so that your hypothesis could be disconfirmed if it is wrong, but also suggest that you are on the right track if it is not disconfirmed. A correlational study ideally seeks to isolate and examine variables to determine how change in one is or is not accompanied by change in another. As a community counselor, you will naturally be involved in research. The idea of being a researcher may not resonate immediately with you. But consider—on a daily basis you will be making hypotheses about what may be happening with a client, collecting data to inform how best to intervene, interpreting these data, and then evaluating your progress to determine future actions. Thus, you are employing the basis of research—the scientific method. But you may be wondering, "What about research in terms of research designs, experimental methods, and statistical analysis? How will I *ever* relate to or use any of that?" We would contend that there are three very important research-oriented roles for you as a community counselor.

First, you are ethically bound to keep abreast of the research in your field. To fully benefit from the professional literature, you will need to know the language, the methodology, and the other nuances involved in conducting research so that you can be a critical reader and evaluator of what is reported. Your own understanding of research principles is the only way to ensure that you are able to critically assess and evaluate the quality of new interventions and theories. Facilitated Communication, which was dealt with in the Defining Moment story, is a good example of a procedure that needed good research efforts and good consumers of the research literature. We have recently heard that, in spite of the fact that numerous studies have proven Facilitated Communication to be useless, some people are still doing it.

Second, there is a tremendous need for partnerships of practitioners and researchers in defining research questions and conducting research. Within a context of accountability and the most effective use of resources, evidence-based counseling requires the integration of research with the best elements of practice, clinical experience, and reliable treatment protocols in our efforts to help our clients. Research is most relevant when it builds upon and involves the people directly affected by it. These partnerships are thus benefited when the experience and knowledge of the practitioner are combined with the expertise of the researcher. So-called "outcome research" to support the efficacy of counseling has long been lacking in our field. With the exception of the behavioral and cognitive behavioral interventions that yield more easily to empirical scrutiny, most techniques in counseling have been based on the counselor's beliefs: We somehow "know" that what we do is helpful to clients, but we have had a hard time convincing those who look for critical evidence.

Finally, and ideally, as you read the literature and develop your practice, you will begin to formulate your own questions that may serve as the basis for conducting your own research. Suppose, for example, you become the director of a counseling center and you need to report to a funding source whether its money is being well spent. Depending on the agreed upon criteria for success, you would need to put together a design that would yield demonstrable results that satisfy the funding source.

Obviously, research is a very broad topic. What we hope to accomplish here is to introduce some of the basic ideas that will give you somewhat of an overview of this area of study. In a simplistic manner, research may be thought of as a systematic approach to asking and answering questions. Research may be divided into two basic approaches: quantitative and qualitative.

Quantitative Research

Quantitative research is a systematic, well-controlled approach to identifying relationships of variables representing constructs (e.g., is performance on the GRE related to performance in a graduate counseling program?) and/or determining differences between or among groups in relation to a variable or variables of interest (e.g., do students with an undergraduate degree in Psychology perform better in graduate counseling programs than students with degrees in English or History?). Although there are many different approaches to conducting quantitative research, they all are characterized by being empirical; being repeatable and public; and striving to be explanatory, predictive, and theoretical (McGrath & Johnson, 2003).

The process of trying to identify relationships through research may involve *nonexperimental* studies—that is, we attempt to observe subjects in order to describe them, as they naturally exist, without any experimental intervention by the researchers. In *experimental* studies, researchers give treatments to groups, try to control other possible factors that might impact the criterion behavior, and then check to see if the treatments caused changes in the criterion behavior. For instance, in an agency a counselor may use a specific group counseling protocol with one group of clients and use a different protocol with another group, and then examine differences between the two groups in an attempt to determine differences in effects of the protocols. Of course setting up this type of experiment becomes complicated as the counselor must respond to practical and ethical issues. We discuss this in more detail later in the chapter.

The overall strategy of research first involves formulating a proposed answer to a question—known as the *hypothesis*. Then the counselor operationally defines how her observations will be conducted—the *research design*. Then, she collects the data and analyzes them using *statistical analysis*. Finally, she arrives at a conclusion regarding her hypothesis and draws inferences as to the broader application, if any, of the findings.

Variables are the way we operationally identify the varying factors of the research design. There are three basic types of variables. *Independent variables* are those that are manipulated by the researcher—e.g., one group is given drug A for headaches and another is given a placebo. The *dependent variable(s)* is the criterion behavior the researcher is interested in affecting—e.g., the headache as defined by some measure of the level of pain endured. Finally, *control variables* are ones the researcher attempts to control by holding them constant or randomizing them so that their effects are neutralized—e.g., headache history of subjects. The key to quantitative research is to be able to be confident in saying that the researcher's manipulation of the independent variable(s) caused the effect observed in the dependent variable(s).

This requires the researcher to control all other extraneous variables or effects that might impact the dependent variable.

Planning for this control is the *experimental design*. The goal of a good experimental design is to maximize differences in the dependent variable due to the manipulation involved in the independent variable while minimizing extraneous sources of differences, called *error variance*. The type of experimental design chosen will depend upon the purposes of the research study. Some of the more common general categories of designs include the following:

- *Historical:* Objectively and accurately reconstruct the past in relation to the tenability of an hypothesis.

- *Descriptive:* Systematically describe a situation or area of interest factually and accurately (e.g., public opinion polls, needs assessments, case study, etc.).

- *True Experimental:* Identify a cause-effect relationship by exposing certain groups to treatments or controls, controlling all other extraneous factors, and then comparing results.

- *Quasi-Experimental:* Attempt to approximate a true experimental design in a situation that does not allow the control and/or manipulation of all relevant factors.

The key to being confident in the conclusions we draw from our research is knowing that our design is valid. As both a researcher and a reader of research, there are some important design validity concepts for you to keep in mind. Think of this as detective work—reading a good who-done-it novel. The question you are trying to answer is whether or not there is some alternative plausible explanation for the researcher getting the results that were obtained. All of the alternatives deal with confounding factors that are not controlled. There are two basic categories of threats to validity. *Internal validity* responds to the question of whether it was really the experimental manipulation that produced the differences in this specific instance. *External validity* refers to the relevance of the experimental condition to the real world.

Qualitative Research

Qualitative research tends to capture more distinctly the postmodern aspects of existence. Rather than providing specific data that can be generalized to many people, qualitative research generates data that are rich in description of an individual's or group of individuals' experience (Denzin & Lincoln, 2000). Qualitative research is therefore expected to delve deeply into a participant's experience and beliefs.

According to Guba and Lincoln's (1989) impressive handbook, the tenets of qualitative research include beliefs that (1) the relationship between the researcher and respondent is interactive; (2) reality is complex and therefore not easily reduced to quantification; and (3) the values of the researcher definitely influence the research itself. Thus, qualitative inquiry is markedly different than quantitative research. Furthermore, rather than emphasizing reliability and validity, qualitative researchers instead focus on goodness (Arminio & Hultgren, 2002). Goodness in qualitative research suggests that the researcher has thoroughly identified the phenomenon that she or he is studying, chosen the methodology intentionally, and clearly delineated the process of data gathering. A good qualitative study would, by definition, lead to improvement in our knowledge base and practice.

Just as there are numerous ways to conduct quantitative research, many distinct forms of qualitative research exist. Grounded theory, hermeneutic phenomenology, and critical theory are specific modes of qualitative inquiry. Although qualitative research may sound more appealing to counselors who feel quantitative approaches are reductionistic, keep in mind that qualitative research can be costly, time-consuming, and very difficult to do well.

Consider Greg's experience. Greg was a fine counselor, but had little interest in research per se. Therefore, when he was planning his graduate thesis he chose to conduct a qualitative study. Greg was required to keep a research journal as a part of his research competency. Excerpts from his journal are in the accompanying box, "No Number-Crunching."

Making Research Decisions

How do researchers decide which approach to use? Ideally, you will use quantitative research when you need to identify specific, quantifiable information that relies on normative data and/or can be generalized to a larger group of people. Determining the relationship between level of acculturative stress and the availability of community mental health services, for instance, may be a research study that would lend itself well to quantitative methods. Qualitative research is most useful when the counselor has sufficient time to thoroughly explore multiple or complex aspects of a person's experience (Ponterotto, 2005). A counselor attempting to gain in-depth knowledge of the experience of surviving sexual assault may find that qualitative methods best suit her research needs. Now, many counselors are turning to mixed method designs that utilize both qualitative and quantitative procedures (Hanson, Clark, Petska, Creswell, & Creswell, 2005). These designs are particularly useful in providing generalizable results that also provide rich detail and description (Creswell, 2003).

In the fairly controlled settings of graduate training, the research process is usually first informed by theory and the research studies that have been developed regarding that theory. Then, as mentioned above, the researcher formulates hypotheses regarding a specific aspect of behavior or experience

No Number-Crunching

Early August

I was really dreading the idea of this research, but now that I'm in my internship and learning the system I'm looking forward to it. I've decided to be very intentional about what I will do for my project. No number-crunching for me. I know I could pick out some instrument and administer it to a bunch of clients (or beginning psychology students) but that's not my style. Too impersonal, and not really relevant for my interests. I've decided I'm going to interview veteran counselors regarding their resolution of countertransference issues.

Late August

I'm meeting with my research chair today to talk about my project. I've identified my respondents (older people who work at my agency), and chosen three open-ended questions I want to ask each of them:

1. What countertransference issues have you encountered?

2. How do you believe these issues affected your counseling relationship?

3. How did you resolve these issues?

   Three strong, open-ended questions. I'm ready to go.

Early September

Well, I'm a little behind. I thought that because I wasn't doing quantitative research I didn't have to go through our institutional review board for permission to survey people. Wrong. Not only that, but my chair told me that I need to be more systematic in choosing who I'm going to interview; I need to base

my interview questions on research; and I have to identify in advance how I'm going to analyze my data. I thought all I had to do was tape my interviews and transcribe the tapes—what analysis am I supposed to do?

Late September

I've refined some of my research study and feel a little better about it, but I still have to figure out what exactly I'm going to do with these interviews once I've finished them. I've completed one interview so far, and it was really a lot different than I expected. I wasn't sure how to best follow-up on some of his [the respondent's] answers, and I lost my focus a couple of times. I had no idea that transcribing the tape would take so long. I'm beginning to wonder if I should just scrap this whole thing and start over with a quantitative study.

Mid-October

I've completed three interviews, so I have two more to go. The interview process has gotten a lot easier for me, and I really am getting some good information. I'm struggling, though, to figure out how to make sense of the themes I'm seeing. How much detail should I provide when I write this up? I haven't even finished transcribing yet, and I can't analyze anything until I've completed all the interviews. Am I ever going to finish?

Mid-November

I've finished all the interviews. I've gotten such amazing information from these people. I feel a strong responsibility to

(continued)

(No Number-Crunching, continued)

make sure I do a good job of writing all this up, but I haven't been able to make sense of the "big picture" yet. No way I'm going to finish this by the end of the semester. Doing a qualitative study was definitely a trade-off. I'm glad now that I've done this, but it certainly seems like more work than some of my classmates have done. I just hope I can produce a good quality report out of all this.

Questions for Reflection

1. What do you see as the specific advantages and disadvantages to using a qualitative rather than quantitative approach to exploring the topic of countertransference?

2. If you were to undertake a qualitative study, how could you avoid some of the problems Greg encountered?

---

relevant to the theory (Heppner, Kivlighan, & Wampold, 1999). Throughout the process the researcher will be weighing the benefits and drawbacks of using qualitative versus quantitative methods. The next step is to develop a research design that will optimize the chance that the researcher will be able to isolate and study the variables of interest. Finally, the researcher analyzes the data and draws conclusions regarding his or her hypotheses. Obviously, this potentially time-consuming process requires the researcher to understand thoroughly the research area of interest, have access to research participants, comprehend the potential benefits of different research designs, and have the capability to measure and then analyze the data received.

Analyzing Research

Research decisions in real life are, unfortunately, often based on the two Es: Expediency and Economy. Whatever approach will quickly get the answers needed, using the least amount of resources (including human resources) will often be chosen. The emphasis on expediency and economy can help explain why people may be duped by procedures such as the one presented in the Defining Moment at the beginning of the chapter. Furthermore, as lay people learn through the mass media about "breakthrough" treatments and remarkable cures, they are likely to clamor for these quick fixes to be applied to themselves. Think about the last time you watched television or thumbed through a popular magazine. How many ads did you see or read promoting pharmaceutical products? Look through again and note how many of those ads are for psychotropic medications. Although these products are well researched and undergo rigorous clinical trials, the rush to put some products on shelves has resulted in recalls of medications and significant concerns about side effects.

Your clients will hear about new research findings and ask for your opinion and guidance. You can begin to enhance your own competence regarding

EXPERIENTIAL LEARNING

Identify a phenomenon of interest to you related to counseling and/or mental health. You may, for instance, wonder how gender affects client self-disclosure. Perhaps you're curious about what factors are most predictive of depression among teenage boys. Develop a possible research question and plan how you might measure the phenomenon in question.

research by ensuring you know how to critically analyze the research you read. You will receive training regarding how to effectively analyze and critique research, so we provide the following as a brief template for you to keep in mind as you read through counseling-related and other journals. Realize, first, that primary publications are peer reviewed. These are the publications that you will rely on for new research findings, suggestions for interventions, or evaluations of protocols or programs. Before an article is accepted for publication, peers in the field review the article and, usually, suggest revision. The reviewers expect the articles they review to be original research that is valid and significant (American Psychological Association, 2001). An article published in a journal such as *The Journal of Counseling and Development* has been reviewed, often several times, by counselors and counselor educators who themselves have a wealth of research experience.

Why, then, should you take the time to analyze the research? No review process is perfect. Every research article includes an explanation of the limits of the study. As a consumer of research, you should ensure that you have read those limitations and understand their implications. While researchers may make significant findings, the findings themselves may not be that important for you in your daily practice. Keep in mind that what sounds like promising significant findings may have limited application to the population with which you work, or for the setting in which you work. Realize that flawed research does get published, either through oversight or misunderstanding. Don't make the mistake of assuming that every article in a peer-reviewed journal represents a well-controlled, well-designed research effort.

To be systematic in your analysis of research, first determine whether the researcher's hypothesis or research statement is clear and specific (Gall, Borg, & Gall, 2002). A study purporting to measure the effectiveness of in-home versus agency counseling services, for instance, is so broad that any data generated would likely be useless. Consider also whether or not the researcher has based her research statement and hypotheses on existing research. Simply thinking that something might be interesting and then choosing to study it is okay for high school term papers. The studies represented in peer-reviewed articles, however, are built on existing research and are designed to fill gaps in what we already know (American Psychological Association, 2001).

As you read, consider the potential bias of the researcher. For instance, does she or he seem to be attempting to make a point through the research? If the researcher is attempting to prove something, rather than to explore or find the answer to something, then the design may be biased (Gall, Borg, & Gall, 2002). Look also at the participants used in the study, and consider whether or not these individuals constitute a representative sample. Are they volunteers? Are they all college students? Is there any diversity in the sample? Sampling errors and limitations can restrict the generalizability and legitimacy of any study.

Also, think about the general complexity of the research question and how it is being measured. Are important variables being overlooked (Gall, Borg, & Gall, 2002)? For instance, in one study of the self-reported multicultural competence of counselors, the researcher failed to determine the participants' previous formal training in multicultural counseling. Since the respondents were self-reporting, there is a chance that those who understood very little about multicultural counseling were rating themselves very highly, while those who had formal training in the field and understood the challenges of multicultural counseling were rating themselves as less competent.

Next, if analyzing a quantitative study, look at the reliability and validity data provided regarding the measurement tools the researcher used. Further, is the measure appropriate for the sample to which it was given? Is the reading level too high or too low, for instance? Has the measure been used with this type of sample before? This question is especially important to consider when analyzing studies in which the researcher has translated an existing instrument into a different language. In these cases the validity of the translated instrument needs to be assessed, and the particular translation must be relevant and appropriate for the intended participants. Mexican dialects and idioms, for instance, can differ from Cuban dialects. If analyzing a qualitative study, consider whether or not the researcher exhibits bias in his or her questions and descriptions. Does the researcher seem to be focusing only on what is consistent with the initial research question and underemphasizing areas that present discrepancies? Do the themes identified by the researcher make sense?

We have heard some counselors confess that they skip over the quantitative results sections of articles and go right to conclusions and recommendations. We encourage you to examine the quantitative data. Do the numbers "add up," meaning do they seem to be consistent with the author's conclusions and recommendations? Are percentages reported without including the number of cases? (Forty percent of 10 people, for instance, isn't much. Forty percent of 200 people, however, may have significant implications.) Do the statistical procedures seem appropriate for the research question? We know that the answer to this question may lie beyond your immediate level of understanding. Further, statistical procedures do go in and out of vogue. However, a quick glance at a statistics textbook may be all you need to determine whether or not the researcher chose her analysis wisely.

Finally, do the researcher's conclusions seem valid, based on what she or he found in the study? What limitations are not mentioned? What implications are missed? What do these conclusions mean for you and your clients? Perhaps most important, what questions remain unanswered after you've read the article? Those questions may suggest your own next research study.

PROGRAM EVALUATION

Certainly one of the activities in which you are very likely to find yourself involved as a community agency counselor is that of program evaluation. Evaluation is generally a process of gaining information about a counseling program. It is intended to judge how effective our interventions are for our specific population. While research focuses on explanation and prediction, evaluation is designed to determine worth and social utility. Research is about testing hypotheses; evaluation may be thought of as measuring attainment of objectives.

Unlike research, evaluation purposefully incorporates values and judgment in determining effectiveness or worth. Thus, program evaluation, although using many of the same tools and techniques of what we think of as research, has a very different context than research. As noted previously, the purpose of research is to explain or predict leading to generalized conclusions. The purpose of program evaluation is to improve by providing useful information for decision making. Program evaluation involves determining the worth or value of actions directed toward specific goals as a means of assessing credibility.

Posavac and Carey (2003) note that program evaluation determines whether a service is needed and likely to be used, whether it is sufficient to meet unmet needs, whether the service is offered as intended, and whether the service actually does help people. The basic elements of program evaluation are:

1. Needs assessment
2. Program planning
3. Implementation
4. Implementation evaluation, including formative and progress evaluation
5. Outcome evaluation

Needs assessment involves describing the current situation or general context—such as the community, the incidence and prevalence rates of a specific concern among the population, the target group, and the social indicators of need—as well as directly assessing the community's need for the service (Cook, 1989). Direct assessment techniques may involve surveys, interviews, and focus groups. The assessment of need should include an assessment of current resources available and the extent of use of these resources. Sometimes the issue is not a matter of needing more resources or new programs; rather, it is a matter of clients having adequate physical or psychological access to existing resources and programs.

If a need is defined, the counselor begins the process of *program planning*. The primary step in program planning is making sure the counselor has the critical stakeholders and decision makers involved. Program evaluation involves judging among decision alternatives, so having the decision makers fully informed regarding the need and program to begin with engages their commitment and acknowledges the value systems that they represent. Once the need is identified, then outcome goals are specified, services are outlined to enhance clients' abilities to meet those goals, resources are carefully analyzed in relation to fully enacting the services outlined, and a specific action plan (who does what, when, and how) is developed. Having the critical stakeholders involved in determining the outcome goals ensures objectivity and clarity about the parameters and data by which the intervention will be evaluated.

The next element involves the actual *implementation* of whatever program the counselor has decided to use to meet the community's needs. This step incorporates the information gleaned from the first two steps in the process and ideally reflects a systematic and comprehensive assessment of the overall situation. Counselors are encouraged to be vigilant during this process, being sure to smoothly incorporate implementation evaluation. *Implementation evaluation* refers to answering the question of whether the program is being offered as planned—assessing the validity of the intervention.

Formative evaluation, a type of implementation evaluation, is designed to monitor the program as it is operating so that decisions can be made along the way to modify the program to make it more effective as, and if, needed. A good counselor does formative evaluation at the end of each session with a client by asking: "Are we making progress? Are we headed in a positive/productive direction?" The same is true for group or larger interventions. One doesn't wait until the end of an eight-week group intervention program to access progress and make changes, especially if it is apparent that the program is not meeting the needs of the group members along the way. Progress evaluation, also a type of implementation evaluation, refers to the progress of clients within the program. In this type of evaluation, the counselor looks closely at how the services are offered and monitors client progress to try and ascertain whether the intervention is meeting overall needs. In progress evaluation, the counselor is likely to examine issues such as accessibility, the presence of sufficient and appropriately trained staff, the receptivity of the atmosphere for clients, costs, and confidentiality/stigma of services.

The final element, *outcome evaluation,* also known as *summative evaluation,* focuses on progress in addressing the pre-specified goals. This component of program evaluation must make the linkages among intervention and progress toward the goals as well as measure the relative efficiency of the program based on the practical limitations of budget and time.

For instance, the counselors in one community agency started a psycho-educational program with a preventive focus for first-time parents. The program was offered in English and Spanish, which required the agency to pay interpreters overtime pay. The agency also provided each participant or couple with a handbook, a pizza dinner after each week's meeting, and a $25 coupon for a local grocery store if the couple or parent completed the training. The outcome evaluation showed that the program was actually very effective, but the agency found that administering the program was too costly. Several counselors at the agency therefore decided to use their extensive outcome data to write a grant to fund future administrations of the program. The counselor's careful, systematic evaluation plan paid off—the grant was awarded. In "How Are We Doing," in the accompanying box, you can read about another counselor's evaluation efforts.

Clearly, if the evaluation process is carefully planned and administered, counseling programs are likely to be improved. Furthermore, effective program evaluation can enable community agencies to provide evidence of their efforts and successes, thereby enabling them to meet the accountability expectations of their funding sources (Steenbarger & Smith, 1996). Clients will be better served as a result.

ETHICAL AND LEGAL ISSUES IN PRACTICE

The ACA Code of Ethics (2005) regarding research specifies that counselors must pay particular attention to several areas. These ethical issues also overlap with legal concerns, in that a breach of client rights in research may be legally as well as ethically actionable. First, in all research endeavors, counselors should ensure that their participants are fully informed regarding their involvement in the research, their rights to stop participating, and the ways in which their responses will be used. The principle of informed consent is vitally important in research and evaluation.

Counselors must also take reasonable precautions to ensure that their participants are not harmed in any way. The use of deception in research, for instance, should be used only when there is no other way to gain the desired information. Even then, the counselor should be able to clearly explain why

How Are We Doing?

Janine had recently begun her first job as a community counselor in a community services agency. She actively attempted to learn more about the town and county in which she lived, and she found that a relatively large number of Cambodian immigrants had recently moved to the area. She suspected that these residents needed mental health as well as social service assistance, but very few Cambodians ever sought help from her agency. Janine therefore decided to evaluate her agency's effectiveness in serving the needs of Cambodian citizens in her community.

She began her program evaluation by contacting the local refugee resettlement office and the immigrant assistance office in her area. With their help, she developed two needs assessment instruments. An interpreter with the immigrant assistant office translated the first assessment instrument designed specifically to ask Cambodian residents about their mental health needs. The other needs assessment instrument was written for physicians, social workers, and school personnel. This instrument asked these groups of people to indicate what they believed were critical mental health needs for the Cambodian population. Janine then distributed the instruments widely, attempting to blanket as much of her community as possible. She struggled to reach a large segment of the Cambodian population, so she sought assistance from proprietors of local stores owned and managed by Cambodians, as well as religious leaders who assisted recent Cambodian immigrants.

As she analyzed the data from her needs assessment instruments, Janine found that many of the Cambodians surveyed indicated that they were hesitant to seek mental health counseling, but they were very interested in information about schools, U.S. parenting styles, and negotiating life in the United State. Janine therefore joined forces with several social service agencies, a physician's office, and a local church to develop a plan. Together, they offered a series of workshops that offered training and tips on the topics of interest. Throughout the program implementation, Janine evaluated not only the effectiveness of the workshops but the quality of the evaluation process. She then developed a plan for refining her workshop series and started an outreach program to help educate members of the Cambodian community about the services her agency offered.

Questions for Reflection

1. Janine's particular program evaluation required a level of multicultural competence. If you were in a similar situation, how could you ensure that you adequately surveyed the population in question?

2. What steps could you take to increase the likelihood that your needs assessment was valid for the distinct groups to which it was administered?

she chose to use this approach, and participants have a right to be informed about the deception at the conclusion of the study. The confidentiality of information gained in research studies must be ensured, and participants must understand in advance any potential limitations of that confidentiality. The ACA Code of Ethics also emphasizes the importance of attending to multicultural and diversity issues in research and provides guidance on how to manage relationships with research participants.

If you are conducting research as a part of your training program, you will likely be required to receive permission from your institution's research review board. Similarly, if you are conducting research through an agency later in your career, seek permission from the agency's human subjects review board or, if no such board exists, seek consultation from researchers who understand research safeguards and procedures, obtain full informed consent from participants, and ensure that you are following the Code of Ethics throughout the research process.

Finally, the ACA Code of Ethics also addresses how counselors report and publish their research findings. Counselors are obligated to fully disclose the conditions of their research, including findings that may shed an unfavorable light on other research or institutions. Furthermore, when publishing a research article, counselors are expected to give credit to others who have assisted with the research study. Any research study that is based primarily on a student's thesis or dissertation should list the student as a principal author. In all other cases, we recommend that all co-authors determine the order of authorship at the beginning of the research study. This is a professional rather than ethical issue, but one that could become important for graduate students who find they have an appreciation for, and interest in, research and evaluation.

We've said it before, but it bears repeating here: As a community counselor you need to stay abreast of current research findings. Begin now to cultivate the habit of regularly reading counseling and counseling-related journals. Critically analyze the articles you read, and continue to explore the questions that remain unanswered. Doing so will help protect you against burnout and will help you practice effectively and ethically.

CONCLUDING THOUGHTS

We have attempted to provide you with an overview of the processes of research and evaluation. Attention to research is critical for counselors, not only for promoting effective practice, but for ensuring the continued vitality and relevance of the field. We challenge you to make systematic, data-driven inquiry an integral part of your counseling training experience and build the effective use of research and evaluation into your counseling work.

RECOMMENDED RESOURCES

We recommend that you keep whatever text you use in your research and evaluation course for use in your work as a community counselor. You can use this text as a source and update it every few years. If you don't like your text or don't find it useful, consider the following:

> Denzin, N., & Lincoln, E. (Eds.). (2000). *Handbook of qualitative research* (2nd ed.). Beverly Hills, CA: Sage.

> Heppner, P. P., Kivlighan, D. M., & Wampold, B. E. (1999). *Research design in counseling* (2nd ed.). Belmont, CA: Wadsworth.

You may also find it useful to look through an overview of research issues in counseling. The following is a helpful compilation of research ideas, trends, and principles relevant for a wide range of counseling practice areas:

> Loesch, L., & Vacc, N. (Eds.). (1997). *Research in counseling and therapy*. Greensboro, NC: ERIC/CASS.

We also recommend that you regularly read and critique the articles in journals such as *The Journal of Counseling and Development.*

Other Resources

To get a sense of the various ways in which people can investigate phenomena, read any of P. D. James' mystery novels. These novels present an example of systematic and focused inquiry that is representative of research in particular.

Movies such as *The Sixth Sense* and *The Others* are excellent examples of ways in which people can be misled into making questionable assumptions. Watch these movies and then reflect what evidence you found yourself relying on to "know" the truth. Did you discover that you were paying attention to hunches or gut reactions? After the movie, did you mentally review the movie for clues regarding the truth or for logical inconsistencies?

Finally, a classic study of research ethics can be explored in the documentary *Quiet Rage: The Stanford Prison Experiment.* The video provides footage and interviews with researchers and students who participated in an experiment conducted by Dr. Phillip Zimbardo in 1971. The implications of the original experiment, and the participants' reactions, are fascinating and raise many relevant questions regarding not only human nature, but research in general.

REFERENCES

American Counseling Association. (2005). *ACA Code of Ethics.* Retrieved August 22, 2005, from **http://www.counseling.org/Content/NavigationMenu/ RESOURCES/ETHICS/ACA_Code_of_Ethics.htm.**

American Psychological Association. (2001). *Publication manual of the American Psychological Association* (5th ed.). Washington, DC: American Psychological Association.

Arminio, J. L, & Hultgren, F. H. (2002). Breaking out from the shadow: The question of criteria in qualitative research. *Journal of College Student Development, 43,* 446–460.

Bligh, S., & Kupperman, P. (1993). Evaluation procedure for determining the source of the communication in facilitated communication accepted in a court case. *Journal of Autism and Developmental Disorders, 23,* 553–557.

Cook, D. W. (1989). Systematic needs assessment: A primer. *Journal of Counseling and Development, 67,* 462–464.

Creswell, J. W. (2003). *Research design: Quantitative, qualitative, and mixed methods approaches* (2nd ed.). Thousand Oaks, CA: Sage.

Davies, P., & Gribbin, J. (1992). *The matter myth: Dramatic discoveries that challenge our understanding of physical reality.* New York: Simon & Schuster.

Denzin, N., & Lincoln, E. (Eds.). (2000). *Handbook of qualitative research* (2nd ed.). Beverly Hills, CA: Sage.

Gall, M. D., Borg, W., R., & Gall, J. P. (2002). *Educational research: An introduction* (7th ed.). Boston: Allyn & Bacon.

Green, G. (1994). Facilitated communication: Mental miracle or slight of hand? *Behavior and Social Issues, 4,* 69–85.

Guba, E. G., & Lincoln, Y. S. (1989). *Fourth generation evaluation.* Beverly Hills, CA: Sage.

Hanson, W. E., Clark, V. L., Petska, K., Creswell, J. W., & Creswell, J. D. (2005). Mixed methods in research designs in counseling psychology. *Journal of Counseling Psychology, 52,* 224–235.

Heppner, P. P., Kivlighan, D. M., & Wampold, B. E. (1999). *Research design in counseling* (2nd ed.). Belmont, CA: Wadsworth.

Hirshoren, A., & Gregory, J. (1995). Further negative findings on facilitated communication. *Psychology in the Schools, 32,* 109–113.

Isaac, S., & Michael, W. (1995). *Handbook in research and evaluation: A collection of principles, methods, and strategies useful in the planning, design, and evaluation of studies in education and the behavioral sciences.* San Diego: Edits.

Margolis, H. (1987). *Patterns, thinking and cognition: A theory of judgment.* Chicago: University of Chicago Press.

McGrath, J. E., & Johnson, B. A. (2003). Methodology makes meaning: How both qualitative and quantitative paradigms shape evidence and its interpretation. In P. M. Camis, J. E. Rhodes, & L. Yardley (Eds.), *Qualitative research in psychology: Expanding perspectives in methodology and design* (pp. 31–48). Washington, DC: American Psychological Association.

Ponterotto, J. G. (2005). Qualitative research in counseling psychology: A primer on research paradigms and philosophy of science. *Journal of Counseling Psychology, 52,* 126–136.

Posavac, E. J., & Carey, R. G. (2003). *Program evaluation: Methods and case studies* (6th ed.). Upper Saddle River, NJ: Prentice-Hall.

Presbury, J. H., & Benson, A. J. (1994). Professional transitioning with expert systems: Beyond the "cognitive" process. *Report to Virginia Center for Innovative Technology, College of Integrated Science and Technology,* James Madison University, 59–72.

Steenbarger, B. N., & Smith, H. B. (1997). Assessing the quality of counseling services: Developing accountable helping systems. *Journal of Counseling and Development, 75,* 145–150.

Chapter 12

Working Behind the Scenes: Consultation and Supervision

It is one of the most beautiful compensations of life, that no man can sincerely try to help another without helping himself.

Ralph Waldo Emerson

GOALS

Reading and exploring the ideas in this chapter will help you:

- Understand the role and importance of consultation for community counselors
- Understand the role and importance of collaboration with professional colleagues
- Appreciate key aspects of counselor supervision
- Gain self-awareness regarding yourself as a consultant and supervisor

---

OVERVIEW

This chapter presents information on the development of consultation as a counseling practice; an exploration of the stages of consultation; models of consultation, collaboration, and supervision; and strategies and applications regarding these practices. Interestingly, when some people conjure up an image of consultants, they picture people from outside an organization arriving to shake up the system. In this image, consultants are often seen as well-paid, snappy dressers who use mysterious lingo, including quite a bit of psychobabble, and then leave as abruptly as they came.

Mental health consultation, in reality, tends to look quite a bit like counseling. The consultant spends much of her time listening, clarifying, and gathering information. She may observe, assess, and recommend, while paying particular attention to the process occurring between herself and the consultee. Thus, if the corporate image of a consultant seems inaccessible to you, take heart. Most counselors do function as consultants, even if they don't label it as such. In fact, many counselors work as consultants out of necessity, as they realize that individual counseling services are insufficient to meet our communities' mental health needs (Sue & Sue, 2003).

As researchers such as Conyne (2000) and Albee (2000) asserted, our communities need more mental health services than we can currently provide. We need more accessible, affordable, and appropriate counseling; more effectively integrated approaches to client care; and certainly more efforts aimed at primary prevention. Although not a cure-all, consultation is one way to work efficiently and effectively.

TOM'S DEFINING MOMENT: Joining Forces

Tom is a community counselor who relies on consultation to help manage his work in family preservation. Because his clients are often facing multiple stressors, Tom believes he can best serve them by working collaboratively with numerous social service agencies to provide comprehensive and preventive treatment. He learned the power of consultation when he was in the second year of his graduate training. That year Tom roomed with Marco, a student in the speech pathology program. Marco was intrigued when Tom began learning about play therapy during his practicum at the on-campus clinic. When describing play therapy, Tom talked at length about the benefits for children who were given a safe space in which to experience their full range of emotions.

"All my speech therapy practicum clients right now are kids," Marco said, "and I really believe that what they need is to be with someone who can listen to them and understand their challenges. Having a speech difficulty or disorder can feel so overwhelming for kids. If they could experience play therapy, they'd have a place where they could express themselves. Maybe I could refer some of these kids to the clinic."

Tom and Marco became increasingly excited as they mapped out a procedure through which Marco's clients could be referred for play therapy. They soon realized, though, that if the speech pathology clients followed through on the referrals, the small on-campus clinic would be unable to accommodate all the new clients' needs. They also acknowledged that some parents would be unwilling or unable to follow through on a referral, and the referral itself may be inappropriate for some children.

"What if," Tom wondered, "I arrange for you to learn some of the basics of focused listening and attending to children? Then you could try it out with your clients. If it works, you'll have a better relationship with your clients and reach a lot more people than I would if I just worked with those who followed through on a referral to the clinic. It wouldn't be therapy, but it could be therapeutic." With this, a consultation relationship was formed.

Tom and Marco developed a basic consultative relationship— one in which a professional lends his or her expertise to another professional regarding a work-related issue. Tom and Marco came to this arrangement from a pragmatic standpoint. They realized that Tom could share his knowledge with more people, albeit indirectly, if he worked directly with Marco.

Questions for Reflection

1. As you envision your work as a community counselor, what consultation relationships do you imagine you'll need to create?

2. Community counselors working as consultants often need to be effective public speakers, trainers, and negotiators in addition to being skilled counselors. What do you expect will be your unique strengths and challenges as a consultant? What can you do now to enhance your strengths and address your challenges?

CONSULTATION DEFINED

Definitions of consultation vary, but consultative relationships usually include the following characteristics (Brown, Pryzwansky, & Schulte, 2001; Caplan & Caplan, 1993):

- Consultation involves three parties—the consultant, the consultee, and the client or client system. In the Defining Moment presented above, Tom is the consultant who works directly with the consultee, Marco, to have a positive impact on children in speech therapy.

- Consultation focuses on a work-related concern of the consultee. Tom and Marco will focus specifically on Marco's ability to listen to and understand his child clients. The consultation process may address personal concerns of Marco's as they relate to his work, but the consultative relationship would not extend to addressing issues such as Marco's relationship with his significant other. That issue would be addressed with a different counselor in a counseling relationship.

- Consultation is a voluntary relationship between peers. Tom and Marco differ in expertise, but neither supervises the other. In fact, they work in different settings. Consultation can occur between two people in the same profession, but even in that case, consultation is a voluntary, non-hierarchical, and nonevaluative relationship that can be terminated by either party at any time.

- The consultant relies on the consultee to carry out the consultant's advice and suggestions. Although Tom may seek permission to observe Marco work with children, Tom probably will not work with those children directly. It will be up to Marco to put Tom's consultation suggestions into practice.

These characteristics suggest a definition for consultation: a triadic relationship in which a consultee seeks the help of a consultant, or specialist, with a work-related problem (Caplan & Caplan, 1993; Kratochwill & Pittman, 2002). We should also address, however, what consultation is not: it is neither counseling nor supervision.

Consultation Versus Counseling and Supervision

The goal of *counseling*, on the most basic level, is to help clients to function at a higher level of personal well-being. The goal of *consultation,* on the other hand, is to help consultees function more effectively in their work with clients. Thus, consultation indirectly helps clients through direct intervention with consultees. Further, the focus of the intervention in consultation is always work (Caplan & Caplan, 1993), rather than personal concerns.

The goal of *supervision,* again on the most basic level, is to enhance a counselor's work performance. At first glance that may sound like consultation. Supervision, however, is usually an ongoing relationship between a senior counselor and a more junior counselor, with the expectation that the supervisor will evaluate the supervisee's performance. The supervisor also has vicarious responsibility for the welfare of the supervisee's client (Bernard & Goodyear, 1998). In a consultation relationship, on the other hand, the consultant and consultee are peers. In some cases, the consultant and consultee are in different professions. Furthermore, the consultant is not usually responsible, either administratively or clinically, for the welfare of the consultee's client.

Consultation is therefore a distinct endeavor. In practice, however, the consultation process may feel like counseling, and it may feel like supervision.

CONSULTATION IN AGENCIES

One of the benefits of consultation is the potential to reach a large audience quickly. The consultant does not have to meet with each client individually, but instead meets with significant community members who will then interact with clients. The scope of intervention is dramatically increased through this process (Caplan & Caplan, 1993).

Examples of typical consultant work include:

Testifying in court about client welfare

Serving as an expert witness regarding a particular issue

Working with school personnel, such as school counselors and psychologists, to provide effective educational services for a child with specific mental health needs

Sharing information with local business leaders regarding relevant community issues such as the stress recent immigrants face when they arrive in the United States

Offering workshops for health professionals on topics such as depression or anxiety

Evaluating a suspected case of child abuse

Informally talking with colleagues regarding effective treatment models

In all of these examples, the consultant is a community counselor who seeks opportunities to inform and empower others in order to better serve clients. Thus, some type of consultation is usually a daily occurrence for most counselors.

Community counselors also often find themselves in the role of consultees seeking the help of consultants (Kurpius & Fuqua, 1993). Members of a community agency's board of directors, for instance, serve a consultative role for the agency. The board members are usually expected to provide a view of environmental factors and trends that will affect the daily practice of the counselors in that agency. Further, many counselors use the services of consultants for tasks such as writing or administering grants or completing comprehensive psychological evaluations. Counselors also rely on consultants to help them learn about cultural considerations affecting clients (Brown, 1997), to explain emerging legal trends that affect client care, and to clarify policy revisions that influence record-keeping and reimbursement issues in agencies. Consultation in community agencies is a fact of life. And, like most human services work, consultation has the potential to get messy.

In "I Want This to Be a Clean Consultation Relationship" (see accompanying box) Cindy discovered that the boundaries around consultation are more blurred than one might expect. One of the most well-known consultation

I Want This to Be a Clean Consultation Relationship

Cindy had undertaken a consultation project while enrolled in a consultation class in graduate school and found the experience engaging and straightforward. She helped a member of the board of directors of the local AIDS network assess the climate of her board meetings and develop an intervention to invite greater participation among board members.

Cindy enjoyed the opportunity to enter into a relationship with a professional, gather data, make suggestions, and then exit the relationship. She felt professional and competent, and the consultation experience was a welcome respite from the ambiguity and complexity she encountered with the clients she was seeing in her counseling practicum.

During her internship the next semester, Cindy was therefore pleased to be offered again the chance to serve as a consultant. One part of Cindy's responsibilities in her internship at the community mental health center was to provide clinical services for a local middle school. Cindy's supervisor asked Cindy to consult with the school counselor and teacher regarding Joe, a young student receiving services at the agency.

Wonderful, Cindy thought. *This will be clean and neat. I'll go in, observe, make recommendations, and not have to deal with anybody's personal stuff. This will give me a break.*

Soon, though, Cindy was knee-deep in personal stuff. It started when Cindy observed the little boy in the classroom. The teacher seemed stiff and uncomfortable with Joe. She rarely made eye contact with him and frequently ignored him when he spoke out in class.

When Cindy met with the teacher at the end of the day, she worried about how to phrase her observations. *Should I just tell her she seemed disengaged,* Cindy wondered, *or should I be honest and say she seemed downright rude to him?* Cindy didn't have time to express either concern, for the teacher quickly launched into an explanation of her lack of patience for "kids like Joe."

"He just puts me over the edge sometimes, you know?" the teacher said.

Oh boy, how to handle this, Cindy wondered. *I have to remember my listening skills.*

"Yes, you do seem frustrated," Cindy said. "How is it that you feel pushed over the edge?"

"Well, good grief!" said the teacher. "He comes to school barely able to speak English. He and the other little Hispanic boys sit around speaking in Spanish, and I know they're talking about me, making fun of me. Then the parents give me grief if I come down on him in the class and tell him to straighten up. Now I'm just not giving him attention at all. I figure that's the best way to handle him."

Before Cindy could respond, the school counselor walked in. "Well," he said, "I hope you got a sense for this zoo. Which kid were you observing?"

Before Cindy could respond, he said, "I need a break from this place. Can we talk about this later?"

(continued)

(I Want This to Be a Clean Consultation Relationship, continued)

"Yeah," agreed the teacher. "I've got so much to do this afternoon. When can you come back and tell us what's going on with Joe? Just let us know if we need to call in the school psychologist to get a special ed evaluation. We'll work out the rest."

Cindy left the school in a daze. *This is unbelievable,* she thought. *One of my consultees is overtly prejudiced, the other is evidently burned out, and I have no idea what to do about it! So much for clean consultation.*

Thankfully, Cindy's supervisor was able to help her strategize how to best respond to her consultees while clarifying Cindy's role as a consultant. Cindy's desire to avoid personal stuff, however, was unfulfilled as she found herself thrown into intense and often personal discussions with both the teacher and the counselor.

Questions for Reflection

1. As you think about Cindy's experience, consider how you would respond to the teacher. What specific concerns would you have about her work with Joe—and perhaps with other students? How would you specifically state these concerns?

2. How would you respond to the teacher's implicit expectation that you were there to evaluate Joe for special education services?

3. How would you plan on involving the school counselor in your attempt to help the school help Joe succeed?

---

models, developed over thirty years ago by Caplan (1970), suggests that consultants address personal issues only as they affect the work relationship, and then only indirectly. More recently, however, some counselors have found that effective consultation requires flexibility and the ability to respond directly to the consultee's needs, including personal issues, in the consultation session (Dougherty, Henderson, & Lindsey, 1997; Sandoval, 1996).

The ambiguity surrounding consultation is also increased by the fact that many counselors do not approach consultation with a specific model or theory as a guide (Brown, Pryzwansky, & Schulte, 2001). Instead, they apply what they know about helping in general to their work with consultees. This trend is likely to continue, for counselors still face a lack of research support for various models and theories regarding consultation.

Cindy, then, would need to draw on an array of skills in order to intervene effectively with Joe's school. In addition to her ability to counsel and advocate for Joe, she needs to understand the school system well enough to empathize with the teacher's and counselor's daily experience. She must be able to articulate that empathic understanding into an effective interaction when she discusses her observations and recommendations. To do so, she must be sufficiently competent and confident to inspire trust. She must be able to anticipate and respond effectively to potential resistance, and she must be able to provide preliminary suggestions to the teacher and counselor regarding actions they can take to help Joe. She also must be able to effectively communicate her work to relevant people such as Joe's caregivers, her own agency, and the school principal. Although Cindy's job is complex, there is a general framework for conceptualizing consultation that can serve as a valuable resource.

CLASSIFYING CONSULTATION BY FOCUS AND SCOPE

Gerald Caplan's (1970) consultation model has undoubtedly been one of the most popular in the field. Caplan was one of the first consultation theorists to suggest that consultation can be used as a preventive measure rather than occurring strictly as a response to the consultee's crisis. Caplan's model was therefore extremely important to members of community agencies, who saw their job responsibilities as offering primary as well as secondary prevention. Caplan's model has been updated and other models have been developed, but many are adaptations of the basic template offered below.

The consultant begins by classifying the type of consultation she or he is about to offer. The consultant first decides if the focus is on a *case* problem, such as intervention possibilities with a client, or an *administrative* problem, such as planning a program. Then the consultant determines whether to offer a solution to the problem, in which case the consultation is *client-* or *program-centered,* or whether to help the consultee come up with a solution, in which case the consultation is *consultee-centered.* The scope and focus of consultation will therefore determine its classification as one of four types of consultation:

1. Client-centered case consultation
2. Consultee-centered case consultation
3. Program-centered administrative consultation
4. Consultee-centered administrative consultation

Client-centered case consultation suggests the consultant is helping the consultee to work successfully with a specific client or group of clients. In this case, the consultant gathers information regarding the case or cases and then makes recommendations to the consultee. For example, an outpatient clinic began to face an increase in the number of adolescent suicide attempts. The director of the clinic sought client-centered case consultation from a counselor educator who was an expert in assessing and responding to adolescent suicide. The counselor educator met with the staff and made specific recommendations regarding prevention and intervention with adolescents in the surrounding community.

In *consultee-centered case consultation,* the consultant also helps the consultee with a specific client or group of clients, but in this case the consultant focuses more specifically on how well the consultee works with the clients. In doing so the consultant will attempt to determine what obstacles or difficulties the consultee faces as she attempts to work with a specific client or client group.

For example, Benji, an intern working as a Head Start counselor, was having difficulty working with African American boys who were referred to him. The Head Start coordinator believed that Benji, as an African American man, would have a unique understanding of the boys and therefore be better able to help them. Benji, however, found himself feeling stiff and uncomfortable with these students. He had difficulty building relationships with them and started to informally refer them to another intern.

After being questioned by his supervisor about making so many referrals, Benji sought the consultative services of an LPC who volunteered with Head Start. The consultant helped Benji uncover some of the sources of his discomfort by focusing on how Benji conceptualized the young boys. Soon, Benji determined that he felt self-conscious as one of the few African American counselors in the area. He secretly wondered if he was destined to be referred only African American youth in the future. Furthermore, he felt angry that the young boys who had been referred to him were probably going to be short-changed by the system as they grew up. He feared becoming overly involved with them and losing his objectivity.

Caplan explored many of the possible factors involved in consultee-centered case consultation, suggesting that psychodynamic concepts were significant issues for consideration. He therefore called for an indirect approach to addressing the consultee's concerns. In Benji's case, however, the consultant preferred to be direct. The consultant asked Benji what it was about these clients that got in his way. This consultant risked stepping into more intense personal territory than a consultant strictly adhering to Caplan's model. Similarly, more recently Caplan's psychodynamic view of consultee-centered case consultation has been revised by practitioners to take a more constructivist approach (Knotek & Sandoval, 2003). With the consultant's interest and help, Benji was able to explore the feelings and concerns that negatively affected his work performance.

The third broad category of consultation, *program-centered administrative consultation* requires the consultant to address problems associated with managing or developing a program. Usually, consultants engaging in program-centered administrative consultation gather information about the program or agency and then make recommendations regarding the best way for agency personnel to proceed. Program-centered administrative consultation is similar to client-centered case consultation, in that the consultant is focusing on a specific issue and offering her or his suggestions. The scope is much broader, however, and requires the consultant to be able to accurately determine the issues that affect the agency at a systemic level. Therefore, consultants who offer program-centered administrative consultation must be adept at understanding group dynamics, systems, and organizational issues (McDowell, 1999).

For example, Rhonda offered program-centered administrative consultation to a local middle school. At the request of the school principal, Rhonda began to assess the prevalence and severity of sexual harassment at the school. This consultation required a significant time investment on Rhonda's part. She recognized that she couldn't simply enter the school, start asking questions of the students, and expect to receive honest answers. Therefore, she worked slowly and carefully to build relationships with, and gather information from, school personnel. She frequented areas where students congregated and established herself as a nonjudgmental adult who would not automatically censor the students' behaviors. Gradually, she built enough rapport with students to hold several group meetings in which she defined sexual harassment and gathered reactions and anecdotes from the students.

Rhonda also took pains from the beginning of the consultation relationship to safeguard students' confidentiality within ethical guidelines and attempted to create as little disturbance in the system of the school as possible. After gathering sufficient information, Rhonda made recommendations to the school staff regarding a plan for combating and preventing sexual harassment.

The fourth type of consultation, according to Caplan's categorization, is *consultee-centered administrative consultation*. This process requires that the consultant help the consultee, or consultees, develop better ways of dealing with the issues and problems in their organization. Consultee-centered administrative consultation is, according to Caplan (1970) and Caplan and Caplan (1993), an extremely demanding type of consultation. In this case, the consultant must not only gather information about the consultee and how she or he (or they, in some cases) functions, but also understand the dynamics of the organization itself. Then, the consultant must put this information together to try to help the consultee(s) find more effective ways of working within that specific organization (Dougherty, 2005).

For example, Dennis was asked to provide consultation to the director of a community mental health center. In this case, the director needed help controlling dissension among her staff, which consisted of licensed and unlicensed counselors and social workers. The predominately unlicensed staff members who offered home services to clients felt undervalued by the predominately licensed staff members who provided clinic-only services. The director tried to ignore the situation, hoping that it would dissipate over time.

However, what started as one or two disgruntled counselors expanded into a full-blown conflict that affected the entire agency. Staff meetings became increasingly contentious as counselors began to air old complaints that had never been directly addressed. Dennis had the difficult task of helping the consultee—the director—examine the series of problems and determine what interfered with the director's ability to effectively manage the situation. Through consultation, the director began to realize that avoiding the issue and ignoring the distress merely added to the staff's sense of frustration.

Caplan acknowledged that significant overlap might exist among the different types of consultation presented above. In addition, within any consultation project, a consultant may assume a number of roles. The roles that consultants take can be categorized from most directive to least directive, or from content-oriented to process-oriented, with an added dimension reflecting the consultant's degree of involvement (Brown, Pryzawansky, & Schulte, 2001).

CLASSIFYING CONSULTATION BY CONSULTANT ROLE

Dougherty (2005) offered a practical model of consultation that emphasizes the roles of advocate, expert, trainer, fact finder, and process specialist.

The consultant who acts as an *advocate* is direct in suggesting that the consultee take a specific action. Consultants in advocate roles, for instance, may ask the consultee to offer certain services for specific clients. A defining feature of advocacy is the consultant's clear stance, based on expertise, about the recommendations that the consultee should take: Advocacy is often seen as an endeavor in and of itself, aside from consultation, and requires significant counselor self-awareness in order to be effective.

The consultant who assumes the role of *expert* usually offers guidance to the consultee regarding a specific problem defined by the consultee. For example, Al, a Latino intern in the campus counseling center, was assigned a female client from Lebanon. Al believed that his gender, as well as his ethnicity, were potential obstacles to his ability to build an effective relationship with his client. Al therefore sought the expertise of Suha, another counseling student who had been born and raised in Lebanon. Suha served as an expert and helped Al build a relationship with his client by focusing specifically on the cross-cultural characteristics of the situation.

Consultants acting as *trainers* offer workshops or other educational experiences, such as in-service training, for consultees. For example, Karen, a counseling student who had undertaken research and training in multicultural counseling, was often asked to provide multicultural workshops for counselors and teachers in the public schools.

Consultants who perform *fact-finding* services usually gather data and then report that information back to the consultee. For instance, counselors who have been trained to administer and interpret certain assessment instruments

EXPERIENTIAL LEARNING

1. Look back through the list of roles and determine which roles might be most comfortable for you.
   - What specific skills do you think each role would require?
   - What can you do now to hone those skills for yourself?

2. Identify a real or hypothetical problem in a community agency. Describe the problem in as much detail as possible, identifying key participants, such as clients, consultant, and consultee(s).
   - Conduct a role-play with your peers in which you each assume the role of someone involved in the hypothetical problem. Ask those who don't have a role to serve as observers. As the consultant in the role-play, attempt to explore the problem as thoroughly as possible so that you can gain a sense of how you might proceed if this were an actual consultation experience. In particular, pay attention to how easy or difficult it may be to build a trusting consultative relationship, gather information, and assess the problem.
   - Based on the information you gather in the role-play, determine what consultation role (e.g., fact-finder, expert, trainer) you would probably assume if you were to actually be the consultant in this situation.
   - Seek feedback from observers regarding your choice of consultant role as well as your overall performance as a consultant.

may assess a client and then report the assessment results back to the client's counselor or therapist.

Finally, the role of *process specialist* requires the consultant to examine how the consultee works. In this case, consultants "focus more on the *how* than on the *what*" (Dougherty, 2005, p. 35). For instance, when Dennis, in the earlier example, undertook consultee-centered administrative consultation, he was required to examine the processes that occurred in the agency. He observed staff meetings. He watched counselors talk with each other in the hallway. He saw how the director failed to directly address problems when they arose, and he noted that the director often lost control of meetings. Dennis then had to share his observations with the director, explaining how he felt the ineffective processes of communication and interaction exacerbated the existing situation.

Numerous other roles exist for consultants, and most consultants adopt more than one role in their work. For example, in the role of *expert* regarding child development, a consultant may also take on the role of *assessor,* assessing a child for possible physical or sexual abuse. Furthermore, some consultants consistently ascribe certain roles to themselves. Many consultants who work with seriously emotionally disturbed children, for instance, see themselves as *advocates* regardless of their specific consultation intervention or role. Other consultants see every consultation intervention as an extension of the role of *evaluator.* These consultants emphasize the importance of assessing all interventions and programs regarding their effectiveness and outcome.

THE PROCESS OF CONSULTATION

The process of offering consultation services, regardless of the focus, often follows a general approach that includes several steps. These steps, adapted from the work of Dougherty (2005), Brown, Pryzwansky, and Schulte (2001), and Caplan (1970) usually include:

- Preparing
- Joining
- Assessing
- Intervening
- Terminating

Ideally, when *preparing* to offer consultation services, the consultant engages in self-exploration to determine what skills she or he has to offer, as well as what work setting the consultant prefers. We say "ideally" because often consultants are community counselors who are asked to help other professionals do their jobs better. In those situations, counselors often do a quick "goodness of fit" test (to borrow from statistics) to determine whether or not they can do what's expected. Then, over time, consultants learn by trial and error how they work best and what they are able to do effectively for their consultees.

Part of the preparation process also includes exploring the work setting of the consultee. As the consultant gathers information about the consultee's work problem, she or he will likewise be gathering information about the system, the clients, and the consultee. This information will then enable the consultant to ease into the next step, *joining,* more easily.

Andre, for instance, was asked to consult with the director of the outpatient mental health unit of a regional hospital. Part of his preparation process included touring the facility, reading the minutes of recent meetings of the unit's staff, and undertaking an in-depth interview with the director. After completing this preparation process, Andre was ready to join with the consultee.

When the consultant *joins* the consultee, she or he attempts to build a strong, therapeutically oriented relationship with clear boundaries and expectations. By using counseling and conceptualizing skills, the consultant enables the consultee to present and explore thoroughly the problem or concern. If the joining process goes well, the consultee will see the consultant as an ally or partner. Furthermore, the system in which the consultee works will accept the presence of the consultant with minimal disruption.

One of the best examples of preparing and joining is provided in videos of Dr. Jane Goodall working with chimpanzees. These videos reveal Dr. Goodall silently watching the chimpanzees from a distance, and then gradually moving closer. Over time, the chimpanzees accept her presence and move about as though she weren't there. Eventually, some of the chimpanzees actually interact with her. Clearly, Dr. Goodall does her homework prior to entering the jungle, and then watches respectfully as she learns the workings of the system. Only when she has a clear sense of how these animals operate, and a definite sense of her own role in the jungle, does she actually enter their community.

The importance of preparing and joining cannot be overstated, for these processes are prerequisites for building trust with the consultee. Consultees are most likely to trust those consultants who understand their own role and who are attempting to understand empathically the consultees' and clients' experience. In this way consultation is much like counseling. The helper cannot effectively help until he is allowed close enough to understand what is happening.

The next step in the process of consultation is *assessing*, in which the consultant attempts to investigate the problem or concern. In actuality, the consultant is usually engaged in assessment throughout the consultation process, from the moment she or he decides to intervene as a consultant. As a formal process, however, after joining the consultant usually spends some time focusing specifically on the issue at hand. Anna, for instance, was consulting with another counselor regarding the use of cognitive behavioral techniques. Anna spent a significant amount of time engaged in role-playing sessions with the consultee, so that she could assess how the consultee worked. Then, she felt better able to provide instruction and information regarding techniques.

After thoroughly assessing the concern, the consultant then moves to the task of *intervening. Intervening* may sound like the most exciting part of the consultation process—the point when the consultant takes action— but the consultant has actually been intervening all along. The processes of joining and assessing always have an effect on the consultee and the issue at hand (Brown, Pryzwansky, & Schulte, 2001), so intervening often feels less like taking action and more like the next logical step in the process. As a result of the information gathered when joining and assessing, the consultant develops a sense of what she or he can provide to improve the consultee's situation. Thus, depending on the focus and scope of the consultation project, the consultant may intervene by offering feedback, suggesting recommendations, teaching, or providing information.

After the intervention process, the consultant and consultee usually agree to end their consultation relationship. At this point, as the relationship is *terminating,* the consultant will often (1) ensure that the consultee is prepared to continue to act on suggestions or plans offered by the consultant, (2) complete a summative evaluation process to assess the consultation, and (3) provide the consultee with follow-up information to enable the consultee to seek additional assistance or clarification in the future.

This process is presented as a general description for what consultation might look like. In everyday practice, consultation varies from a clear-cut enterprise driven by contracts and agreements to casual meetings between counselors before or after staff meetings. Whether formal or informal, however, effective consultation efforts tend to share several themes.

Consultant self-awareness. At this point you've undoubtedly discovered that counselors must understand themselves before they can effectively intervene in *any* setting.

Consultant understanding of consultee. Effective consultants understand the needs of their consultees and have a sense for how the consultee's agency or work setting operates.

Community assessment. Community counselors are expected to understand how the community, the client's overall environment, influences the client. Effective consultants can answer questions such as, What community obstacles are in the client's way? What community resources currently exist to help the client? What needs are currently unmet in this community? How can my agency intervene?

Ongoing evaluation. In order to ensure that their efforts are hitting the mark and effecting positive change for the consultee, consultants must continually evaluate the progress *and* the process of consultation.

Consultee empowerment. The best consultants work hard to make sure that their consultees do not become dependent on them (Sandoval, 1996). Instead, they build on their consultees' strengths. Thus, rather than doing things for the consultee, the consultant encourages the consultee throughout the process. Even in Caplan's model, in which the consultant is less transparent than we've proposed, the consultant is encouraged to avoid "undue dependency" by building on the strengths of the consultee (Caplan & Caplan, 1993, p. 59). By empowering the consultee, the consultant essentially works her- or himself out of a job.

The image of a consultant as a high-power professional with fancy jargon would suggest that the consultant keeps her secrets to herself. She enters a system, meets with the consultee, works her magic, and leaves. The best consultants, however, share their magic. They explain what they see, what they think, and how they work. As a result, the consultee learns about the consultation process as she or he works with the consultant. In this way, there's a greater chance that the next time a problem occurs the consultee will be able to address the concern independently or, if necessary, will be more likely to seek consultation.

CONSULTATION SKILLS

What does it take to be an effective consultant? Good consultants can listen, communicate understanding and empathy, conceptualize issues, plan and implement interventions, and ensure appropriate termination and follow-up. In addition, the best consultants are able to:

- *Collaborate.* Consultation interventions that incorporate the feedback, opinions, and concerns of the consultee, and if possible the client system, are more likely to succeed than those that are conceived only by the consultant. The most effective consultants, those who can build and maintain effective relationships, work diligently to include the consultee throughout the process. Thus, decisions are shared, and the consultee's sense of ownership is enhanced. We discuss the art of collaboration in more detail later in the chapter.

- *Foresee outcomes.* Because consultants are seen as experts, their decisions and suggestions often carry a great deal of weight. Therefore, consultants must ensure that they've gathered sufficient information, thoroughly conceptualized the issues at hand, and anticipated the consequences of their actions prior to formally intervening.

- *Be assertive.* Consultants are usually invited into a system just when the people within that system are experiencing problems. At that point people may feel desperate for help. They may be struggling with their sense of self-efficacy as professionals or may feel frustrated and at a loss regarding how to proceed. In these situations, counselors usually find that they need to be clear and confident regarding their professional boundaries. Consultants must be able to explain what they can, as well as what they can't, do for their consultees.

- *Negotiate.* Consultation, like private practice work, may require the counselor to set a price for his or her skills. Consultation is also often based on contractual agreements that specify what's delivered and for how much. For counselors who rely on secretaries and avoid money talk with clients, the negotiation aspect of consultation may take some practice.

- *Feel confident.* Many counselors enter the profession having taken numerous counseling courses and only one course in consultation. They often don't see themselves as consultants, but weave consultation skills into their counseling work. As a result, when counselors first begin working as consultants, they often suffer from self-doubt. Some, especially those working with organizational issues, may feel over-whelmed by the scope of their power.

In addition to their effective counseling skills and the abovementioned process-oriented skills, consultants need to be cognizant of numerous relevant content areas, including the following:

- *Organizational and Systems Theories.* Consultants need to understand models regarding how change occurs, and how it is best managed within organizations and systems.

- *Multicultural and Diversity Competencies.* Effective consultants are multiculturally competent counselors who understand issues such as oppression, discrimination, and privilege. They are then able to enact this understanding by modeling sensitive and appropriate practice (Brown, 1997).

- *Communication and Personal Interaction Models.* Counselors often pride themselves on their ability to listen and respond, but many fail to acknowledge or utilize the broad base of studies that highlight how we communicate most effectively. Studies regarding group communication are especially relevant. See, for instance, Johnson and Johnson (2003) and Beebe, Beebe, and Redmond (1999).

- *Assessment and Program Evaluation.* Consultants are often expected to assess the effectiveness of services and programs. A rudimentary knowledge of statistics and research methods is insufficient. Instead, effective consultants understand principles of program evaluation and assessment including measurement skills, test administration and interpretation skills, and the ability to interpret and report data.

- *Community-specific knowledge regarding systems and subsystems.* In order to effect lasting change, consultants must understand how they and their agencies interact with other groups in the community. This skill requires the consultant to understand the roles of professionals such as social workers, probation officers, nurse practitioners, home health workers, and a wide array of other individuals who impact the client's life. Only through a thorough understanding of the complex web of community interrelationships can the consultant provide comprehensive, effective intervention.

Carol's Consultation Catastrophe

Carol recently received her counseling license and was asked to consult with a family resource center regarding staff development. The project seemed straightforward, so Carol agreed. When she first met with her consultee, the agency administrator, Carol said, "You have much more experience than I do with this kind of thing. Why don't you just tell me what you want me to do and I'll do it."

Fortunately for Carol's learning process, the administrator was unwilling to assume that role. She let Carol know that she preferred that Carol investigate the workings of the agency, assess staff morale, and make suggestions regarding continuing education and staff development.

When Carol heard "morale," she quickly decided that the easiest way to proceed, while appearing professional, was to use a basic morale inventory. In her need to establish her sense of credibility, Carol developed the inventory herself one evening and then administered it to the staff. She realized that she felt a little over her head, but she was afraid that if she asked her supervisor for help, she would look incompetent.

Soon, Carol discovered that one of the staff members she surveyed, Joan, felt that her supervisor was racist. Joan was the only person of color on the staff. During their interview, Joan informed Carol that she planned to take her concerns to the NAACP in order to publicize what she perceived as the hypocrisy of the agency. She requested, however, that Carol keep her survey responses and comments confidential.

Several other staff members also mentioned experiencing different problems with the same supervisor. Tension among these several staff members regarding the supervisor was clearly contributing to the dissatisfaction among staff, but Carol had promised all the survey respondents that she would protect their anonymity when reporting survey results.

How could she protect Joan's identity when sharing her survey results with the agency administrator? What responsibility did she owe Joan, and for that matter, the agency, regarding Joan's claim of racism? Was she obligated to inform her consultee, the agency administrator, that Joan was planning to publicize her complaints of racism?

To make matters worse, in Carol's rush to develop a morale survey, she neglected to consider basics of survey construction. Her quantitative results were so confusing to interpret that the only usable data she obtained from the surveys were from her discussions with the staff members.

Questions for Reflection

1. Starting from the beginning, what could Carol have done to avoid getting herself in this situation?

2. What would you do with the information provided to you about potential racism within the organization?

EXPERIENTIAL LEARNING

1. Interview a mental health consultant.
   - Based on the interview, identify factors that you believe constitute effective practice.
   - Ask the person to share his or her most powerful learning experiences.

2. Interview a consultee.
   - Find out what consultant skills and behaviors were most and least helpful.

In "Carol's Consultation Catastrophe" in the accompanying box, more planning prior to intervention would have improved Carol's situation. Carol needed to ensure, before beginning, that she felt confident enough to work with this system. She also needed to spend sufficient time observing and gathering information to avoid jumping to conclusions and hastily suggesting interventions. As a result of her fear of looking incompetent, Carol ended up facing a dilemma that could have affected her credibility as a counselor as well as a consultant.

This fear of appearing incompetent is a phenomenon that affects most counselors, if they're honest about it, and can hit especially hard for counselors serving as consultants. When working as a consultant, the "client" is another professional—perhaps one who's been in the business longer than the consultant. Thus, it's not surprising that consultants can feel anxious about their first consultation projects. Many beginning consultants worry, "What if the consultee figures out I'm a phony?"

As we mentioned in Chapter 4, Clance and Imes (1978) studied this feeling of "phoniness," calling it the *imposter phenomenon.* In their work with over one hundred successful women, they found that these women tended to attribute their successes to being lucky, working hard, or being able to get along with others. They did not, however, feel their success was related to their ability or competence. They thus gave away much of their personal power. Later studies revealed that men apparently experience the imposter phenomenon as well (Clance & O'Toole, 1988).

Although feeling like an imposter may not necessarily impede success (Clance & O'Toole 1988), it can create such anxiety and skewed reasoning that the individual suffers unnecessary self-doubt. Then he or she may avoid taking appropriate risks. Unless we occasionally push ourselves and take risks, however, we'll have a tough time developing a healthy sense of self-efficacy.

As you imagine yourself taking on a consultation project, what concerns might you have about your competence as a consultant? What can you do now to address those concerns?

INTERPROFESSIONAL COLLABORATION

A distinct form of consultation is Interprofessional Collaboration. Many of the examples we've offered have presented counselors in consultation with other mental health professionals, but counselors also often consult with other professionals, such as business and industry leaders, school personnel, health professionals, and criminal justice officers. The current needs of our communities demand that we adopt innovative intervention efforts. Therefore, we as counselors should expect to reach out to other professionals to establish helping networks that can serve preventive functions across a broad sector of our communities.

This type of consultation sometimes takes the form of interprofessional collaboration—a coordinated effort among professionals to plan, implement, and evaluate programs for individuals, families, and communities (Staton & Gilligan, 2003). Unlike our traditional view of consultation, in collaboration, resources and power, as well as responsibility for the outcome of interventions, are shared by the collaborators (Idol, Nevin, & Paolucci-Whitcomb, 1995). Thus, the consultant, or interprofessional collaborator, does not pass responsibility for client care back to the consultee. Instead, the consultant is a partner in a multidisciplinary team and shares responsibilities with his or her collaborators. Read "I Forgot I Was a Counselor" in the accompanying box to learn about Tracy's experience working as a collaborator.

Interprofessional collaboration may include working with the court system to help a family learn to adequately care for their children. It may mean meeting regularly with social workers and psychologists to develop educational programs for mental health providers in the community. Interprofessional collaboration may also take the form of community counselors working with school personnel and the police department to provide comprehensive community programs to stop gang-related violence. Providing this type of consultation service demands that the consultant/collaborator be skilled in cultural competency, team-building skills, systemic thinking, and professional behavior (Staton & Kiyuna, in press).

Cultural competency can be defined two ways in interprofessional collaboration. First, effective collaborators are multiculturally competent in their work. They understand themselves and the worldview of their collaborators and clients, and they can draw from a range of culturally appropriate resources and strategies. They understand environmental factors such as racism and oppression, and they are willing to work as advocates to confront barriers to client potential (Lewis & Arnold, 1998).

Collaborators also need cultural competence in their ability to build interprofessional teams. They understand that different professions have

I Forgot I Was a Counselor

Tracy, who participated in a community collaboration team focusing on substance abuse prevention, was dismayed to find that the team members seemed to work *against* each other more than *with* each other. The school personnel ignored the police and listened only to the counselor. The school resource officer deferred to the medical representatives but downplayed the contributions of the social worker. The social worker seemed pessimistic about the entire endeavor, and the police representatives didn't seem to listen to anyone.

As Tracy thought about her team's struggles, she realized that several issues were complicating the process. First, no one had taken the time to explain the unique perspectives and skills of the various professions represented on the team. Instead, at the first meeting the team members had taken for granted that they each knew why everyone else was there. Second, no clear leader or group of leaders had emerged to help guide the group's direction. At each meeting several people seemed to jockey for leader position. Perhaps not surprisingly, the jockeying seemed based on degree of extroversion. Finally, no one ever talked about the process that was occurring at the group meetings. The same dance seemed to happen every time the team met, and any real

progress that was made came about because of individual, rather than united, effort.

When Tracy discussed this group dynamic with her supervisor, the supervisor congratulated her on her conceptualization. Then she asked, "So what's stopped you from intervening in this process? As the counselor there, it sounds like you're the ideal person to step in and talk about what's happening."

Tracy looked at her supervisor with surprise. "It didn't enter my mind!" she said. "It's almost as though I forgot I was a counselor. I've compartmentalized myself into counselor when I'm with clients and consultant/collaborator when I'm with the team."

Tracy's experience is not unusual. Negotiating our way in the presence of other professionals takes sensitivity and skill. The effectiveness of any consultation or collaboration relies on the counselor's ability to use counseling skills while focusing on the broad issues involved with the consultees and client system.

Questions for Reflection

1. If you were Tracy, how would you intervene with the team?

2. What would you say to them regarding the process you saw occurring?

different cultures, and they are able to respond accordingly (Wood, 1996). The culture of a community mental health agency, for instance, is likely to be very different from the culture of a public school. Collaborators must therefore learn to understand, if not necessarily appreciate, the need to work through structures that may feel more hierarchical, paternalistic, or bureaucratic than their own agencies. They may also need to handle with grace the demands by others to be called by professional titles or to work through clerical staff rather than to communicate directly.

Collaborators also need to have team-building skills. Ideally, they will genuinely value teamwork and look forward to the opportunity to hear and learn from the unique perspectives of the various professionals involved. One potential obstacle for many interprofessional collaboration teams is the lack of a clear leader. Effective collaborators can anticipate this issue and use their group counseling skills to keep both the collaboration process and product in mind.

The most effective collaborators are able to think and conceptualize systemically. They understand the complex relationships and networks that exist among professionals and agencies, and they can envision the best ways in which to capitalize on strengths and minimize weaknesses. This type of vision takes time to cultivate. One of the first steps in facilitating this process is to ensure that each collaborator in any project understands the role of each individual participating, as well as the mission of each individual's agency.

Finally, effective collaborators behave professionally. They respect the contributions of others, keep confidential information confidential, and refrain from splitting groups or forming secret alliances with subgroups. They also keep adequate records and live up to the promises they make to others. By working to maintain honesty and transparency throughout the process, collaborators can improve their chance of success.

GUIDING FRAMEWORKS FOR CONSULTATION AND COLLABORATION

Interprofessional collaboration and consultation can take a variety of forms and will be directly influenced by the counselor's values and orientation. The consultant may take a behavioral approach to consultation, an organizational focus, or emphasize a specific theoretical orientation, such as Adlerian or systemic (Dougherty, 2005). Regardless of the consultation situation or approach of the consultant, we recommend two broad strategies that have the potential to enhance the practices of consultation and collaboration: working collaboratively and working in a solution-focused manner.

Assuming a Collaborative Stance

As we described above, the processes of collaboration and consultation are usually distinguished by the amount of responsibility the consultant or collaborator has over the outcome (Brown, Pryzwansky, & Schulte, 2001; Dougherty, 2005). However, the counselor can always assume a collaborative stance in her or his consultation endeavors, regardless of the amount of responsibility the counselor has for the final product.

Using a collaborative approach to helping requires the counselor to begin any consultation or collaboration endeavor with a fundamental respect for the parties involved. Taking a collaborative approach suggests that the counselor believes in her consultees' or fellow collaborators' strengths and trusts their opinions. Further, working collaboratively enables the consultant to systematically empower the consultee, thereby enhancing the consultee's sense of self–efficacy. Also, by seeing consultation and collaboration as a partnership, or perhaps as a team endeavor, the consultant will likely improve the legitimacy of any interventions. In this case, too many cooks may not necessarily spoil the soup, especially if the consultant is prepared to use his or her counseling skills to effectively hear and conceptualize consultee concerns. Finally, collaborating during consultation and collaboration is likely to improve the integrity with which interventions are applied. If consultees feel they have been respected and included in the problem-definition and problem-solving processes, they are more likely to understand interventions, more willing to implement them, and better able to respond to follow-up and termination issues (Dougherty, 2005).

Assuming a collaborative stance will likely come quite naturally to many counselors, especially those who are accustomed to taking a respectful, "not-knowing" approach to their clients. Working collaboratively does remove some of the positional and expert power of the consultant, though, which may feed the consultant's ego a little less than more traditional stances may. We believe that the trade-off will be well worth it, as the consultant is rewarded by stronger consultative relationships and more comprehensive and relevant interventions.

Looking Toward Solutions

Consultation and collaboration can be effective ways to provide primary and secondary prevention efficiently to large groups of people. As community agencies and mental health centers struggle with budgetary constraints, consultation will likely become an even more popular intervention for many counseling administrators. It's not surprising, then, that some counselors are now integrating brief and solution-focused counseling skills into their consultation work.

The brief and solution-focused movements emerged from the work of numerous theorists (see Presbury, Echterling, & McKee, 2002) and have been heavily influenced by the tenets of postmodernism. Postmodernism suggests, among other things, that multiple truths exist because each person has a unique subjective reality. When applied to counseling, this idea gives great power and respect to the client's experience. When applied to consultation, this idea can serve to broaden the scope of conceptualization and intervention for consultant and consultee.

Brief and solution-focused approaches, combined here for the sake of convenience, rely on several assumptions:

- People's successes are as important as their failures.
- People are the experts on themselves, their lives, and their problems.
- Exceptions to every problem exist.
- Change is constant.
- Envisioning a solution is more effective than defining the problem.

The list continues, but the gist is that consultants can work efficiently and effectively by attending to consultee strengths and using the dynamic forces of change to the consultee's advantage. This solution-focused approach is especially relevant for conceptualizing change in communities and agencies, in which entropy may falsely suggest that viable solutions don't exist. Consultants can, for instance, look for exceptions to the problem to see what these exceptions suggest about the system, the consultee, and their untapped potential. Consultants can help consultees formulate specific goals that will guide their collaborative efforts. Consultants can work deliberately, using the given of change to their advantage, as they help their consultees navigate their way toward new skills.

SUPERVISION

Although supervision and consultation are distinct practices, they do share several common features. Similar to consultation, supervision is a relationship focused on improving work-related performance. Also, effective supervision demands many of the same skills as effective consultation. Good supervisors know how to assess, conceptualize, be direct, and intervene appropriately (Bernard & Goodyear, 1998). We include supervision in this chapter because, like consultation, whether or not they feel prepared for it, many community counselors are likely to be thrust into the role of supervisor. Furthermore, we feel it is important for beginning counselors to have an understanding of their responsibilities as supervisees. Community counselors are typically expected to have a period of postgraduate experience in which they participate in formal supervision arrangements. After licensure, counselors are expected to engage in ongoing consultative relationships in which they receive guidance and feedback from their peers. In one way or another, supervision is a vital part of the life of most community counselors.

Working as a Supervisee

Imagine your ideal supervision situation. What do you picture? When asked what they want from supervision, most counselors in training say they want to work with supervisors who are supportive, accessible, and able to provide constructive feedback (Baird, 2002). Fortunately, most counselor training programs involve moderate to intensive supervision expectations, so that by the time they graduate most students have been videotaped and observed with numerous clients over a significant period of time. In internships and paid positions, however, supervision may become less intense. Supervision may be held only in group settings, supervisors may have little or no supervision training, and observation and taping may be difficult or even impossible to provide.

We therefore encourage all counseling students to become prepared to make the most of the supervision they are offered by fully understanding their professional rights and responsibilities as supervisees. First, supervisees have the right to know what to expect of supervision, including the format (individual or group), the frequency of supervision sessions, the duration of the sessions, and the charge, if any, for the supervisor's services. Many community agencies ask an experienced, licensed counselor on staff to provide supervision and do not expect beginning counselors to pay for the service. However, all such parameters of the supervisory relationship should be clarified at the beginning of the relationship (Haynes, Corey, & Moulton, 2003).

When entering any supervision relationship, supervisees also have the professional right to know their supervisors' credentials, years of experience, and supervision training (Cohen, 2004). In fact, recording this information is critical for counselors who plan to pursue licensure. Some states have stringent requirements governing who can serve as an approved supervisor. In some cases, for instance, state licensure boards may require a certain number of supervised hours be provided by licensed professional counselors. Other states have more lenient restrictions and allow for a significant number of supervision hours to be provided by licensed clinical social workers or licensed psychologists. Take time now to visit the ACA website at **www.counseling.org** to check the supervision requirements in your state. Be prepared to keep accurate and detailed records of your supervision experiences.

Third, supervisees have the professional right to receive competent and timely supervision and to work in settings in which supervision is readily available in times of crisis. In a perfect world, every supervisor would be a

EXPERIENTIAL LEARNING

We present these supervisee rights as professional rather than legal rights—there is not necessarily a legal requirement for agencies to comply with these expectations. However, as a counselor in training you are expected to be able to know your own needs, advocate for yourself, and address problematic work situations.

- Spend some time creating a list of your rights as a supervisee.
- What will be easiest for you to ask for? What will be hardest?
- What actions could you take if you found yourself working with an incompetent supervisor?
- Discuss your list and the answers to these questions with your peers.

well-trained, ethical professional. In the real word, though, we come across supervisors who are incompetent, mentally ill, or inappropriate. We have heard of supervisors who neglect their duties and leave supervisees feeling alone and unsupported. We know of at least one instance in which a supervisor acted unethically and encouraged a supervisee to do the same. Ideally, supervisees will be able to identify inadequate or inappropriate supervision, seek consultation from other professionals, and act immediately to address problematic situations. These types of problems put the supervisee in the unfair position of having to confront a professional who is in a superior role, but nevertheless, the supervisee may be the person who has to take action. In these cases, supervisees are encouraged to seek consultation.

Supervisees also have responsibilities within the supervision relationship. These responsibilities will likely be determined between you and your various supervisors, but we suggest you consider at minimum the following:

1. Supervisees are responsible for being prepared to begin the supervision relationship. They are responsible for knowing themselves, including their strengths and weaknesses, and for being able to identify, with their supervisor's assistance, their own learning goals. Counselors in training are often expected to "hit the ground running" in internships and in their first jobs. Therefore, supervisors usually expect their supervisees to have an accurate and fairly complex level of self-understanding.

2. Supervisees are expected to be prepared for each supervision session. Supervisees should be able to readily identify every client's diagnoses, relevant issues, and treatment goals. They should be prepared to ask for direct feedback regarding problematic aspects of sessions, and they should be able to take the initiative to direct the focus of the

supervision session in order to meet their clinical needs (Baird, 2002). This is not to suggest that the supervisee should not defer to the supervisor's guidance regarding the process and focus of sessions. However, supervisees who enter supervision sessions feeling aimless and without direction week after week are very likely failing to take clinical responsibility for their own work.

3. Supervisees are expected to keep accurate, detailed records of client sessions and follow-up actions, in accordance with the guidelines of their agencies. We recognize that the paperwork aspect of counseling is often the counselor's least favorite job. However, failure to document sessions is a breach of the ACA Code of Ethics and can result in not only ethical but legal trouble for the counselor and supervisor.

4. Supervisees have the responsibility to let their supervisors know immediately of any crisis situations with clients or of any instances that may require breaking the client's confidentiality. Most supervisors will provide their supervisees with contact information to make sure the supervisee always has someone to call if crisis hits. If the supervisee feels out of his or her level of competence in dealing with a crisis, the supervisee has the responsibility and the right to seek assistance. Imagine, for instance, how you might feel when you have to call Child Protective Services to report child abuse. How will you respond if you have to hospitalize a suicidal client? What will you do if a client threatens to harm someone else and then runs out of your office? In these and many other potentially volatile situations, supervisees need assistance. Asking for help when you need it is critical for your ongoing professional development.

Receiving supervision may be one of the most profound and meaningful experiences in your counselor training (Baird, 2002). Being prepared for supervision, and taking your role as a supervisee seriously, can help build the framework for ongoing professional development and competent practice. Ideally, you will also find that your relationships with supervisors will, over time, result in enduring, supportive, and meaningful relationships with colleagues.

Providing Supervision

We invite you now to think ahead to the time when you will be called on to serve as a supervisor in a community agency. The supervision counselors provide in agencies is usually either *clinical* or *administrative*. Clinical supervision focuses on the counseling services that the supervisee (the counselor) provides to clients. Administrative supervision is centered on the supervisee's role as an organizational employee (Bradley & Kottler, 2001). Community counselors provide both administrative and clinical supervision, often in the same supervisory session (Haynes, Corey, & Moulton, 2003), and many find that the same skills apply to both types of supervision.

The role of the supervisor is complex, as she or he must attend to several issues. First, supervisors are responsible for their supervisees' actions. Thus, if a supervisee is performing inappropriately, the supervisor may be ethically and legally accountable for that behavior (Falvey, 2002). Supervisors are also expected to be familiar with every case their supervisees are handling, and to provide feedback and evaluation to every supervisee. Further, most supervisors are expected to document their supervision sessions and to provide their supervisees with a written explanation of their scope of responsibilities and expectations for performance. Supervisors are also often expected to coach and socialize their supervisee into professional growth and development (Bernard & Goodyear, 1998). They are also expected to ensure appropriate due process procedures, especially during those times when a supervisee is not performing to a supervisor's or agency's expectations.

Effective supervision is clearly a challenging endeavor. Supervisors therefore assume numerous roles within sessions, including roles such as teacher, mentor, consultant, administrator, or evaluator (Bernard & Goodyear, 1998). Building an effective supervisory relationship is much like building an effective counseling relationship. Skills such as empathy, effective communication, and conceptualization are critical (Haynes, Corey, & Moulton, 2003).

The need to provide evaluative feedback, however, is a unique demand of supervision. Further, unlike counseling, most agency supervisors work side by side with their supervisees on a daily basis. They become team members, or perhaps friends with their supervisees. Shifting roles as a supervisor can therefore be challenging, especially when supervisors are called on to confront supervisees regarding issues such as ineffective client care, shoddy record keeping, or administrative issues such as tardiness.

An additional challenge for supervisors is the fact that many agency supervisors have not had formal supervision training. They recall their experiences as supervisees and then replicate (or work hard *not* to replicate) that experience. Unfortunately, untrained supervisors are likely to provide "idiosyncratic and uneven" supervision (Bernard & Goodyear, 1998, p. 5). Although many untrained supervisors doubtless do a fine job, the lack of requirements for systematic training sends a message that supervision, which is a vital, foundational skill, is less important than other counselor functions.

Thankfully, organizations such as the Association for Counselor Education and Supervision, a division of ACA, is a resource that has highlighted the relevance and importance of competent supervision and adequate supervision training. The development of supervision theories and models, such as the classic Discrimination Model (Bernard, 1979), the Systems Approach (Holloway,

1995), and Solution-Oriented Models (Presbury, Echterling, & McKee, 1999; Thomas, 1994) may be indicative of the field's dawning recognition that supervision is a critically important practice. These models also provide helpful suggestions for community counselors who are struggling to integrate the role of supervisor into their existing roles as counselors and consultants.

Providing a comprehensive overview of supervision is beyond the scope of this chapter. Rather, we provide below a template for the beginning supervisor to consider.

First, whether you are providing administrative or clinical supervision, or both, ideally you will begin by identifying your own supervisory philosophy and approach. We encourage you to further develop this approach by writing a professional disclosure statement in which you specify, at the very least, your experience and scope of practice; your contact information, including emergency contact information; and your expectations of your supervisees. A sample professional disclosure statement is provided on page 426.

Next, identify the scope of supervision. Is it primarily administrative or clinical? If administrative, ensure that you understand agency policies, including informal expectations such as dress code, work schedule, and communication patterns. Plan how to initiate the relationship, including identifying, or even practicing, how you plan to explain your role to your supervisee. Document conversations with your supervisees, including suggestions and outcomes.

If you're providing clinical supervision, develop a descriptive log for each supervisee. The log should include supervisee contact information as well as a list and description of all of the supervisee's clients. Each week, indicate on the log relevant client information such as treatment plan, progress toward goals, collateral contacts, and critical concerns such as suicidality or child/elder abuse. Clearly identify your and your supervisee's actions regarding any issues that concern you, such as potential for client violence or suicide. Your supervision will become very important to your supervisee if she is pursuing counselor licensure, so keep your supervision log up to date and stored in a secure location.

Finally, realize that developing helpful and dynamic supervisory relationships takes time and practice. The best supervisors assess their supervision effectiveness, learn from their mistakes, and take seriously their commitment to serve clients and counselors by providing supervision.

ETHICAL AND LEGAL ISSUES IN PRACTICE

Ethical practice for consultants, just like ethical practice for counselors, is critical. The practice of consultation is covered in the ACA Code of Ethics (2005), although these types of codes and standards usually do not adequately capture

Sample Professional Disclosure Statement—Clinical Supervision

Supervisor Name and Contact Information,
including emergency contact phone numbers

I welcome you as a supervisee and look forward to working with you. This form is intended to provide you with information about my background and approach to supervision as well as inform you of my expectations regarding our relationship.

I received my M.S. in counseling psychology in 1992. I received formal training in clinical supervision through twelve hours of professional development experiences. I have also conducted research regarding clinical supervision and continue to investigate this area. As a counselor, I provide individual, marriage, family, and child counseling as well as group counseling services. I therefore focus my supervision in those areas as well.

I rely on a developmental model of supervision, in which I first assess your needs, capabilities, and preferred learning style and then work with you to create a supervisory experience that is specifically designed to facilitate your professional growth. My goals in supervision are to ensure that (1) your clients receive high-quality care, (2) you receive helpful feedback and guidance regarding your clinical work, and (3) you gain increased competence and proficiency in your role as a counselor. In order to ensure that we meet those goals, I ask that you (1) come to our supervision sessions prepared to discuss your cases; (2) when possible, bring to our sessions video or audiotapes cued to significant segments of the tape; (3) when possible, provide me with complete video or audiotapes so that I can review entire sessions; (4) notify me immediately if you encounter a client concern that involves the potential for harm to self or others, including specifically the possibility of client suicidal intent, child abuse, or elder abuse; and (5) keep accurate and current records of your work with clients.

During our supervision sessions we will watch or listen to your tapes if such tapes are available, discuss your progress and concerns, and strategize plans for both your clients and for you. At our first meeting we will discuss the specific minimum expectations for satisfactory performance, as well as the grievance policy for situations in which supervisees disagree with the supervisor's evaluation. If I feel that you are not meeting those criteria at any time I will notify you immediately. I will evaluate your progress in the areas of client conceptualization, process skills and intervention, and professional and ethical behavior. In addition to our discussions during our supervision sessions, I will provide you with written feedback approximately every eight weeks. I will also keep accurate records for your use in pursuing your professional licensure. I will attempt to provide specific feedback in order to ensure

(continued)

(Sample Professional Disclosure Statement—Clinical Supervision, continued)

that you understand my evaluation and are equipped with the tools necessary for continued professional growth. I do consult with colleagues in this agency regarding my supervision, so I will inform you if and when I discuss with others my supervision of you.

Everything you discuss with me will be kept confidential by me, except on those occasions when I consult, as mentioned above, and in matters pertaining to (1) suicide and harm to another person; (2) physical/sexual abuse or neglect of minors, persons with disabilities, and the elderly; (3) legal activity resulting in a court order; and (4) anything else required by law. For those matters, legally and/or ethically I would have to break confidentiality and involve others. Further, if your performance warrants a review of your employment status, I will reveal information necessary to allow the agency to make an informed decision. In order to enhance the potential for learning, my intention would always be to assist you as you work through these important concerns and ensure that you understand your ethical and legal obligations.

Our supervisory relationship is a part of your professional experience in this agency. Therefore, I am compensated by the agency for my supervision services. I do hope, however, that you will make the most of our relationship by having high expectations for yourself and for me. At the end of our relationship I will seek written feedback from you regarding your perceptions of our working alliance. If you have questions about any of this information, please feel free to ask me at any time. Please make special note of the contact information listed on the first page and below, and do not hesitate to get in touch with me as you have questions or concerns. I believe supervision can be a professionally and personally meaningful experience.

I adhere to the American Counseling Association's Code of Ethics, the code of ethics established by the National Board for Certified Counselors, the Approved Clinical Supervisor Code of Ethics, and the Center for Credentialing and Education's Standards for the Ethical Practice of Clinical Supervision. I expect you to read, understand, and adhere to the American Counseling Association Code of Ethics. Your signature below indicates that you have read and understand the expectations described above.

_____

Signature   Date

---

the complexity of consultation (Newman, 1993). Perhaps the most salient ethical issue regarding consultation is the fact that consultation interventions typically affect a "hidden client" (Robinson & Gross, 1985). Although clients are not directly included in planning consultation, they are undoubtedly affected by it. Thus, consultants have a responsibility to anticipate the consequences of their actions not only on the consultee and agency, but on the client as well (Brown, Pryzwansky, & Schulte, 2001; Newman, 1993).

EXPERIENTIAL LEARNING

Interview a community counselor who serves as a clinical or administrative supervisor. Then, begin to develop or refine your own supervision philosophy, and write your own professional disclosure statement. We realize that it may be several years before you actually practice as a supervisor. However, thinking now about what you plan to offer as a supervisor will help you clearly articulate your needs and expectations as a supervisee.

Consultants also have unique considerations regarding issues such as confidentiality. Consultants frequently gather information that is then shared with the court system, schools, agency personnel, and other health care providers (Brown, Pryzwansky, & Schulte, 2001). However, the ACA Code of Ethics limits the counselor's ability to share confidential information. Again, the consultant is required to "think ahead" and anticipate the potential consequences of every action prior to sharing any client information.

In general, consultants are encouraged to think like counselors when it comes to engaging in ethical practice. Communicating the limits of confidentiality, not practicing outside of the scope of one's expertise, being alert to potential complications of dual relationships and conflicts of interest, and appropriately representing the profession are all reasonable standards of care for not only consultants, but supervisors as well.

The ACA Code of Ethics (2005) addresses counselor supervision in regard to client welfare, counselor credentials, informed consent, supervisor competence, supervisor responsibilities, and the supervisor's general role in supervision, evaluation, remediation, and endorsement. The Code is fairly explicit in delineating the need for supervisors to understand the scope and complexity of their role prior to undertaking supervision responsibilities. The Code of Ethics also clearly indicates that ethical practice in supervision requires ongoing vigilance in overseeing supervisee competence while attending to client welfare. Ethical guidelines for supervisors have also been developed by the Center for Credentialing and Education. These guidelines supplement the ACA Codes of Ethics and include expectations such as the supervisor will (1) ensure clients have been informed of their right to confidentiality, (2) establish procedures for handling crisis situations, and (3) intervene in situations in which the supervisee is impaired. These guidelines, available at

www.cce-global.org/acs.htm, pertain to the Approved Clinical Supervisor credential but are relevant for all practicing supervisors.

Interestingly, counselors have faced fewer legal battles when working as consultants than when providing therapy services (Brown, Pryzwansky, & Schulte, 2001). However, consultants can be charged with malpractice for issues such as negligence, misrepresentation, and breach of contract. Consultants, like counselors, are also likely to be called to testify in court regarding their work with families and individual clients. In these situations, consultants can take several steps to protect themselves and facilitate their ability to provide effective service.

First, engage in active and thorough record-keeping. Use written contracts and keep accurate records (Dougherty, 2005; Rivas-Vazquez, Blais, Rey, Gustavo, & Rivas-Vazquez, 2001). Second, discuss fees at the beginning of the relationship, and identify as clearly as possible the limits of confidentiality and the scope of the consultation. Encourage open communication at all times, and seek the services of a consultant, supervisor, attorney, and/or the American Counseling Association as needed.

Just knowing ethical guidelines is not enough to ensure ethical practice and to avoid legal difficulty. Appropriate professional behavior always depends on our ability to know ourselves accurately, and then to act on that knowledge. Many community counselors find that one of the most efficient and effective methods of responding to ethical and legal questions is to consult with trusted colleagues. The consultation process when exploring ethical and legal issues is much as we've described in this chapter, although usually less formal: Counselors seek the assistance of another professional, in this case another counselor or mental health professional, regarding a work-related problem. Consultation regarding ethical and legal issues may be informal or formal, long-term or formed on an as-needed basis. Regardless of the format, counselors typically find that sharing their concerns with trusted colleagues in a confidential setting is a useful and rewarding practice that can enhance the competence of the consultant and the consultee.

CONCLUDING THOUGHTS

In some settings, calling in a consultant suggests desperation. For community counselors, however, consultation can suggest empowerment and facilitation of consultee strengths. After all, consultation is the ultimate act of prevention. Effective consultation can help people discover (or rediscover) their strengths, find solutions, circumvent problems, and perhaps most important, learn valuable skills that can then be transferred to more and more people.

RECOMMENDED RESOURCES

In addition to the texts on consultation included in the reference list, we recommend:

Schein, E. H. (1999). *Process consultation revisited: Building the helping relationship*. Upper Saddle River, NJ: Prentice Hall.

The special edition of the *Journal of Educational and Psychological Consultation, 14*(3&4), also contains several helpful articles.

Community counselors working in organizational consultation may want to consider refreshing their understanding of principles of industrial/organizational psychology. Texts such as Ott, J. S., Parkes, S. J., & Simpson, R. B. (2003). *Classical readings in organizational behavior* (3rd ed.) may be enlightening.

Comprehensive texts on supervision include:

Bernard, J. M., & Goodyear, R. K. (1998). *Fundamentals of clinical supervision* (2nd ed.). Needham Heights, MA: Allyn & Bacon.

Bradley, L. J., & Ladany, N. (Eds.). (2001). *Counselor supervision: Principles, process, and practice* (3rd ed.). Philadelphia: Brunner-Routledge.

In addition, *Counselor Education and Supervision,* the journal established by the Association for Counselor Education and Supervision will undoubtedly be a valuable resource to you, as will the ACES webpage at **www.acesonline.net/**.

Other Resources

Written resources include the book upon which the movie *Dead Man Walking* is based—*Dead Man Walking*: *An Eyewitness Account of the Death Penalty in the United States,* by Helen Prejean. We mentioned the movie in Chapter 5 as relevant for exploring a nonjudgmental, helping relationship. The book reveals much more about Prejean's experiences as an advocate while working within many subsystems. Also, we break our rule of not mentioning textbooks in this section and recommend that you peruse the *Handbook of Positive Psychology,* edited by Snyder and Lopez. This book provides relevant, current information regarding what consultants, supervisors, and collaborators do best: building on strengths to empower others.

In this chapter, we mentioned Jane Goodall. The documentary *Jane Goodall: A Life in the Wild* is a wonderful account of Goodall's work with the chimpanzees of Gombe Stream National Park in Tanzania. You can certainly enjoy the film at the level of a nature study, but it's fascinating to appreciate the care that Goodall takes in preparing for and joining with a chimpanzee colony. Besides, many human organizations have a lot in common with chimpanzee colonies!

If you prefer Westerns, then *Dances with Wolves*, the 1990 Academy Award–winning movie, explores similar dynamics of an outsider gaining the trust of members of a system. The movie takes place in the wilderness of the Dakota territory during the Civil War. Lieutenant John Dunbar's encounters with a wolf and a local Sioux tribe mirror the consultation process.

REFERENCES

Albee, G. W. (2000). Commentary on prevention and counseling psychology. *The Counseling Psychologist, 28,* 845–853.

Baird, B. N. (2002). *The internship, practicum, and field placement handbook* (3rd ed.). Upper Saddle River, NJ: Prentice Hall.

Beebe, S. A., Beebe, S. J., & Redmond, M. V. (1999). *Interpersonal communication: Relating to others* (2nd ed.). Needham Heights, MA: Allyn & Bacon.

Bernard, J. M. (1979). Supervisor training: A discrimination model. *Counselor Education and Supervision, 19,* 60–68.

Bernard, J. M., & Goodyear, R. K. (1998). *Fundamentals of clinical supervision* (2nd ed.). Needham Heights, MA: Allyn & Bacon.

Bradley, L. J., & Kottler, J. A. (2001). Overview of counseling supervision. In L. J. Bradley & N. Ladany (Eds.), *Counselor supervision: Principles, process and practice* (3rd ed., pp. 28–57). Philadelphia: Brunner-Routledge.

Brown, D. (1997). Implications for cross-cultural consultation with families. *Journal of Counseling and Development, 76,* 29–35.

Brown, D., Pryzwansky, W. B., & Schulte, A. C. (2001). *Psychological consultation: Introduction to theory and practice* (5th ed.). Boston: Allyn & Bacon.

Caplan, G. (1970). *Theory and practice of mental health consultation.* New York: Basic Books.

Caplan, G., & Caplan, R. B. (1993). *Mental health consultation and collaboration.* Prospect Heights, IL: Waveland.

Clance, P. R., & Imes, S. A. (1978). The imposter phenomenon in high achieving women: Dynamics and therapeutic intervention. *Psychotherapy: Theory, Research and Practice, 15,* 241–247.

Clance, P. R., & O'Toole, M. A. (1988). The imposter phenomenon: An internal barrier to empowerment and achievement. *Women and Therapy, 6,* 51–64.

Cohen, R. I. (2004). *Clinical supervision: What to do and how to do it.* Belmont, CA: Thomson Brooks/Cole.

Conyne, R. K. (2000). Prevention in counseling psychology: At long last, has the time come? *The Counseling Psychologist, 28,* 838–844.

Dougherty, A. M. (2000). *Psychological consultation and collaboration in school and community settings* (3rd ed.). Belmont, CA: Wadsworth.

Dougherty, A. M. (2005). *Psychological consultation and collaboration in school and community settings* (4th ed.). Belmont, CA: Thomson Brooks/Cole.

Dougherty, A. M., Henderson, B. B., & Lindsey, B. (1997). The effectiveness of direct versus indirect confrontation as a function of stage of consultation: Results of an exploratory investigation. *Journal of Educational and Psychological Consultation, 8,* 361–372.

Falvey, J. E. (2002). *Managing clinical supervision: Ethical practice and legal risk management.* Pacific Grove, CA: Brooks/Cole.

Haynes, R., Corey, G., & Moulton, P. (2003). *Clinical supervision in the helping professions: A practical guide.* Belmont, CA: Thomson Brooks/Cole.

Holloway, E. L. (1995). *Clinical supervision: A systems approach.* Thousand Oaks, CA: Sage.

Idol, L., Nevin, A., & Paolucci-Whitcomb, P. (1995). The collaborative consultation model. *Journal of Educational & Psychological Consultation, 6,* 347–361.

Johnson, D. W., & Johnson, F. P. (2003). *Joining together: Group theory and group skills* (8th ed.). Boston: Allyn & Bacon.

Knotek, S. E., & Sandoval, J. (2003). Current research in consultee-centered consultation. *Journal of Educational and Psychological Consultation, 14*(3&4), 243–250.

Kratochwill, T. R., & Pittman, P. H. (2002). Expanding problem-solving consultation training: Prospects and frameworks. *Journal of Educational and Psychological Consultation, 13*(1&2), 69–95.

Kurpius, D. J., & Fuqua, D. R. (1993). Fundamental issues in defining consultation. *Journal of Counseling and Development, 71,* 597–597.

Lewis, J. A., & Arnold, M. S. (1998). From multiculturalism to social action. In C. C. Lee & G. R. Walz (Eds.), *Social action: A mandate for counselors* (pp. 51–66). Alexandria, VA: American Counseling Association.

McDowell, T. (1999). Systems consultation and Head Start: An alternative to traditional family therapy. *Journal of Marital and Family Therapy, 25,* 155–168.

Newman, J. L. (1993). Ethical issues in consultation. *Journal of Counseling and Development, 72,* 148–156.

Presbury, J., Echterling, L. G., & Mckee, J. E. (1999). Supervision for innervision: Solution-focused strategies. *Counselor Education and Supervision, 39,* 146–155.

Presbury, J., Echterling, L. G., & McKee, J. E. (2002). *Ideas and tools for brief counseling.* Upper Saddle River, NJ: Merrill/Prentice Hall.

Rivas-Vasquez, Blais, R. A., Rey, M. A., Gustavo, J., & Rivas-Vazquez, A. (2001). A brief reminder about documenting the psychological consultation. *Professional Psychology Research and Practice, 32,* 194–199.

Robinson, S. E., & Gross, D. (1985). Ethics in consultation: The Canterville ghost. *The Counseling Psychologist, 13,* 444–465.

Sandoval, J. (1996). Constructivism, consultee-centered consultation, and conceptual change. *Journal of Educational and Psychological Consultation, 7,* 89–97.

Schlozman, S. C. (2003). Innovative models for school consultation. *Educational Leadership, 60,* 87–89.

Staton, A. R., & Gilligan, T. D. (2003). Teaching school counselors and school psychologists to work collaboratively. *Counselor Education and Supervision, 42,* 162–176.

Staton, A. R., & Kiyuna, R. (in press). Interpersonal collaboration: A process for meeting community needs. *The Virginia Counselors Journal, 29.*

Sue, D. W., & Sue, D. (2003). *Counseling the culturally diverse: Theory and practice* (4th ed.). New York: Wiley.

Thomas, F. N. (1994). Solution-oriented supervision: The coaxing of expertise. *The Family Journal: Counseling and Therapy for Couples and Families, 2,* 11–18.

Wood, G., (1996). An analysis of professional values: Implications for interprofessional collaboration. In J. McCroskey & S. Einbinder (Eds.), *Universities and communities: Remaking professional and interprofessional education for the next century* (pp. 26–43). Los Angeles, CA: University of Southern California.

Name Index

Subject Index